Accessing the E-book edition

Using the VitalSource® ebook

Access to the VitalBook™ ebook accompanying this book is via VitalSource® Bookshelf — an ebook reader which allows you to make and share notes and highlights on your ebooks and search across all of the ebooks that you hold on your VitalSource Bookshelf. You can access the ebook online or offline on your smartphone, tablet or PC/Mac and your notes and highlights will automatically stay in sync no matter where you make them.

1. **Create a VitalSource Bookshelf account at** *https://online.vitalsource.com/user/new* or log into your existing account if you already have one.

2. **Redeem the code provided in the panel below to get online access to the ebook.**
Log in to Bookshelf and select **Redeem** at the top right of the screen. Enter the redemption code shown on the scratch-off panel below in the **Redeem Code** pop-up and press **Redeem**. Once the code has been redeemed your ebook will download and appear in your library.

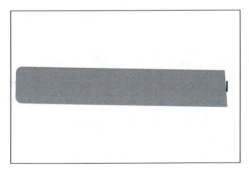

No returns if this code has been revealed.

DOWNLOAD AND READ OFFLINE

To use your ebook offline, download BookShelf to your PC, Mac, iOS device, Android device or Kindle Fire, and log in to your Bookshelf account to access your ebook:

On your PC/Mac

Go to *https://support.vitalsource.com/hc/en-us* and follow the instructions to download the free **VitalSource Bookshelf** app to your PC or Mac and log into your Bookshelf account.

On your iPhone/iPod Touch/iPad

Download the free **VitalSource Bookshelf** App available via the iTunes App Store and log into your Bookshelf account. You can find more information at *https://support.vitalsource.com/hc/en-us/categories/200134217-Bookshelf-for-iOS*

On your Android™ smartphone or tablet

Download the free **VitalSource Bookshelf** App available via Google Play and log into your Bookshelf account. You can find more information at *https://support.vitalsource.com/hc/en-us/categories/200139976-Bookshelf-for-Android-and-Kindle-Fire*

On your Kindle Fire

Download the free **VitalSource Bookshelf** App available from Amazon and log into your Bookshelf account. You can find more information at *https://support.vitalsource.com/hc/en-us/categories/200139976-Bookshelf-for-Android-and-Kindle-Fire*

N.B. The code in the scratch-off panel can only be used once. When you have created a Bookshelf account and redeemed the code you will be able to access the ebook online or offline on your smartphone, tablet or PC/Mac.

SUPPORT

If you have any questions about downloading Bookshelf, creating your account, or accessing and using your ebook edition, please visit *http://support.vitalsource.com/*

OBESITY
Evaluation and Treatment Essentials

SECOND EDITION

OBESITY
Evaluation and Treatment Essentials

Edited by

G. Michael Steelman, MD, FASBP
American Society of Bariatric Physicians
The Steelman Clinic
Oklahoma City, Oklahoma, USA

Eric C. Westman, MD, MHS
Lifestyle Medicine Clinic
Duke University Medical Center
Durham, North Carolina, USA

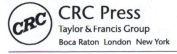

CRC Press
Taylor & Francis Group
Boca Raton London New York

CRC Press is an imprint of the
Taylor & Francis Group, an **informa** business

CRC Press
Taylor & Francis Group
6000 Broken Sound Parkway NW, Suite 300
Boca Raton, FL 33487-2742

Printed on acid-free paper
Version Date: 20160229

International Standard Book Number-13: 978-1-4822-6207-0 (Pack - Book and Ebook)

Library of Congress Cataloging-in-Publication Data

Names: Steelman, G. Michael, editor. | Westman, Eric C., editor.
Title: Obesity : evaluation and treatment essentials / [edited by] G. Michael
Steelman, Eric C. Westman.
Other titles: Obesity (Steelman)
Description: Second edition. | Boca Raton : Taylor & Francis, 2016. |
Includes bibliographical references and index.
Identifiers: LCCN 2015039007 | ISBN 9781482262070 (alk. paper)
Subjects: | MESH: Obesity--therapy. | Obesity--prevention & control.
Classification: LCC RC628 | NLM WD 210 | DDC 616.3/98--dc23
LC record available at http://lccn.loc.gov/2015039007

Visit the Taylor & Francis Web site at
http://www.taylorandfrancis.com

and the CRC Press Web site at
http://www.crcpress.com

Contents

Foreword

Obesity, the word itself doesn't conjure up many positive emotions from people at large, or from busy doctors. Perhaps being fat was a good thing in the year AD 1000 when our ancestors were running around, and when there were no supermarkets on the corners. Who survived when there was a famine and passed their gene pools down to us? Generally, it wasn't the skinny ones. Significant corpulence was out of vogue by the 1860s, at the time of our Civil War. William Banting, a 5′ 5″, 202-lb undertaker in merry old England tried nearly everything to lose weight without much success. A hearing problem led him to see Dr. William Harvey, an ear, nose, and throat doctor of some renown. Dr. Harvey thought Banting's hearing problem might be related to his obesity and suggested a reduced carbohydrate diet (with still a few spirits allowed). Low-carbohydrate diets were used to treat diabetes in the pre-insulin era. Following this eating plan, Banting lost weight nicely and kept it off. He was so happy that he wrote and distributed a pamphlet about his success. This stirred up considerable discussion at the time, and, by the early 1900s, some people, instead of saying, "it's time to diet," were saying, "it's time to Bant." No, I wasn't there then, but I do remember the "Great Depression" (what was so *great* about the depression of the 1930s?). Anyway, in the 1950s and 1970s, curbing the intake of carbs was more in vogue than keeping the dietary fat down. Yudkin, in England, advocated a low-carbohydrate diet and wrote extensively in this regard in the 1970s. Then the "experts" came along, telling us to keep the fat down and load up on nonrefined carbohydrates, etc. Low and behold, we've continued getting fatter. They've been fattening Iowa hogs with a nonrefined carbohydrate, namely corn, for decades. The last I checked, they weren't using the fibrous veggies, such as cabbage or zucchini.

So, it's nice to have a book, *Obesity: Evaluation and Treatment Essentials*, which covers it all. It's written primarily by practicing bariatricians who make their living treating patients with obesity problems. There are also chapters by academicians who have been doing research involving human obesity for quite some time and also chapters by experts on exercise, behavior modification, and nutrition. Overall, you have an outstanding group of experts who bring it all together. This book is an excellent read for those of us who have been treating the obese for years and need to be updated. It's especially beneficial for doctors who have got into, are getting into, or thinking about getting into bariatric medicine. In essence, this book is a must read for practicing bariatricians. Let me give you a short history regarding appetite suppressants. Starting in 1969, I led the American Society of Bariatric Physicians (ASBP), from a group comprising 35 obesity-treating, dues-paying physician members to a burgeoning group of approximately 450 physician members by 1974. Currently, the ASBP has more than 1000 members. In the late 1960s and early 1970s, the mothers of America were crying for the feds to take the amphetamine appetite suppressants off the market, so their kids wouldn't be abusing them.

I flew back to Washington, DC, and spent time at the Food and Drug Administration (FDA) presenting the ASBP's position that at least some of the appetite suppressants should remain available for the treatment of obesity. Barrett Scoville, MD, a career FDA bureaucrat involved with the issue, said he had reviewed the studies submitted in the 1960s to get approval for the nonamphetamine appetite suppressants and that, over the 12-week study periods, those getting the appetite suppressants lost about a pound a week and those taking the placebos lost about one-half pound a week.

To him that wasn't a significant difference. Therefore, he opined that all appetite suppressants should be taken off the market. I made the ASBP's position clear that we strongly opposed such action. Charles Edwards, MD, was another physician working at the FDA at the time. He had a little cooler head. After much discussion, the upshot was that the amphetamines moved up to schedule II (no appetite suppressant use) and the other three, phentermine, diethylpropion, and phendimetrazine, went into schedule III or IV, with the "few week" limitation being put in the package insert material. So, we do have them and most of us bariatricians use them "off label." I do, and I've had patients on them more or less continuously for 30 years. I saw a patient a few weeks ago who is still fighting the weight battle at age 69; she was 27 years old when I first saw her. Certainly, this doesn't make me feel any younger. Obviously, she wouldn't be coming back to see me if she wasn't needing and getting ongoing help.

So, let's get back to the FDA and the Bureau of Narcotics and Dangerous Drugs (now Drug Enforcement Administration). I asked Barrett at the time to define what a "few weeks" meant. He said they weren't going to do that. I had my appetite suppressants, so, "be gone." Over the next several years, "a few weeks" came to be interpreted as 12 weeks, the length of time for which most studies were done to get these drugs approved by the FDA in the 1960s. I've had patients come in and say "I didn't think the medication was helping but, boy, when I didn't have it...." If the appetite suppressants continued working like they do in the first few weeks, we wouldn't have much of an obesity problem—but they don't, even with long-term usage, they only help to keep the hunger levels down enough to enable patients to make intelligent food choices. If they do, the patients won't be so hungry. I've always said "You won't keep very many patients, if they're very hungry, very long." So, I welcome the way this book covers the appetite suppressants plus much, much more. Thanks to G. Michael Steelman, MD, FASBP, and Eric Westman, MD, MHS, the editors of *Obesity: Evaluation and Treatment Essentials*, and thanks also to all chapter contributors for doing a fine job covering the other aspects of the obese state, its treatment, and what may be in store for bariatricians and their patients in the not too distant future. In short, I highly recommend *Obesity: Evaluation and Treatment Essentials*. On winding down my history lesson, I'm reminded of the story of a seven-year-old boy in church who kept looking around and generally appeared bored. On his way out, the pastor, who had noted the boy's behavior, shook the boy's hand and asked if there was anything he could help him with. The seven-year-old asked "What are those plaques on the wall with the name and dates on them?" The pastor replied, "Son, those are our members who have died in the service." To this, the young lad asked, "In the 8 o'clock service or the 10 o'clock service?" Thus, I wind down my commentary before the readers start asking, "... the 8 o'clock or the 10 o'clock?"

W. L. Asher, MD, FASBP
Past President, ASBP
Littleton, Colorado

Preface to the first edition

It is clear that obesity is one of our nation's biggest health care challenges. It is associated with our most common causes of mortality and morbidity as well as with considerable psychosocial discomfort. The incidence of this killer disease has been steadily increasing and has reached epidemic proportions. Most physicians receive little or no training in nutritional matters or the treatment of obesity. Perhaps because the treatment of obesity is less glamorous and more frustrating than the treatment of other conditions, too many physicians are unable or unwilling to deliver effective medical assistance to overweight patients. Too often, this void is filled by commercial interests more focused on "the bottom line" rather than on the health of the consumer. The treatment of obesity has been hindered by myths, misconceptions, and prejudices about its causes and consequences. The obese individual is not simply a lazy, metabolically normal adult with too much adipose tissue; rather, he or she is a metabolically complex individual who may respond differently to nutritional intake and exercise/activity. The causes of obesity are complex and multifactorial. Its treatment therefore must be multimodal and tailored to meet the individual needs of the particular patient. This book will discuss the essential clinical guidelines and standards of each treatment option, from dietary interventions to bariatric surgery, as well as the bariatrician's role in this treatment option. Dietary intervention is the mainstay of bariatric treatment. In order to individualize treatment, the physician needs to be familiar with various approaches, including low calorie diets, low-carbohydrate diets, and very-low–carbohydrate diets (VLCD). It is our hope that nutritionists and dieticians will benefit from the detail and level of discussion of these dietary interventions in addition to the bariatric physician. Exercise is an important part of weight loss efforts and is probably essential for long-term weight maintenance. It provides numerous benefits in addition to its effect on weight. While patients are willing to follow almost any diet plan, it is often difficult to get them to initiate and sustain a meaningful exercise regimen. Weight loss and maintenance require that individuals make changes in the way they interact with their environment. In this effort, they battle with a culture that, on one hand, values being fit and trim and, on the other, promotes obesogenic food patterns and sedentary lifestyles. To succeed, the overweight individual must be armed with effective strategies to deal with internal and external forces that favor the overweight state. Various pharmaceutical agents have been used to help facilitate weight loss. Anorectic agents have been in use for over four decades and have been shown to be both safe and effective. Newer agents that inhibit the absorption of fat or carbohydrate are also available. Various other pharmaceuticals and some natural substances may also play a role in helping with the process of weight management. On the other hand, there are many common medications that promote weight gain, and replacing these with ones that are similarly effective but less likely to impact weight negatively can often bring rewarding results.

We must also consider, when treating the bariatric patient, that children represent a special population with special needs. The increasing incidence of obesity (and attendant type II diabetes) in this population is alarming. Clearly, something must be done to stem this tide or, as has been suggested, today's generation of children will be the first generation of Americans with a life expectancy less than that of their parents. The chapter on Childhood Obesity clearly identifies the special needs of children and outlines approaches for managing the obese child. For some individuals, obesity and its comorbidities advance to such a degree that their life is at considerable risk. For them, bariatric surgery may be warranted. It is essential that they be properly evaluated before surgery, skillfully treated during surgery, and followed appropriately afterwards. The bariatric physician plays an important role in treating the patient preoperatively if bariatric surgery is a determined method of treatment for a particular patient. Those of us who have developed a special interest and specialize in the field of bariatric medicine find great satisfaction in the work we do and the role we play in helping our patients live healthier, happier, and longer lives. We are excited about the potential for better understanding of this complex and fascinating disease and for the development of better weapons to use in its treatment. To our colleagues engaged in academic and clinical research, we offer our sincere appreciation for your efforts and eagerly await the fruits of your labor.

To our colleagues engaged in clinical practice who are awakening to this field and want to improve their skills and expertise in the medical management of obese patients, we extend our heartfelt encouragement and support.

G. Michael Steelman, MD, FASBP
Eric C. Westman, MD, MHS

Preface to the second edition

A lot has changed since I graduated from medical school in the mid-1970s. We were taught that obesity, except in rare cases, was simply a matter of caloric imbalance and that adipose tissue functioned only to store triglycerides and to offer some protection to the skeletal and thermo-regulatory systems.

There were few serious researchers and few skilled clinicians approaching the problem of obesity. On the academic side, Stunkard, Bray, and Blackburn are notable. Skilled and compassionate clinicians who helped mentor me and hundreds of others included Peter Lindner, James T. Cooper, Bill Asher, and Robert Johnson. These are the giants on whose shoulders we stand today as the field expands exponentially.

In this edition we have updated pertinent chapters. The chapters on the legal aspects of bariatric medicine and residential treatment of obesity have been dropped, and a new chapter on binge eating disorder and an appendix containing a portion of the American Society of Bariatric Physicians *Algorithm for the Treatment of Obesity* have been included.*

Now that the research community and a rapidly increasing number of clinicians are diligently attacking the disease of obesity (or adiposopathy), it is our fervent hope that this book will play a role in helping promote serious and ultimately more successful understanding and treatment of this fascinating but stubborn disease.

G. Michael Steelman, MD, FASBP

---

* As this book was being prepared for printing, the American Society of Bariatric Physicians (ASBP) changed its name to the Obesity Medicine Association (OMA) which can be accessed online at http://obesitymedicine.org/ (as of December 2015).

This organization is referenced several times in various chapters and a small portion of The ASBP Algorithm for Obesity Treatment is included as Appendix C. This appendix includes only the initial few pages of a much more detailed document which can be accessed at http://obesitymedicine.org/obesity-algorithm/ (as of December 2015).

We apologize for any confusion caused by this change.

Contributors

Ralph Carson
FitRx Binge Eating Disorder
Treatment Facility
Brentwood, Tennessee

Erin Chamberlin-Snyder
American Weight Loss Center
Indianapolis, Indiana

John B. Cleek
Carolinas Weight Management &
Wellness Center
Charlotte, North Carolina

James T. Cooper*
Private Practice
Marietta, Georgia

Frank L. Greenway
Pennington Biomedical Research Center
Louisiana State University System
Baton Rouge, Louisiana

Ed J. Hendricks
Center for Weight Management
Roseville, California

Deborah Bade Horn
Private Practice
Houston, Texas

Jeffrey D. Lawrence
Private Practice (Retired)
Williamsburg, Virginia

Larry A. Richardson
Doctor's Weight Control Center
Spring, Texas

Scott Rigden
Private Practice
Chandler, Arizona

Harold C. Seim
Weight Management
Stillwater, Minnesota
University of Minnesota
Minneapolis, Minnesota

Steven R. Smith
Molecular Endocrinology Laboratory
Pennington Biomedical Research Center
Louisiana State University System
Baton Rouge, Louisiana

G. Michael Steelman
Private Practice
The Steelman Clinic
Oklahoma City, Oklahoma

Mary C. Vernon
Private Practice
Lawrence, Kansas

Eric C. Westman
Lifestyle Medicine Clinic
Duke University Medical Center
Durham, North Carolina

James A. Wortman
First Nations and Inuit Health Branch
Health Canada
Vancouver, British Columbia, Canada

* Deceased.

xiii

Editors

G. Michael Steelman, MD, FASBP, graduated from the University of Oklahoma School of Medicine, Oklahoma City, in 1973 and after completing his postgraduate training, practiced family medicine for 10 years. During that time, he became interested in obesity and spent more than 30 years in specialized practice of clinical bariatric medicine as the founder and medical director of The Steelman Clinic Weight Loss in Oklahoma City.

Dr. Steelman served two terms as president of the American Society of Bariatric Physicians and was elected as a Fellow of the ASBP. He is one of the few physicians to have been awarded the Bariatrician of the Year by the ASBP twice, in 1993 and 2006. Dr. Steelman has been a frequent speaker at continuing medical education meetings and has published several articles. He was a member of a committee formed by former US Surgeon General C. Everett Koop to develop guidelines for the treatment of obesity in adults.

Eric C. Westman, MD, MHS, received his MD from the University of Wisconsin-Madison, completed an internal medicine residency and chief residency at the University of Kentucky, Lexington, and completed a General Internal Medicine Fellowship at Duke University, Durham, North Carolina, which included a master's degree in clinical research. At Duke, since 1990, he is director of the Duke Lifestyle Medicine Clinic, and has carried out clinical research and clinical care regarding lifestyle treatments for obesity and diabetes. Dr. Westman has over 90 peer-reviewed publications. He is currently the chairman of the board of the Obesity Medicine Association (formerly the American Society of Bariatric Physicians) and a Fellow of the Obesity Medicine Association and the Obesity Society. He is co-author of the New York Times' best seller *The New Atkins for a New You* (2010, Touchstone), *Cholesterol Clarity* (2013, Victory Belt) and *Keto Clarity* (2014, Victory Belt).

Obesity: The scope of a growing problem

HAROLD C. SEIM

It is common knowledge that obesity has reached epidemic proportions in the United States and worldwide and that we come across obese people in every walk of life. In the United States, Dr. C. Everett Koop, former Surgeon General (1982–1989), said, "Except for smoking, obesity is now the number one preventable cause of death in this country." So what has caused this epidemic and what remedial action is taken to prevent it?

CAUSE

Early studies in the 1950s and 1960s were interpreted to show that eating fat caused heart disease, leading to a public health effort to curtail fat in the diet, an effort that remains to the present day. Unfortunately, the low-fat diet has been a major contributor to the fattening of people in the United States. When fat is removed from a food product, sugar or another carbohydrate is added in its place. Many people, especially those who are insulin resistant, are unable to process sugar and other easily digested carbohydrates for energy. Insulin is released when sugar is eaten, and it helps convert sugar into triglyceride that is stored in the fat cells.

In addition, when insulin is present, we become hungry and eat more carbohydrates and thus put more fat on our bodies. Insulin is also a very atherogenic hormone that causes inflammation in the cells of the body, a response that, over time, could lead to diabetes and to cardiovascular and kidney diseases (1).

As our society has become more urban and more affluent, diets high in complex carbohydrates have decreased, and now we eat a higher proportion of saturated fats and sugars. Also, there has been a shift to less physical work and less activity in our leisure time. Americans eat large amounts of food at meals; plates are larger than they were 50 years ago and we tend to fill them. We see this overindulgence especially when eating out.

Fast foods have been a large contributor to this epidemic, and supersizing makes the situation worse. Fast foods are high in carbohydrate calories and high in fats. Calories do count, and for persons who are insulin resistant, carbohydrate calories are a worse choice. For example, drinking one soda a day for a year (150 cal) will add 15 extra pounds to your weight.

RESULTS

Children in America

Our children have become obese as they have been immersed in high-calorie, high-carbohydrate eating patterns and are now developing type 2 diabetes—a disease that was formerly seen only in obese adults (2).

World Health Organization (WHO) statistics on children estimate that approximately 22 million children younger than 5 years old are overweight. In the United States, the percentage of overweight children (5–14 years) has increased from 15% to 32% over the past 30 years (3). A National Health and Nutrition Examination Survey (NHANES) is conducted periodically by the National Center for Health Statistics using measured heights and weights. These surveys show that the prevalence of obesity among children and adolescents (Table 1.1) and adults (Table 1.2) has been increasing over the years (4–6).

Must et al. (3) noted the following serious health problems in children associated with excess weight: high blood pressure, 3 times more prevalent; type 2 diabetes, 13–18 times more common among the heaviest individuals; gall bladder disease, 21 times more common; heart disease 3–5 times more prevalent; and osteoarthritis, 30 times more common.

Adults in America

A study conducted by the Centers for Disease Control and Prevention found that from 1971 to 2000, obesity in the United States increased from 14.5% to 30.9% (7), with a calorie increase of 335 cal per day (1542–1877) for women and 168 cal per day (2450–2618) for men. This increase was mainly due to an increase in carbohydrate consumption rather than fat consumption (7). By 2010, the prevalence of obesity in adults had increased to 36% (8).

Worldwide

Obesity is not just a problem in the United States; it is also increasing at an alarming rate worldwide. The WHO estimates that there are 1.6 billion *overweight* people in the world. Ironically, this number is about the same number of people who go to bed hungry each night. It is estimated that there are more than 400 million *obese* people worldwide (www.who.int), and obesity is becoming an increasing problem in many developing countries. Studies have

Table 1.1 Prevalence of obesity among US children and
adolescents (percentage)

Year	Age (years) 2–5	6–11	12–19
1963–1970 NHES I		4.2	4.6
1971–1974 NHANES I	5.0	4.0	6.1
1976–1980 NHANES II	5.0	6.5	5.0
1988–1994 NCHS	7.2	11.3	10.5
1999–2000 NCHS	10.3	15.1	14.8
2001–2002 NCHS	10.6	16.3	16.7
2003–2004 NCHS	14.0	18.8	17.4
2005–2006 NCHS	11.0	15.1	17.8
2007–2008 NCHS	10.1	19.6	18.1
2009–2010 NCHS	12.1	18.0	18.4
2011–2012 NCHS	8.4	17.7	20.5

Source: Center for Disease Control and Prevention (CDC). Health, United States,
2013, Table 64. Data from the National Health and Nutrition Examination
Survey (NHANES). www.cdc.gov/nchs/data/hus/hus13.pdf#064
Note: NCHS, National Center for Health Statistics; NHANES, National Health
and Nutrition Examination Survey; NHES, National Health Examination
Survey.

Table 1.2 Age-adjusted prevalence of overweight and obesity among
US adults aged 20 and older (percentage)

Year	Overweight or obese (BMI 25+)	Obese
1971–1974 NHANES I[a]	46.8	14.5
1976–1980 NHANES II[a]	47.1	15.0
1988–1994 NCHS	56.0	22.9
1999–2000 NCHS	64.5	30.5
2001–2002 NCHS	65.6	30.5
2003–2004 NCHS	66.4	32.3
2005–2006 NCHS	66.9	34.4
2007–2008 NCHS	68.1	33.7
2009–2010 NCHS	68.8	35.7
2011–2012 NCHS	68.6	34.9

Source: Center for Disease Control and Prevention (CDC). Health, United States,
2013, Table 64. Data from the National Health and Nutrition Examination
Survey (NHANES). www.cdc.gov/nchs/data/hus/hus13.pdf#064
Note: BMI, body mass index; NCHS, National Center for Health Statistics;
NHANES, National Health and Nutrition Examination Survey.
[a] NHANES I and II did not include individuals over 74 years of age.

found that the prevalence of obesity varies from less than 5% in rural China, Japan, and some African countries to as high as 75% in urban Samoa. In the United States, where 65% of people are overweight, there are also large differences in obesity between people of different ethnic origins.

PREVENTION: SO WHAT IS BEING DONE ABOUT THIS EPIDEMIC?

Several government agencies have weight loss campaigns designed for use in schools. There is a move in schools to have less soda and more water and milk in vending machines. Fast-food concessions are disappearing from schools, and less high-carbohydrate, government-surplus foods are being served. Most magazines at the grocery store checkouts have articles about losing weight to raise awareness about the problem.

In addition, exercise is being promoted in schools and by local gyms. Some parents have started to limit the time their children spend on computers, Internet games, and TV. People are walking more often than in the past.

The following are the American Medical Association Expert Committee recommendations for childhood obesity (paraphrased):

- Address the issue of weight once yearly at the child's clinical visit. Assess dietary habits, especially the consumption of sweetened beverages; physical activity habits; readiness to change lifestyle habits; and family history of obesity and related illnesses.
- Limit sweet drinks and fast food, eat breakfast, and have family meals most days of the week. Limit screen time and engage in physical activity for 60 minutes daily.
- Do a lipid profile, liver profile, and blood glucose for children in the 85th to 94th percentile with comorbidities. Add kidney function tests for those above the 95th percentile (9).

The WHO has suggested the following actions to help prevent obesity:

- Creating supportive population-based environments through public policies that promote low-fat, high-fiber foods and provide opportunities for physical activity.
- Promoting weight loss by eating more fruit and vegetables, nuts, and whole grains.
- Cutting the amount of fatty, sugary foods in the diet, moving from animal-based fats to unsaturated vegetable oil–based fats, and engaging in physical activity for 30 minutes daily.
- Establishing clinical programs to aid losing weight and avoid further weight gain (www.who.int).

SOCIAL IMPLICATIONS

Obesity is the only remaining issue in our society in which discrimination seems to be acceptable. Obese persons have been thought of as being gluttonous and slothful. People say, "Why don't they take care of themselves?" There is discrimination in the workplace.

In Japan, a national law mandates that a waist circumference of 33.5 in. for men and 35.4 in. for women is where health risks begin. Those exceeding the limit will get dieting help if they do not lose weight by themselves after three months. Further education will be given after six months if they have not met the goal.

A survey in the United States found that the average waist size of men was 39 in., just under the 40 in. threshold of the International Diabetes Federation. The average waist size of women was 36.5 in., 2 in. above the threshold of 34.6 in.

COST OF OBESITY

Cost to society

In 2003, the annual US obesity-attributable medical expenditures were estimated at $75 billion, and about one-half of these expenditures were financed by Medicare and Medicaid. If all these obesity-attributable medical expenditures had been financed by federal taxes, the cost would have been approximately $350 per adult to cover the cost. This figure would be reduced by one-half if limited to expenditures financed by Medicare and Medicaid (10).

The cost of obesity-related expenditures had risen to $147 billion by 2010 (11). Costs are estimated to reach $344 billion in 2018 if rates continue to increase at current levels (12).

Costs to insurance companies

The Milliman Research Report in 2004 presented findings from an examination of a large 2001 database from a single plan employer/employee group coverage (13):

- Per-person claim costs for obese persons were triple those for the average member.
- Hospital admission rate for obese was 350 per 1000 contrasted to 50 per 1000 for an average population.
- Cesarean section rate was 50% of deliveries of obese mothers, more than double that of a typical insured population.

Employers bear most of the costs associated with treating obesity-related conditions, primarily in terms of lost productivity; paid sick leave; and the increased cost of health, life, and disability insurance. Obese employees are twice as likely to have high-level absenteeism (seven or more absences in 6 months) and 1.5 times more likely to have moderate absenteeism (six absences in 6 months) (14).

Thus, there are many prevention programs in place, but how do we help the 65% of Americans who are obese? When reanalyzing the past 50 years of "research," it becomes obvious that true scientific evidence that eating fat causes heart disease is lacking. Academicians over the years have challenged the fat–heart disease issue; however, going against accepted medical practice is deadly to future funding and the ability to get their research published. When organized medicine owns up to a failed 50-year experiment on what we should eat, society will be healthier. I predict within the next 10 years the tide will turn and fats will be on our tables and sugar and other carbohydrates will be on the "no-eat" list and obesity and diabetes will become rare (15–19). For now, the best treatment of obesity and its comorbidities is the subject of this book, written by experienced bariatricians, and physicians who are devoted to, and specialize in, the treatment of individuals with obesity.

REFERENCES

1. Curb JD, Marcus EB. Body fat and obesity in Japanese Americans. *Am J Clin Nutr* 1991; 53: 1552S–1555S.
2. Ogden CL, Flegal KM, Carroll MD, et al. Prevalence and trends in overweight among US children and adolescents, 1999–2000. *JAMA* 2002; 288: 1728–1732.
3. Must A, Hollander SA, Economos CD. Childhood obesity: a growing public health concern. *Expert Review of Endocrinology and Metabolism* 2005; 1: 233–255.

4. Flegal KM, Carroll MD, Ogden CL, et al. Prevalence and trends in obesity among US adults, 1999–2000. *JAMA* 2002; 288: 1723–1727.
5. Ogden CL, Carroll MD, Curtin LR, et al. Prevalence of overweight and obesity in the United States, 1999–2004. *JAMA* 2006; 295: 1549–1555.
6. Center for Disease Control and Prevention (CDC). Health, United States, 2013, Table 64. Data from the National Health and Nutrition Examination Survey (NHANES). www.cdc.gov/nchs/data/hus/hus13.pdf#064, accessed July 31, 2014.
7. Centers for Disease Control and Prevention (CDC). Trends in intake of energy and macronutrients, United States, 1971–2000. *MMWR Morb Mortal Wkly Rep* 2004; 53(4): 80–82.
8. May AL, Freedman D, Sherry B, et al. Obesity—Unites States, 1999–2010. *MMWR Surveill Sum* 2013; 62(3): 120–128.
9. Rao G. Childhood obesity: Highlights of AMA expert committee recommendations. *Am Fam Physician* 2008; 78(1): 56–63.
10. Finkelstein EA, Fiebelkorn IC, Wang G. State-level estimates of annual medical expenditures attributable to obesity. *Obes Res* 2004; 12(1): 18–24.
11. Finkelstein EA, Trogdon JB, Cohen JW, et al. Annual medical spending attributable to obesity: Payer-and service-specific estimates. *Health Aff (Millwood)* 2009; 28(5): w822–w831.
12. United Health Foundation, American Public Health Association and Partnership for Prevention. The future costs of obesity: National and state estimates of the impact of obesity on direct health care expenses. 2009. www.americashealthrankings/2009/spotlight.aspx
13. Fitch K, Pyenson B, Abbs S, et al. *Obesity: A Big Problem Getting Bigger*. Milliman Research Report. New York; 2004.
14. Tucker LA, Friedman GM. Obesity and absenteeism: An epidemiologic study of 10,825 employed adults. *Am J Health Promot* 1998; 12(3): 202–207.
15. Teicholz N. *The Big Fat Surprise: Why Butter, Meat and Cheese Belong in a Healthy Diet*. New York: Simon & Schuster; 2014.
16. Taubes G. *Good Calories, Bad Calories: Fats, Carbs and the Controversial Science of Diet and Health*. New York: Knopf; 2007.
17. Taubes G. *Why We Get Fat and What To Do About It*. New York: Anchor Books; 2012.
18. Westman EC, Phinney SD, Volek JS. *The New Atkins for a New You*. New York: Simon & Schuster (Fireside); 2010.
19. Lustig RH. *Fat Chance: Beating the Odds against Sugar, Processed Food, Obesity and Disease*. New York: Penguin; 2012.

2

Etiologies of obesity

LARRY A. RICHARDSON

INTRODUCTION

Khalil Gibran said, "Perplexity is the beginning of knowledge." This claim seems appropriate when dealing with the quest to define and categorize the myriad etiologies relating to overweight and obesity. Wherein we once were taught that the fat cell (adipocyte) was just a simple storage vessel for excess fat, we have now discovered a microcosm of energy regulation and other physiological functions via its endocrine, paracrine, and autocrine activities.

The historically underappreciated adipocyte has now been elevated well beyond the simplistic roles of body insulation and organ protection imparted in medical education just a few decades ago.

By similar inference, many researchers and health personnel were taught that overweight and obesity were simply due to an energy imbalance: too much eating (excess calories in) and too little exercise (not enough calories burned) (1). It therefore seemed logical for health providers to view obesity as a result of gluttony and slothfulness and all too often dispense the advice, "Just push yourself away from the table and exercise." Often this does not solve the problem because weight regulation is not governed by a uniform tally of calories in–calories out (2).

The etiologies of obesity described in this chapter can be considered, on a foundational level, to serve as insight for our continually expanding knowledge and understanding of the complexities of excessive adipose tissue. If lean body mass remains stable and energy output is less than energy intake, body fat does increase. It would be simple if the explanation stopped here, but it does not. This chapter examines the multifaceted keys to susceptibility for obesity that are strongly influenced by genetic, behavioral, environmental, biological, circadian, and other factors. A visual representation of the complex interactions between 108 variables thought by experts to contribute to obesity causation, the Foresight Obesity System map (3), was developed by the UK government in 2007 and gives a good oversight of the multiple interactions among some of the elements discussed later in this chapter.

Family and twin studies show genetics determines a moderate portion of weight variation, but the almost exponential increase in US obesity prevalence over the past several decades cannot be blamed on sudden genetic changes. New insights into epigenetics through genome-wide association studies (GWASs) and identification of single-nucleotide polymorphisms (SNPs) are offering additional data to help map this part of the puzzle.

In 2008, the World Health Organization estimated that 1.4 billion people worldwide are overweight and more than 500 million of them are obese (4). Although these current numbers are staggering, the fact that they continue to rise mandates that we better understand the various factors influencing adiposity and devise new and innovative medical alternatives and social strategies to stem this true, worldwide pandemic.

As seen in the Foresight Obesity System map, there are numerous classification schemes that can be used to organize causative adipogenic factors into a useable framework. This chapter uses the major categories of (1) global and community influences, (2) personal characteristics, and (3) behavioral factors. Each of these major divisions comprised many smaller segments that are also briefly described. Since some elements may fall under more than one subcategory, they may be referenced throughout this chapter. Information presented herein has either been proven to be causative for obesity (longitudinal studies) or has been strongly associated with (cross-sectional studies) influencing adiposity.

GLOBAL AND COMMUNITY INFLUENCES

It is readily apparent that food and societal environments are large stimuli in promoting what is termed an "obesogenic environment," the sum of influences that the surroundings, opportunities, or conditions of life have on promoting obesity in individuals or populations (5). They have a major impact on inducing food acquisition, eating, and lifestyle habits.

Food environment

The food environment encompasses several factors beyond just food itself, such as economics, industrialization, and governmental policies. Technical advances in both food production and transportation, coupled with the global marketing of modern commerce, have led to the introduction of relatively cheap, energy-dense foods into the domestic food markets of many developing countries. The cost of energy-dense foods high in fat, sugar, and salt has fallen, whereas that of healthier options has increased in relative terms (6). Commodity subsidization (e.g., grains, fat and oils, dairy, and cattle) by the government has contributed to an American food diet that is very favorable to the overconsumption of high-calorie foods (7). Note that highly palatable high-fat and high-sucrose diets blunt the signals of the satiety neuropeptides (i.e., those that are supposed to decrease appetite) insulin and cholecystokinin (CCK). As if this were not enough to promote overeating, such palatable food also activates a brain reward system that reinforces the eating behavior.

One of the most controversial areas of obesity research is the role of diet composition upon body weight (8,9). Both high-fat and high simple carbohydrate diets affect metabolism (10). These two macronutrients were the primary source of the increase in food energy of the North American diet from 1980 to 2009. This food energy increase is reflected by a per capita increase of 10 kg per year in fat and almost 5 kg per year in caloric sweeteners. A majority of the increased fat and sugar consumed was added during food processing. The increased sugar intake is largely from the increased consumption of sweetened beverages, including those containing high-fructose corn syrup (HFCS) (11). At the high doses ingested by most Americans, HFCS has pathological consequences. Unlike glucose, which is stored as glycogen, fructose metabolites are stored as triglycerides in the liver (12).

Changes in dietary composition can produce obesity in genetically normal animals, independent of an increase in calorie intake. When animals fed a high glycemic index (GI) diet were food restricted to prevent excessive weight gain, they still gained substantially more fat (70%) than animals on a low GI diet and also exhibited adverse changes in cardiovascular disease risk factors (13).

Even as investigation continues into the contribution of various macronutrients (protein, carbohydrate, and fat) in promoting obesity, the spotlight has fallen on micronutrients (vitamins, minerals, trace elements, phytochemicals, and antioxidants). As part of some countries' governmental policies, fortification of food with vitamins became popular. This approach led to national increases in the consumption of many vitamins, especially fat synthesis–promoting B vitamins, that were often added to ready-to-eat cereals. Emerging evidence suggests that this excess vitamin intake might play a role in the increased prevalence of obesity.

It seems more than a coincidence that in countries that prohibit flour fortification there is low prevalence of obesity compared with countries that have high flour fortification standards. Animal studies suggest that the supplemental dose for niacin to achieve maximum weight-gain effect may be about 60 mg/kg diet. This dose is similar to that used in wheat flour fortification in some countries, such as the United States. Further supplementation with niacin or a niacin-containing multivitamin may offset the weight gain effect due to increased toxic effects, such as hepatotoxicity and oxidative tissue damage (14).

The average US caloric intake increased 500 kcal per day between 1970 and 2000. This increased intake included increased consumption of sweetened beverages by young adults to constitute almost 20% of their daily calories. The consumption of energy-dense foods and beverages typically results in greater energy intake, because many people respond to the volume of food consumed rather than to the energy content of the food itself. High-carbohydrate or high-fat foods (e.g., sugar-sweetened beverages [SSBs], salad dressings, sauces, cooking oils, and gravies) can be low volume but energy dense.

There are many factors leading to an increase in the consumption of energy-dense foods and dietary sugars and fats. The commercial food environment influences these increases through numerous small changes, including the following:

- Increased, inexpensive, energy-dense foods: soft drinks, cheese, fat, and sugary foods
  - Up-regulation of hunger and blunting of satiety signals by processed foods
- Numerous convenient eating sites promoting non–home-cooked meals (see also built environment in Community dynamics section)
  - Neighborhood fast-food restaurants
  - Delivery options (pizza)
  - Convenience marts and gas stations
  - Sports venues (snack bars)
  - Movie theaters, playhouses, and concerts
  - Snack and soda machines (airports, hotels, schools, and offices)
- High variety of foods at mealtime
  - Especially high-energy content but low nutrient density foods
  - Increased fatness and food intake seen with more choices of entrees, sweets, snacks, and other refined carbohydrates (i.e., "cafeteria diet")
- Unreasonably large portion sizes
  - Omnipresent food and larger portion sizes translate into greater intake of food and beverages (seen in affluent societies).
  - There is strong evidence supporting genetic determination of obesity set point in response to high-fat and high-sucrose diets (10). Overconsumption of such palatable food leads to shift in set point similar to adaptation in drug addiction.

Socioeconomic status

Socioeconomic status usually entails income, education, occupation, or a composite. The prevalence of obesity in most developed countries, including the United States, seems to be negatively correlated with socioeconomic class; that is, it predominantly affects the most socioeconomically disadvantaged groups. Lower income, minority urban neighborhoods, and rural areas ("food deserts") may have limited access to food choice. Food insecurity has been identified as a major determinant of food selection and a contributor to obesity in these areas. Food-insecure families identified price as the most salient factor influencing their purchases. Nutrient-dense foods (e.g., fruits, vegetables, whole grains, nonfat or low-fat milk, and lean meats) cost significantly more per calorie than energy-dense foods (e.g., soft drinks, salty and sugary snacks, pastries, and packaged and frozen foods), leading to greater availability of obesogenic foods in the home. Children in such households experience poor diet quality and subsequent accumulation of body fat in adulthood (15).

In contrast, in less developed countries obesity most frequently affects the most well-off socioeconomic groups who, perhaps, can afford more of the processed and refined items, particularly those individuals who have incorporated western lifestyles (16). Besides food consumed, there is also an association with increased ownership of televisions, cars, and computers by wealthier citizens in such countries, leading to trends of increased sitting, dietary energy intake, body mass index (BMI), and waist circumference (WC) and to decreased physical activity (PA) (17).

Family structure variations

Family structure variations include the subsets of cultural influences and parenting behaviors. Cultural factors can influence through attitudes, beliefs, and behaviors. They can shape values and norms about dietary intake, PA, and body weight itself that, in turn, can influence body weight and weight change of individuals through societal modernization, migration, and acculturation. Such influences are thought to contribute to the higher than average risk of obesity among children and youth of US ethnic minority populations (18) as each child is trained to shape his or her eating behavior according to the culturally appropriate pattern (19). Some of the culturally defined contributors to body size and shape that are conveyed from parents to their children include the following:

- Types and amounts of food and beverages
  - Among African American populations in the southeastern United States, consumption of food high in fat is a part of cultural practice (20).
- Textures, flavors, and food combinations
- Traditional uses and symbolic meanings of food
- Foods used to create social interactions as well as pleasure and punishment
  - Food has now taken on new social roles—eating for enjoyment and amusement—beyond solely survival (21).
  - Social networks may also contribute to the increasing prevalence of obesity. One study showed that a person's chance of becoming obese increased by 57% if he or she had a friend who became obese in a given interval. A similar phenomenon was observed among adult siblings and married couples (22).
- Conceptualization of which foods are healthful, harmful, or protective (23)
  - Hispanic parents may be more likely to hold on to cultural beliefs that their children need to be heavier for them to be healthy (24).
- Dietary celebration of various holidays
  - Behavioral holiday changes contribute to winter seasonal weight gain.
  - Holiday changes can contribute up to one-half of an individual's annual weight gain.
  - Many influences (including major physiological factors such as hunger and nonphysiological factors such as number of people present) exert a small, but significant, effect on the size of an eating event (19).
- Media influence
  - Media influences all cultures to promote enhanced food intake.
  - Media enhances "addiction" to excessive fat and sugar intake.
  - Media can influence body-image attitudes and desires to avoid or accept overweight or obesity. Compared to white women, ethnic minority women and adolescents have, on average, a greater acceptance of overweight and report higher rates of body-image satisfaction, independent of body weight (25).

Even some governmental policies display a cultural tone when dealing with certain ethnic groups. Subtle societal influences on energy intake and expenditure can foster the development of obesity. One such example involves the Pima Indians in Arizona. Due to US-imposed dietary modifications and altered manual labor and hunting activity resulting from reservation life, they have developed tremendous rates of diabetes and obesity compared to their genetically identical clan in Mexico.

Parenting is indeed a subset of family structure variations and includes maternal attributes, feeding practices, and monitoring activity. Behaviors associated with parenting are a culmination of the family's food and physical environments, family resources (structure, parental education, and income), and beliefs and norms reinforced through kin and nonkin groups. Even after correcting for genetic influences, parental beliefs, attitudes, and practices correlate with children's weight.

Maternal obesity itself is one of the epigenetic (see also Genetic influences section) exposures that can influence the weight and health of future children. Children born after maternal weight loss have a lower risk for obesity than do their siblings born before maternal weight loss (26). Malnutrition and overnutrition during pregnancy can exert deleterious effects on the fetus, suggesting that maternal weight demonstrates a U-shaped effect in relation to fetal programming and adult diseases (27).

Feeding practice initially consisting of postnatal nutrition, received indirectly through the maternal lactational diet or directly through infant feeding, can modulate the risk of obesity later in life. Rates of weight gain have been shown to be lower in breast-fed than formula-fed infants. Breast-fed infants consume not only less energy than formula-fed infants but also disproportionately less protein and fewer micronutrients. Breast-fed children present with lower risk for overweight and obesity (16). However, it has been shown that formula feeding and micronutrient-fortified human milk feeding can lead to rapid infant weight gain, a known major risk factor for children developing obesity (14). Since human milk is exquisitely designed for optimal infant growth and development, breast-feeding should be promoted regardless of its modest influence on later obesity. Early weaning has been associated with greater risk of overweight in adolescence, and the nature of the maternal diet during breastfeeding can modulate subsequent food preferences and appetite control (28).

When infants are weaned to foods, those who are parentally spoon fed preferred sweet foods and have a higher rate of obesity in early childhood than those who self-feed (29). As the child ages, when they self-select their own food portion size, their consumption is usually reduced. Current child feeding practices by parents seem to be creating diets that promote excessive weight gain during the first years of life.

During childhood and adolescence, dietary predictors of increased adiposity include increased energy intake and greater percentages of energy supplied by fat and refined carbohydrates. Preferences and selections of foods, along with regulation of energy intake, are affected by parental feeding practices, including the foods made available to them, portion sizes, frequency of eating occasions, and the social context in which eating occurs. For example, larger portion size leads to higher energy intake in both children and adults within eating events (30).

Patterns of eating are an integral part of feeding practices within families. One healthy model includes regular high-order (i.e., more regimented) meals by the family characterized by sharing meals with one another at prescribed times and locations, with menus comprising more traditionally prepared (vs. processed) foods. This model contrasts with low-order eating whereby families rarely eat together, eat at different times and locations, and have menu choices that are more flexible and quicker to prepare (e.g., microwave meals, fast foods, sports and energy drinks, and sodas) (5).

Although some longitudinal studies are neutral on the topic, others show significant correlation between snacking and body weight increase. Given the increased convenience of the food supply providing greater opportunity to eat more frequently and evidence that eating frequency is positively associated with energy intake and weight gain, it seems to be important that healthy snacks be readily available to children and adults. Some noteworthy information regarding snacking includes the following:

- Observational trials in humans indicate that eating more often than three times a day may play a role in overweight and obesity (31).
- Consumption of "snacks" in addition to meals has been viewed by many experts as a major contributor to the rise in overweight and obesity (19). This view is supported by large prospective studies demonstrating that frequent snacking may lead to weight gain (32).
- Periods of fasting between meals may be even more important than the composition of the diet (33) (circadian effect).
- In obese children and adults, in addition to selecting energy-dense foods, eating in the absence of hunger in response to external nonphysiological cues, in an irregular manner, in ways that do not favor attention to the act of eating, might be crucial factors determining the nutritional effects of snacking.
- In families with at least one overweight parent, the increased snacking in girls who watched more television was associated with higher intake of fats from energy-dense snack foods, and this behavior predicted an increase in BMI from ages 5 to 9 years.
- Children, adolescents, and adults in various parts of Europe and America snack at least once and often several times a day.
- The latest data reveal that American children are moving toward three snacks per day, accounting for more than 27% of daily energy. The major sources of energy from their snacks are desserts, sweetened beverages, salty snack foods, and candy (19).

Monitoring of activity and sleep quantity is another integral subset of parenting influences on childhood weight. These activities include computer use, video gaming, TV watching, and the encouragement of PA (e.g., biking, swimming, and sports). The amount of TV watched seems to have some correlation with overweight. Children and adolescents (8–18 years old) spend up to 4.5 hours per day watching TV or related media (34). Some of this time displaces PA time and encourages increased snacking due to advertising of snack items. Increased TV viewing and computer and Internet use during adolescence have been shown to be associated with higher odds of consumption of sweetened beverages, especially at the upper tail of the BMI distribution between ages 14 and 18 years.

Parents need to be role models for healthy eating and activity as culturally determined attitudes may influence PA and inactivity levels. In children, general levels of PA are negatively correlated with weight status. Even ensuring adequate sleep for their children and themselves influences weight within the entire family. Sleep duration has been identified as a risk factor for adolescent and child overweight (see also Nontraditional factors section).

Community dynamics

The term "built environment" has been coined to try to summarize the living and working conditions that are collectively created by societies and are key determinants of both restrictions and opportunities for food consumption and for PA. To reverse currently unhealthy trends in these areas, major changes in urban planning, transportation, public safety, and food production and marketing need to occur. As an example of societal working conditions, there is evidence to suggest that low-energy-expenditure occupations are now the norm and that workers engaged in these types of occupations are at increased risk of obesity. Energy expended at the typical worksite declined by more than 100 cal per day over the past 50 years in the United States, and this decline has been associated with concomitant population levels of weight gain over the same period (35).

Other factors relating to the dynamics of the community and how it interplays with eating behavior and PA within that community include the following:

- Population density—urban living is associated with lower energy demands than rural life
- Street connectivity—impedes or facilitates access to travel and acquisition of food
  - Poor connectivity encourages more vehicle use versus walking or biking. In places where governments have invested heavily in building cities and towns that are conducive to walking and bicycling, obesity rates are lower than in places that are more car dependent (36).
- Access to fast-food restaurants, supermarkets, or nutritious food sources
  - In a sample of 5688 community-dwelling adults aged 50 to 74 years, densities of fast-food establishments and storefronts (convenience stores, bars, and small grocery stores) were positively associated with obesity (37).
  - The lower density of full-service supermarkets and higher density of fast-food restaurants in food deserts have been associated with poorer diets and a higher prevalence of obesity (38).
  - In a review of the association between the built environment and childhood obesity, weight gain was found to be more likely to occur when convenience stores were more accessible and when PA facilities were less accessible (39).
- Access to parks and recreational facilities—importance of walking paths and sidewalks
  - Limited access to open space, playgrounds, and sidewalks has affected the amount of opportunities available to children for outdoor activity, and, in turn, has been shown to significantly contribute to child PA levels (40).
- Public transportation systems
  - Transportation policies have been shown to impact population levels of PA and obesity. Countries with the highest levels of active transportation (bike, walk, and public transport) tended to have the lowest obesity rates (41).
- Schools
  - As the child's experience moves beyond the family into school and peer environments, these new settings assume greater influence over diet and activity patterns.
  - Features of schools believed related to childhood and adolescent obesity risk include the following:
    - Nutritional content of foods made available in schools, including cafeterias and vending machines offering sodas and snacks
    - Availability of (and requirements for) regular physical education classes and involvement in organized sports
    - Patterns of transportation to and from school (the number of US children walking or biking to school was 48% in 1969 compared to 13% in 2009, but rose to approximately 20% in 2012) (42)

Health care

PREGNANCY

This section focuses on potential causes of obesity during pregnancy as well as iatrogenic or secondary factors leading to obesity. Studies show the importance of good nutritional counseling and monitoring during all trimesters of pregnancy in regard to risk factors (and outcomes) for obesity in the offspring.

Reduced, increased, or imbalanced growth during gestation and early postnatal life due to abnormal perinatal environments (e.g., malnutrition and maternal diabetes) can result in the permanent programming of physiological systems that will predispose individuals to develop obesity and diabetes. Both maternal undernutrition and overnutrition can induce persistent changes in gene expression and metabolism (43), resulting in epigenetically mediated fetal programming that is currently seen as an important contributor to the pathogenesis of obesity and metabolic disease (44).

It has been assumed that environmental exposure during gestation and infancy has the potential to alter the regulatory circuits that control feeding and metabolism, thereby playing a critical role in phenotype determination (45). Exposure to a high-fat diet in utero might cause a metabolic syndrome–like phenomenon through epigenetic modifications of adipocytokine, adiponectin, and leptin gene expression (46). The effects of prenatal development on subsequent obesity risk are clearest with respect to accelerated fetal growth (macrosomia), a condition that is associated with an increased risk for obesity in later life (16). Macrosomia is most often related to excessive gestational weight gain, maternal hyperglycemia, or diabetes. Gestational weight gain, irrespective of prepregnancy body mass, is positively associated with obesity in offspring at 3 years (26).

There is also evidence that fetuses with low birth weights who were malnourished in the first and second trimesters of pregnancy compensate after birth with enhanced growth in childhood. These children are similarly predisposed to adult obesity and type 2 diabetes mellitus. Furthermore, this compensatory rapid growth in infancy and childhood is another risk for adult obesity (47).

Besides affecting adipocytes and peripheral targets, these prenatal nutritional factors affect development of the central nervous system (CNS). Several epidemiological studies have highlighted the role of fetal nutrition in the development of the CNS early in life. Developmental abnormalities rooted in abnormal in utero conditions provide evidence that environmental factors related to inadequate nutrition affect brain development in ways that will predispose to obesity. The first clearly defined example of this abnormality came from studies of effects of long-term starvation on the development of the fetus in pregnant women during the Dutch famine in the winter of 1944 to 1945. Some of the findings from these studies are as follows:

- High prevalence of obesity and comorbidities (e.g., diabetes mellitus) later in life
  - Hypothesized mechanism was that altered fetal brain development shifted fetal CNS regulation of energy homeostasis toward favoring enhanced energy storage to compensate for deficient nutrition.
  - Additional theories assigned changes in hypothalamic circuitry toward supporting positive energy balance through increased food consumption during times of improved nutrition, leading to obesity and its comorbidities.

Other than nutritional effects, maternal smoking during pregnancy and lactation were also associated with an increased long-term risk for overweight and obesity in childhood and adult life (16). Children whose mother smoked during pregnancy had a 50% increased risk for overweight compared with children whose mothers did not smoke during pregnancy (48).

Table 2.1 Drugs that may promote weight gain

Psychiatric and neurologic medications

Antipsychotics: olanzapine, clozapine, resperidone, quetiapine, aripiprazole

Antidepressants

    Tricyclics: imipramine, amitriptyline

    Triazolopyridines: trazodone

    Serotonin reuptake inhibitors: paroxetine, fluoxetine, citalopram

    Tetracyclics: mirtazapine

    Monoamine oxidase inhibitors

Antiepileptic drugs: gabapentin (higher dose), valproic acid, carbamazepine, divalproex

Mood stabilizers: lithium, carbamazepine, lamotrigine, gabapentin (higher doses)

Steroid hormones

Progestational steroids

Corticosteroids

Hormonal contraceptives

Antidiabetes agents

Insulin (most forms)

Sulfonylureas

Thiazolidinediones

Antihistamines

Commonly reported with older agents; also oxatomide, loratadine, and azelastine

Antihypertensive agents

α- and β-Adrenergic receptor blockers

Calcium channel blockers: nisoldipine

Highly active antiretroviral therapy

Source: Data from Jensen MD. Obesity. In: Goldman L, Schafer A, eds. *Cecil Textbook of Medicine*, 24th ed. Philadelphia, PA: Saunders Elsevier; 2012, pp. 1409–17.

MEDICATIONS

One of the principles of the Hippocratic Oath is "first, do no harm." However, in an attempt to treat other issues, health care providers often use treatments and pharmacological agents that can contribute to obesity, the so-called iatrogenic or secondary factors. Many of the psychotropic medications, diabetic treatments, antihypertensives, steroid hormones, contraceptives, antihistamines, and protease inhibitors (22) promote appreciable weight gain. Examples are provided in Table 2.1 (49).

Nontraditional factors

The last category of Global and Community Influences examined herein is termed the nontraditional factors. They include the following:

- Ambient temperature variability reduction
  - In humans, the thermal neutral zone (TNZ) is approximately 25°C to 30°C, a range of ambient temperatures across which energy expenditure is not allocated toward maintaining a constant body temperature (26).

- Average indoor temperatures have stabilized and increased in the past 50 years, another weight-contributing factor (44). There is a clear correlation between the use of heating and artificial temperature control mechanisms and obesity (50).
- The metabolic rate in humans is lower within the current temperature ranges as compared to temperatures that were historically the norm (26). Exposure to temperatures above or below the TNZ increases energy expenditure, which, all other things being equal, decreases energy stores (i.e., fat).
- Reduced sleep time (see also Hypothalamus section)
  - Decreases leptin, thyroid-stimulating hormone, and glucose tolerance.
    - Leptin levels are reduced and energy intake is increased during short sleep durations in humans (51).
    - During partial sleep deprivation, thyroid-stimulating hormone levels and the duration of its secretion have been found to be blunted (26).
    - Even limiting a single night to 4 hours of sleep led to decreased peripheral insulin sensitivity by 20% to 25% and increased hepatic insulin resistance.
  - Increases ghrelin, sympathetic nervous system (SNS) activity, evening cortisol level, catecholamine levels, and proinflammatory cytokines.
    - Hormonal imbalance may explain increased appetite for snacks, fat, and carbohydrates, ultimately leading to weight gain.
  - Delays nighttime secretion of growth hormone.
    - May adversely influence glucose regulation, leading to transient insulin resistance, a decrease in glucose uptake, and elevated blood glucose (52).
  - May alter circadian chronobiological systems.
    - It is possible that the shift in circadian rhythm may be a key factor in disturbing resting metabolic rate (RMR) in healthy individuals.
  - Some studies link poor sleep quality, not just quantity (duration), with increased hunger and uncontrolled and emotional eating, as well as decreased cognitive restraint (53).
  - Sleep debt and weight association is most prominent in children and young adults (52).
- Environmental xenobiotic chemicals termed obesogens have an overlap with endocrine disrupting chemicals (EDCs) and deserve special attention as they have become more identified as a major potential pathway for much of the global obesity observed today. There are now nearly 20 obesogenic chemicals shown to cause long-term weight gain and metabolic dysfunction in humans or animals. The effects of early life obesogen exposure are permanent and transgenerational, increasing the risk of future generations developing obesity and related disorders. Chemical exposure during the pubertal period is linked with early menarche in females and delayed sexual maturation in males. These changes in sexual maturation are risk factors for obesity later in life.

  Endocrine disruptors are environmental chemical compounds produced by human activity that were originally designed for a specific purpose such as a pesticide, plasticizer, or solvent (54). An accumulating body of evidence suggests that EDCs may be linked to the obesity epidemic (55). As these links unfold, they become even more ominous when one realizes there are close to 800 chemicals with reported EDC properties (56).

  Types of chemicals with EDC properties

- Synthetic organic compounds (45)
  - Pesticides
    - Organochlorines—chlordane
    - Organophosphates

- Fungicides
  - Organotins—tributyltin (55)
  - Triflumizole
- Pharmaceutical drugs
  - Diethylstilbestrol
- Chemicals used for the polymerization of plastics and resins
  - Bisphenol A and bisphenol A diglycidyl ether
  - Phthalates
- Dioxins
- Polychlorinated biphenyls
- Polybrominated biphenyls
- Butyltins
- Flame retardants (polybrominated diphenyl ether)
- Natural phytoestrogens
  - Genistein
  - Daidzein
- Polyfluoroalkyl chemicals
- Solvents
- Heavy metals (55)
- Home and industrial products
  - Tetrafluoroethylene (Teflon®)
  - Perfluorooctane sulfonate (Scotchgard™)
- Foods and food additives
  - Soy
  - Monosodium glutamate
  - Fructose
    - At the high doses ingested by most Americans, fructose has pathological consequences.
    - Creates de novo lipogenesis in the liver, stimulating inappropriate storage of fat in the liver, as opposed to the adipocyte (12).
- Most common pathways through which obesogens and EDCs lead to overweight or obesity
  - Increase the number of adipocytes by altering the basal metabolic rate (BMR; metabolism) to favor energy storage.
  - Interfere with the endocrine system and neurotransmitters that control appetite and satiety (10).
  - Mimic or block hormonal actions (such as estrogen and androgen) and alter the synthesis of a hormone or modulate its breakdown (26).
  - Modify the epigenome of multipotent stromal stem cells, biasing them to the adipocyte lineage. This modification is of special concern in the fetus as it may result in enlarged white adipose depots.
  - Disrupt some epigenetic, structural, and functional mechanisms that control energy homeostasis, lipid metabolism, appetite regulation, and adipogenesis.
  - Change weight-controlling hormones (e.g., leptin, ghrelin, and neuropeptide Y [NPY]).
  - Alter SNS activity (55).
  - Activate peroxisome proliferator-activated receptor γ (PPAR-γ), the master regulator of fat development (57).

- Smoking cessation is associated with weight gain in 80% of cases.
  - Nicotine has both thermogenic and appetite-suppressant effects.
    - RMR decreases after smoking cessation by about 200 kcal per 25 cigarettes (58).
    - Subsample of National Health and Nutrition Examination Survey III showed weight gain caused by stopping smoking to be 4.4 kg in males and 5 kg in females who quit within past 10 years (16). Smoking acts as a behavioral alternative to eating or snacking.
- In women, nicotine also has an antiestrogenic effect that favors android fat distribution. Therefore, despite lower BMI, smokers tend to have higher risk of abdominal visceral fat deposition and abdominal obesity compared with nonsmokers (59).
- Increasing gravida age.
  - A large British prospective cohort study found that the mothers of obese children were on average 3.5 years older at the time of birth than the mothers of normal-weight children.
  - In a multivariable model, researchers calculated that each 5-year increment in maternal age increased the likelihood for obesity by >14%.
  - Older women are at risk for giving birth to infants at both ends of the birth weight distribution, both large and small for gestational age. Both of these groups are more likely to develop obesity (26).
- Gut microbiome. Although technically a microbiological "community influence" within humans, this evolving field certainly falls under the broad categories of nontraditional factors that have been discussed herein. The human gastrointestinal tract is estimated to host up to 10^{14} microorganisms (predominately bacteria), 10-fold the number of human cells (46). In essence, we are 90% microbial cells (gut microbiota) and 10% human cells. There are some generalities associated with linkage of this microcosm with adiposity, and they include the following:
  - Overall bacterial population of the human gut is determined basically by two bacterial phyla: Bacteroides and Firmicutes (60). Lactobacillus was found at a high concentration in the feces of obese patients.
  - Changes in diet have shown important effects on the composition of the intestinal microbiota. In a controlled-feeding study with humans consuming a high-fat/low-fiber or low-fat/high-fiber diet, notable changes were found in gut microbiota in just 24 hours, highlighting the rapid effect that diet can have on the intestinal microbiota.
  - In the obese mouse model, there is usually a significant reduction in Bacteroides and an increase in Firmicutes (61). The reverse is true in lean mice (26). Microbiota transplantation from either lean or obese mice into the gut of germ-free mice resulted in, respectively, less or more body fat, even when the caloric intake remained the same.
  - High intestinal *Bacteroides fragilis* and low *Staphylococcus* concentrations in infants between 3 weeks from birth and 1 year were associated with a higher risk of obesity later in life. This study suggests that early differences in the composition of the intestinal microflora precede the development of obesity in children.
  - It may be important to modify the microbiota of pregnant women to influence the first inoculum and the transfer of microbiota to the infant, because it may have a significant effect on the later health of the infant (60).

Biological Functions and Proposed Mechanisms of Intestinal Microbiota

Digestion

- Extraction of nutrients
  - Suggestion of higher energy harvest in obese patients
  - Conversion of dietary fiber to short-chain fatty acids

Metabolism

- Nutrient and drug metabolism

Regulation of energy balance and weight

- Central effects on satiety.
- Effects on gut-hormone production.
- Obese mice fed a Western diet shift gut microbiota in favor of carbohydrate fermentation.
- Composition of gut flora significantly affects the amount of energy extracted from the diet.

Synthesis and bioavailability of several vitamins

Immunomodulation (61)

- Epithelial cell proliferation
- Prevention of pathogen colonization
- Immune system and barrier function
  - Triggering systemic inflammation.
  - Increased intestinal permeability causing elevated systemic lipopolysaccharides.
  - Gut microbiota links gut permeability to low-grade inflammation and insulin resistance through GLP-2 and endocannabinoid system–dependent mechanisms (62).

Promoting fat deposition

- Fermentation by microbiota promotes short-chain fatty acid production and absorption.
- Increased hepatic de novo lipogenesis due to substantial elevation in serum glucose and insulin from increased glucose uptake through microbiota colonization.

May modify locomotor activity

Before ending this section, note that humans carry two sets of genes: one set encoded by our own genome and another set encoded by the microbiota genome (microbiome). The human genes are about 23,000 in number and the microbiota genes are about 3 million. Therefore, humans inherit only 1% of total genetic material from their parents, and the remaining 99% is mainly acquired from the immediate environment when they are born, and in particular from their mothers' birth canal and breast milk (60).

PERSONAL CHARACTERISTICS

A second major category of etiologies of obesity falls under the heading of personal characteristics. In this section, the impact of genetic, biological, psychological, inflammatory, and infectious causes of excess adiposity is discussed.

Genetic influences

Multiple twin studies have demonstrated that the impact of genetic influences contributes approximately 70% to the tendency toward a specific body habitus, whereas the remaining

30% derives from nongenetic environmental contributors (44). Direct genetic linkage is implicated with the risk of obesity being about 2 to 3 times higher for an individual with a family history of obesity. The risk of extreme obesity (BMI ≥ 45) is about 7 to 8 times higher in families of extremely obese individuals (63). Some of the environmental contributions can be exemplified by the fact that genetic variations can predispose individuals to disease, whereas diet and other factors can decrease or exacerbate this risk. As one noted obesity researcher stated, "Genes load the gun and environment pulls the trigger."

Many of the new insights being gleaned on genetic promoters of obesity have come from GWASs. Through huge meta-analyses, researchers are able to examine interactions between millions of SNPs and the phenotypic trait of interest (e.g., obesity) (56). To date, GWASs have identified 141 suggestive loci for obesity and closely related traits (e.g., BMI, WC), of which 57 loci reach genome-wide significance (10). Of note is that each obesity allele (genetic loci) has a different phenotype depending on the ethnic group (27).

SNPs cause subtle alterations in the functions of the proteins they regulate, although each individually contributes only a small amount (<1%–3%) to the total genetic propensity toward obesity, thus implicating hundreds, and possibly thousands, of contributing genes (44). Some metabolism-regulating and clock gene SNPs related to obesity have also been discovered (64). These SNPs have helped to connect genetics, chronodisruption, and obesity through such things as sleep reduction, changes in ghrelin values, alterations of eating behaviors, and evening preference for energy intake (65).

Literally meaning "above genetics," epigenetics is the thread that is currently tying together genes, SNPs, nutrition, PA, obesogens, fetal and early life exposures, developmental plasticity, and environmental influences regarding the susceptibility to obesity and associated phenotypes (26). Epigenetics refers to the study of changes in gene expression (usually transient, but some are transgenerational) that are not because of changes in DNA sequence, but are under regulation of two major mechanisms at the transcriptional level (66). Common obesity is postulated to result from the interaction of several polymorphisms and epigenetic modifications (27).

The difference between genetics and epigenetics can be compared to the difference between having all the letters of a text (the DNA sequence) and knowing how to space and punctuate them to provide meaningful sentences (epigenetic modifications) (46). Thus, epigenetic mechanisms can essentially turn genes on or off. For example, PA may act as an epigenetic regulator by affecting DNA methylation and histone modifications of candidate gene regions in various tissues (10). The overall hypothesis in this field is that interindividual epigenetic variation contributes to individual variation in adiposity.

Among biological pathways linked with adiposity through genetic influences are the following:

- Metabolism
  - Resting metabolic rate
  - Thermic effect of food (TEF)
  - Energy use
  - PA energy expenditure and tolerance
  - Energy expenditure changes in response to overfeeding
  - Sedentary time
- Feeding behavior
  - Appetite (hunger, satiety)
  - Caloric and macronutrient intake

- Pattern of fat distribution—16 genetic loci identified affecting sites of storage
  - Lipoprotein lipase activity
  - Hepatic lipogenesis
- Basal rate of lipolysis and substrate oxidation (6,44)

Obesity can be classified into two primary categories on the basis of genetic etiology: monogenic (including pleiotropic syndromes) and polygenic. In contrast to the monogenic animal models of obesity and rare genetic syndromes of human obesity, predilection toward the common types of obesity seen in current societies stems from the interplay of multiple susceptibility genetic loci (polygenic) that can affect expenditure of energy, use of fuel, characteristics of muscle fibers, and even taste preferences. All of these factors, in turn, influence our behavioral responses to the environment.

The overall consensus of the scientific community is that excessive body fat is the end result of interactions among environmental, behavioral, genetic, and epigenetic factors. For example, it is estimated that approximately 40% of the variance in daily energy expenditure (excluding vigorous PA) is attributable to genotype. Genes have also been implicated in one-third of the variance in total caloric intake. Genome-wide linkage studies have linked obesity markers to every chromosomal region except Y (67).

Monogenic obesity is primarily caused by gene mutations in single genes and accounts for a small number of extreme early-onset obesity cases. Target risks identified to date primarily affect the functions of genes involved in the leptinergic–melanocortinergic pathway. Disruption of this pathway results in decreased satiety and increased food intake and energy storage, which ultimately leads to obesity (10).

In 1992, the first obesity gene characterized at a molecular level was the *agouti* gene. *Agouti* is expressed in various tissues, including adipose, suggesting that it may be involved in the regulation of energy homeostasis. However, since then, a better-known gene mutation was discovered. This mutation involves the satiety hormone leptin and its receptors ob and db (68).

Although there are a reported 1663 genes associated with obesity or phenotypic parameters (e.g., BMI, WC, abdominal visceral fat, and waist-to-hip ratio), many of them are still undergoing verification and confirmation (69). Table 2.2 lists some of the more well-known genes that have been identified and verified (70). Mutations of the first four genes have been associated with juvenile-onset morbid obesity. Melanocortin 4 receptor (*MC4R*)–related obesity is the most frequent type of monogenic obesity, responsible for ≤5% of early-onset and severe childhood obesity. It is also the only locus contributing to a significant proportion of cases of severe adult monogenetic obesity (71).

To date, there have been several hundred different human obesity cases associated with single gene defects. Some examples include the following (72):

- Autosomal dominant—achondroplasia, Albright hereditary osteodystrophy, Angelman syndrome, insulin resistance syndromes
- Autosomal recessive—Alstrom–Hallgren, Cohen, and Fanconi–Bickel syndromes

Pleiotropic syndromes are clinical syndromes whereby obesity is one of the many constellations of symptoms. There have been approximately 30 of these Mendelian disorders categorized to date, with several of these mutations (if not all) affecting the central or peripheral pathways controlling weight (27).

- Prader–Willi syndrome—the most common (prevalence 1:25,000) and best characterized human obesity syndrome. Includes progressive obesity, reduced fetal activity, hypotonia

Table 2.2 Verified candidate genes associated with obesity phenotype

Gene	Phenotype
Food intake	
Leptin (*LEP*)	BMI, body weight, leptin secretion
Leptin receptor (*LEPR*)	BMI, fat mass, lean mass
Proopiomelanocortin (*POMC*)	Early-onset obesity, hypocortisolism, red hair in Caucasians
Melanocortin 4 receptor (*MC4R*)	BMI, WHR, resting energy expenditure, obesity
Energy metabolism	
Uncoupling protein 1 (*UCP1*)	BMI, WHR, body fat, resting metabolic rate
Uncoupling protein 2 (*UCP2*)	BMI, glucose oxidation, resting energy expenditure, obesity
Uncoupling protein 3 (*UCP3*)	BMI, fat mass, lean mass
β3-Adrenergic receptor (*ADRβ3*)	BMI, fat mass, obesity
G protein β3 subunit (*GNβ3*)	BMI, lipolysis, fat mass
Adipogenesis	
Peroxisome proliferator-activated receptor γ (*PPARγ*)	BMI, WC, fat mass, WHR, obesity
Adiponectin	BMI, WC, obesity
Tumor necrosis factor α (*TNFα*)	BMI, WC, body weight, fat
β2-Adrenergic receptor (*ADRβ2*)	BMI, WHR, lipolysis, fat mass
Lipase hormone sensitive (*LIPE*)	BMI, WHR, body fat, lipolysis
Glucocorticoid receptor (*NCR3C1*)	BMI, WHR, abdominal visceral fat, lean mass

Source: Data from Shriner D, et al. Genetic contributions to the development of obesity. In: Akabas S, Lederman S, Moore B, eds. *Textbook of Obesity: Biological, Psychological, and Cultural Influences.* West Sussex, UK: Wiley-Blackwell; 2012, pp. 79–86.
Note: BMI, body mass index; WHR, waist-to-hip ratio.

at birth, short stature, mental retardation, behavioral abnormalities, hypogonadism, small hands and feet, and hyperphagia usually developing between 12 and 18 months (73).

- Bardet–Biedl syndrome—also known as Laurence–Moon syndrome (prevalence <1:100,000). Includes polydactyly, developmental delay, impaired vision, hypogonadism, central obesity, and renal abnormalities.
- Cohen syndrome—dysmorphic features, developmental delay, visual problems, and late childhood or adolescent truncal obesity.
- Borjeson–Forssman–Lehmann syndrome—mental retardation, obesity, and hypogonadism.
- Wilson–Turner syndrome—mental retardation, gynecomastia, and childhood onset obesity.

Polygenic obesity results from the synergy of a large number of genes, with each having a small, linear (additive) effect that has a Gaussian (normal) distribution. They are then acted upon by a permissive environment and are thought to constitute more than 90% of human obesity seen today (1). It seems that no single genotype will cause common obesity, with the exception of the monogenic mutations (74).

Research continues to look for candidate genes that can be identified based on their putative roles in relevant metabolic pathways. Some of these candidate genes may pertain to body mass, body fat, or fat distribution, whereas others can be defined from their potential contributions to the regulation of energy intake, energy expenditure, or nutrient partitioning. Others can come from our present understanding of other metabolic, physiological, or behavioral phenotypes involved in the predisposition to obesity (73). One emerging discipline investigating this predisposition is nutrigenetics, the study of the different physiological responses to diet depending on the genotype(s) of each individual (46).

Another proposed genetic–environmental pathway for obesity that is being explored is that of a genetic switch from cold to heat adaptation due to ancestral migration thousands of years ago. It is thought this may explain the propensity for obesity in US inhabitants of Native American ancestry. To date, findings indicate that various elements involved in thermogenesis may shape overall obesity susceptibility in relation to brown adipose tissue function, not only uncoupling protein 1 (50).

Lest we need a reminder of the intricacies of human physiology, obesity and genetic interaction does not exist in a vacuum. For example, genetic variation at the fatso/fat mass and obesity associated gene (*FTO*) locus contributes to the etiology of obesity, insulin resistance, and increased plasma leptin levels. *FTO* also plays a role in controlling food intake (via ghrelin) (10), energy expenditure, and energy homeostasis (75). Of note is that the appetite effect is stronger in sedentary versus physically active individuals (6). *FTO* was the first compelling example of a common variant impacting on variation in weight and fat mass and on the individual risk of obesity (71). Research has recently shown that some of the obesity associations of *FTO* are mediated through functional connections with a distant gene, IRX3 (76).

Biological factors

Obesity arises as a consequence of how the body regulates energy intake, energy expenditure, and energy storage, that is, energy balance. Interestingly, the regulation of energy balance may be biased; negative energy balance may be defended against more strongly than positive energy balance. Our biology is geared to protect more strongly against weight loss than against weight gain (77).

AGE

Our first subset of biological factors to consider is age. Some specifics associated with varying stages of life are as follows:

Young

- Early maturation increases the risk of subsequent obesity, since numerous biological mechanisms support significant increases in body fatness in the postpubertal period (78).
- Children, and particularly adolescents, who are obese have a high probability of becoming adults who are obese (1).

Middle aged

- Increasing age is associated with an increase in obesity. Changes in body weight and composition are attributable, in part, to the natural declines in growth hormone, DHEA, and testosterone with aging.
- The prevalence of obesity in adults tends to rise steadily from the ages of 20 to 60 years, but does not increase and, in fact, begins to decrease in later years (49).

Elderly

- There is evidence suggesting that the optimal BMI range for adults ≥65 years of age is higher than the range for younger adults.

Besides the hormonal alterations affecting weight that are associated with age in the perinatal, pubertal, midlife, and later years of life, age also has a role in influencing human metabolism. RMR generally declines every decade of life after the mid-20s. This reduction alters energy balance and can contribute to weight gain (79). Hill (77) noted metabolic susceptibility with fat-storing tendencies and differences in skeletal muscle composition with aging (77).

In addition to age and hormonal effects on metabolism, other factors also lead to reduced metabolic rate, such as marked food restriction, maintenance of a weight-reduced state, activity diminution, and smoking cessation.

SEX

Differences in patterns of weight gain, as well as the development of overweight and obesity, are apparent between the sexes. Onset of menarche is usually earlier in obese than in nonobese adolescents. Some studies have shown that girls with early menarche (<11 years) are twice as likely to become obese adults compared to those that mature at a later age (>14 years) (16). Also, 70% of obese adolescent males normalize their body weight at a later stage compared to only 20% in obese adolescent females.

These patterns, as well as others, are partially attributable to hormonal differences between males and females during puberty and before menopause (i.e., testosterone vs. estrogen effects) and to hormonal changes in women during menopause. During the peri- and postmenopausal periods, many women experience alterations in body weight, total body fat, and body fat distribution (79). Such alterations can occur also with pregnancy.

RACE AND ETHNICITY

The prevalence of being overweight and becoming overweight at any age during adolescence is approximately twice as high among African and Hispanic Americans compared to European American children. It is believed that inherent ethnic differences in metabolism and fat accumulation in combination with the obesogenic environment may put different population segments at greater risk for disease. Genetic background contributes to racial and ethnic differences in obesity and metabolic risk factors, independent of social and financial aspects (80).

Certain ethnic and racial groups appear to be particularly predisposed to obesity. The Pima Indians of Arizona and other ethnic groups native to North America have a particularly high prevalence of obesity. In addition, Polynesians, Micronesians, Anurans, Maoris of the West and East Indies, African Americans in North America, and the Hispanic populations (both Mexican and Puerto Rican in origin) in North America also have particularly high predispositions to developing obesity (1).

Ethnicity is associated with differences in food-related beliefs, preferences, and behaviors. Cultural influences may contribute to the higher risk of obesity among children and youth in the US ethnic minority populations (18).

CIRCADIAN SYSTEM

The Circadian system is deserving of special attention, especially since it may be somewhat modifiable in preventing or reducing obesity (46). Circadian rhythms are those biological rhythms whose frequency is close to a day (period between 20 and 28 hours). It is accepted that 10% to 30% of the human genome is under the control of circadian molecular clocks (65). Recent work has suggested that circadian rhythms, and disruption of these rhythms by light, shift work, timing of food intake (feeding and fasting), social contacts, PA, and sleep deprivation, could also be a major contributor to the susceptibility of an individual to develop obesity (51,64,65,81).

A substantial percentage of active genes expressed in adipose tissue in both humans and animal models follows a specific temporal order. They entrain adipokines such as leptin, adipsin, resistin, adiponectin, and visfatin. These patterned cytokines appear to be crucial for adipose tissue to exclusively either accumulate fat or to mobilize fat at the proper time, a phenomenon known as temporal compartmentalization. Peripheral circadian clocks (synchronized by rhythmic feeding) (64) dominate local physiological processes, including glucose and lipid homeostasis, hormonal secretion, xenobiotics, the immune response, and the digestive system (51).

WELL-KNOWN HORMONAL AND PHYSIOLOGICAL PATHWAYS

Although we are capable of limiting our food intake for short periods, the control mechanisms for long-term regulation of body weight are well beyond our conscious control (44). Multiple central and peripheral factors are important for regulation of energy balance between fed and fasting states. These factors include orexiants and anorexiants, the CNS, multiple hormones and receptors, uncoupling proteins, catecholamines, and heat production (82).

Textbooks are written about some of these factors, so only a cursory overview of a few of their properties is presented here. Although there are more factors than listed here, this representative example illustrates the varieties and intricacies of these adiposity contributors.

- Thyroid
  - The active component of thyroid is triiodothyronine (T3). There is a decline in active T3 activity with aging and weight reduction.
  - Hypothyroidism can lead to fluid retention, reduced metabolism, and weight gain.
  - Physiologically relevant variations in thyroid status are only likely to have modest effects on RMR, but in the long term such variations could have an appreciable effect on energy balance.
- Growth hormone deficiency
  - Decreased lean body mass
  - Increased fat mass, especially visceral
- Testosterone
  - Male hypogonadism can predispose to central weight gain.
  - There is an inverse relationship between testosterone levels and insulin resistance.
  - There is a strong association with obesity, type 2 diabetes mellitus, and metabolic syndrome.
- Estrogen
  - Inhibits the actions of PPAR-α on obesity and lipid metabolism
- Leptin
  - Fat-derived, anorexigenic hormone that acts at the arcuate nucleus of the hypothalamus to regulate energy homeostasis (82).
    - Reduces food intake by signaling satiety (in parallel with insulin) (81)
    - Increases activity of thermogenetic components of the SNS (83)

- Of the six different isoforms of this receptor, the isoform OB–RB is expressed in the hypothalamic nuclei, where leptin initiates inhibition of food intake and stimulation of energy expenditure.
- The overwhelming majority of obese humans are not leptin deficient. Obesity results in high plasma leptin concentrations. Recent studies suggest that leptin is physiologically more important as an indicator of energy deficiency than energy excess (84).
- Obese individuals overeat despite elevated leptin levels, suggesting that hypothalamic leptin resistance plays a central role in their susceptibility to weight gain (44). Both hypo- and hyperleptinemia are associated with reduced leptin entry into the brain. Excursions from the normal pattern can extinguish target response due to receptor down-regulation.
- Animal data suggest that leptin's appetite suppressant effect may be overridden by access to highly palatable, energy-dense foods, possibly through reactive gliosis. Obesity promoting permanent changes in the hypothalamus has been seen with overconsumption of a fat-rich diet (81).
- Weight loss, whether from dieting or starvation, leads to decreased postprandial peak leptin levels that, in turn, decrease postprandial satiety. This scenario leads to a compensatory increase in food intake over weeks and months, assuming food is available, thus restoring adipose tissue mass (44).
- Evidence suggests that extended periods of central leptin insufficiency orchestrate pathophysiological consequences that include
  - increased rate of fat accrual
  - decreased energy expenditure and general activity level
  - hyperinsulinemia
  - hyperglycemia
  - neuroendocrine disorders
  - osteoporosis
  - metabolic syndrome
  - impaired learning and memory (85)
- Ghrelin
  - Gut hormone that mediates sense of hunger
  - Levels increased in diet-induced weight loss
  - Evidence of ghrelin elevation with sleep deprivation
  - When administered intravenously, decreases fat oxidation and increases food intake and adiposity
  - Even in the absence of effects on nutrient intake, affects nutrient partitioning and increases adiposity, with direct effects on adipocytes (86)
  - May be a regulator of long-term energy balance (83)
- Cushing's disease
  - Adenoma in the pituitary gland, producing large amounts of adrenocorticotropic hormone (ACTH) that, in turn, elevates cortisol, causing weight gain.
  - Cushing's syndrome (hyperadrenocorticism) is an endocrine disorder caused by high levels of cortisol in the blood.
- Polycystic ovarian syndrome (PCOS)
  - Usually associated with central obesity, insulin resistance, hyperinsulinemia, diabetes, and excess testosterone.

- Thought to be caused by insulin resistance, associated with obesity, triggering the development of PCOS in susceptible individuals (49).
- Debate remains as to whether factors contributing to PCOS cause obesity or whether obesity and its predisposing factors can lead to the development of PCOS. (Classic which-came-first question: the chicken or the egg?)
- Metabolic syndrome (MetSyn)
  - Usually includes dyslipidemia and insulin resistance
  - May predispose to truncal obesity and diabetes, but not absolute
    - WC often a key criteria for MetSyn diagnosis
- Central melanocortin (MC) system
  - Involved in body weight regulation through its role in appetite and energy expenditure via leptin, ghrelin, and Agouti-related protein.
  - Two receptors complement each other: MC4R influences food intake and MC3R regulates fat stores by an exclusive metabolic pathway (82).
    - Mutations in the *MC4* gene are described as a monogenic cause of obesity in humans.
    - Impact and contribution of *MC3R* variants to increased adiposity vary among ethnicities (66).
- PPAR
  - Group of nuclear receptor proteins that function as transcription factors, regulating the expression of genes
  - Plays crucial role in the pathogenesis of obesity because it is central to adipocyte differentiation and fat disposal (27)
  - Includes three isoforms (α, δ, γ):
    - PPAR-γ, expressed highest in adipose tissue
      - Important therapeutic target in management of obesity and diabetes
    - PPAR-α, involved in energy balance
      - PPAR-α ligands are reported to regulate adipose tissue metabolism through fatty-acid oxidation, as well as increasing uncoupling proteins in brown adipose tissue, liver, and skeletal muscle.
- Peripheral satiety signalers
  - Stomach stretch receptors
  - Travel to the brain via vagus nerve or the systemic circulation (see Table 2.3) Peripheral signals indicating the size of adipose tissue stores as well as circulating factors, indicating current nutritional status are received and integrated within the CNS (87)
- Lipoprotein lipase
  - Known as the fat-storage enzyme
  - Stimulated in the climacteric by testosterone and cortisol, unopposed by decreased progesterone and estradiol, causing increased visceral fat deposition (88)
- Cannabinoids
  - Genetic variations at the endocannabinoid type-1 receptor gene are reported to be associated with obesity phenotypes.
  - PPAR and endocannabinoid-receptor polymorphisms alter the course of metabolic homeostasis.
  - Endocannabinoids are produced by human white adipose tissue. *N*-Palmitoylethanolamine is the most abundant cannabimimetic compound produced by the human adipocyte, and its levels can be down-regulated by leptin.

Table 2.3 Suggested biological modulators of food intake

Peripheral signal	Proposed effect on food intake
Vagal	−
Cholecystokinin	−
Apolipoprotein A-IV	−
Insulin	−
Glucagon-like peptide 1	−
Other glucagon-related peptides	−
Leptin	+ when leptin ↓↓
Ghrelin	+
Tumor necrosis factor α	−
Obestatin	−

- Peptides that stimulate appetite
  - Proopiomelanocortin (POMC) is the polypeptide precursor of ACTH.
  - Regulation of body weight is linked to the action of Nhlh2 on prohormone convertase mRNA levels, supporting a direct role for transcriptional control of neuropeptide processing enzymes in the etiology of adult-onset obesity also seen in thyroid patients (82).
  - Factors known to regulate eating behavior include several brain–gut peptides, along with more than a dozen neuropeptides expressed in the CNS.
    - NPY
      - NPY is the most potent central appetite stimulant known. It also reduces thermogenesis in brown adipose tissue, thereby further promoting positive energy balance (83).
      - NPY was the first orexigenic factor from the hypothalamus to be identified. NPY may be a redundant signaling molecule in weight regulation (68).
    - Melanin-concentrating hormone
      - Maintains feeding and mediates feeding-related functions via the hormone orexin, which provokes hyperphagia (83)
    - Orexin A/B
      - Found in lateral hypothalamus
      - Increases food intake
      - Up-regulated by fasting
    - Galanin
      - Stimulates feeding (fat intake > carbohydrate)
      - Reduces energy expenditure by inhibiting sympathetic activity
- Hypothalamus
  - Obesity can be caused by structural damage of which craniopharyngioma is the most common.
  - The arcuate nucleus is considered the primary site within the hypothalamus for reception of bloodborne signals of nutritional status (87).
  - A primary site of convergence and integration for redundant energy status signaling, which includes central and peripheral neural inputs as well as hormonal and nutritional factors (89).

- The key energy regulator resides in the CNS. This tightly regulated network resides within the hypothalamus. Two different neuronal populations exist:
  - A population that synthesizes NPY and agouti-related peptide
  - Another population that synthesizes α melanocyte-stimulating hormone from POMC neurons that impact MC4R receptors and thus affect energy intake and expenditure
- Affected via emotions through depression
  - Factors that affect emotional behavior include psychologically induced stress that causes depression. Such depression stimulates the hypothalamic appetite centers to increase food intake, as well as parasympathetic input into the upper gut that enhances fat storage.
- Hunger-increasing neuropeptides
  - Opioids
    - Released in response to intake of highly palatable foods that enhance appetite—maintain ingestion
    - Interact with cannabinoids to enhance food palatability
  - Dopamine
    - The availability of dopamine D2 receptors is decreased in morbidly obese individuals (BMI ≥ 40) in proportion to their BMI.
    - Deficit in dopamine D2 receptors may promote eating as a means to compensate for decreased activation of dopaminergic reward circuits.
  - Offset (−) by satiety neuropeptides insulin, serotonin, and CCK (47)
- Insulinoma
  - Rare: Approximately 4 cases per million per year.
  - Insulinoma is usually seen with patients consciously eating to prevent spells of low blood sugar and eventually developing weight gain.
- Adipocyte
  - Obesity results from abnormal accumulation of fat deposits, leading to an excessive storage of triacylglycerol within adipocytes located within subcutaneous tissue and intra-abdominal viscera.
  - Adiponectin is the most abundant adipokine, and it causes increased insulin sensitivity and decreased tumor necrosis factor α (TNF-α)–induced changes. In obesity, adiponectin levels are decreased.
  - In addition to their storage function, adipocytes serve as endocrine cells by secreting hormones and growth factors that regulate fat metabolism through feedback mechanisms (79).
  - The adipokines, which affect metabolic functioning of fat cells and influence other tissues throughout the body, have been documented to mediate fat metabolism and obesity (80).
  - The adipocyte, which is the cellular unit of obesity, is increasingly found to be a complex and metabolically active cell. Among the products of the adipocyte that are involved in complex intermediary metabolism are cytokines, TNF-α, interleukin (IL)-6, lipotransin, adipocyte lipid-binding protein, acyl-stimulation protein, prostaglandins, adipsin, perilipins, lactate, adiponectin, monobutyrin, and phospholipid transfer protein.
  - Among critical enzymes involved in adipocyte metabolism are endothelial-derived lipoprotein lipase (lipid storage), hormone-sensitive lipase (lipid elaboration and release from adipocyte depots), acylcoenzyme A synthetases (fatty acid synthesis), and a cascade of enzymes (beta oxidation and fatty acid metabolism).

- Another area of active research is investigation of the cues for the differentiation of preadipocytes to adipocytes. This process occurs in both white and brown adipose tissue, even in adults. Its potential role in the development of obesity and the relapse to obesity after weight loss has become increasingly important. Among the identified factors in this process are PPAR-γ; retinoid-X receptor ligands; perilipin; adipocyte differentiation–related protein; and CCAAT enhancer-binding proteins α, β, and δ (1).

Psychological considerations

Less well-defined causes of obesity may be related to psychosocial factors that often have cultural roots (mentioned above) or factors that reflect behavioral expressions that cause excessive food intake, altered body image, and depression. Emotional stress appears to involve multiple brain centers that influence vagal input into the enteric neuromuscular system and its neurotransmitters that affect visceral hypersensitivity (47).

Several lines of evidence indicate that emotional modulation of food intake differs between lean and obese individuals (83). Since many patients who are obese have eating disorders, it is important to screen for these disorders in the history (1).

RESTRAINT DISINHIBITION

Restraint disinhibition involves the inability to refrain from overeating when there is an abundance of food (47). On a genetic level, *CLOCK 3111 T/C SNP* specifically interacts with disinhibition, a principal component of emotional eating behavior. This relationship suggests that high disinhibition is the main driver for this gene–environment interaction (90). Also note that neurobiological processes relating to overindulgence in food overlap with those involved in substance abuse and addiction (91).

Intertwined with restraint disinhibition, emotional and stress eating go hand in hand. Consumption of energy-dense, nutrient-poor foods seems to be associated with emotional eating (90), even in the absence of metabolic need or hunger. Studies show that the stress system and cortisol release through the hypothalamic–pituitary–adrenal axis can be a cause of obesity, thereby representing a mechanism that is initiated in advance of weight gain (92).

ABUSE

Another important psychological aspect for obesity is abuse. Abuse can take the form of emotional, physical, or sexual abuse, especially in women. Some of the long-term adverse consequences of abuse include obesity, both as a result of stress eating and sometimes to provide for protection against unwanted sexual attention (49). One environmental risk factor for binge eating disorder (BED) appears to be childhood maltreatment (93).

EATING PATTERNS AND DISORDERS

Modern society facilitates excessive consumption, and dietary patterns contribute substantially to the development of obesity. Specific eating disorders, such as the overeating syndromes BED, bulimia nervosa, and night eating syndrome (NES), can contribute significantly to overweight and obesity (1,47). The two eating disorders most closely linked with obesity are BED and NES.

BED is the consumption of an objectively large amount of food within a 2-hour period, while feeling a loss of control. Prevalence estimates in obese patients seeking treatment range from 8.9% to 18.8%. In those seeking bariatric surgery, there is a reported prevalence range from 4% to 50%.

NES is characterized by an abnormally increased food intake in the evening and night-time (79). According to proposed criteria, individuals with NES must ingest at least 25% of their daily food intake after the evening meal and/or experience nocturnal awakenings that are associated with eating (i.e., nocturnal ingestions) at least two times per week for at least 3 months. Prevalence ranges from 10% to 15% in those seeking medical obesity treatment and from 2% to 55% in bariatric surgery candidates.

NES typically first appears in the late 20s, and onset may be related to stress. Younger individuals with NES do not appear consistently to have higher rates of obesity, but older individuals with NES do appear to have higher rates of obesity than non-NES counterparts (94).

Inflammatory state

Another characteristic associated with obesity is the inflammatory state of the body. A mild inflammatory response process plays a role in stimulation of weight gain. Studies show association of obesity with the presence of a chronic, mild state of inflammation (95). It is known that overweight individuals have elevated levels of C-reactive protein (CRP). There is also evidence to suggest that the features of metabolic syndrome, including obesity and type 2 diabetes, have a common inflammatory basis.

Central visceral sites of white adipose tissue secrete inflammatory adipokines, such as TNF-α, IL-1, and IL-6 (92), that are the precipitating and/or aggravating factors that contribute to the comorbid conditions of obesity, such as diabetes mellitus with insulin resistance (47). TNF-α causes decreased adipose cell differentiation, increased lipolysis, and increased free fatty acids.

Some adults recruit new adipocytes more readily than others do and thus gain weight more from adipocyte hyperplasia than from hypertrophy. Those who gain fat with enlarging adipocytes are more likely to display inflammatory responses, both in adipose tissue and systemically (increased CRP) (49). As the adipocytes enlarge, they begin to secrete proinflammatory cytokines and attract macrophages into the adipose tissue, thereby initiating a low-grade chronic inflammation. Osteopontin is secreted by the swelling adipocyte and recruits an increasing number of macrophages that, in turn, recruit even more macrophages (96).

Just as obesity can cause inflammation, modest evidence shows that inflammation can precede obesity. Consumption of a saturated fatty acid–rich diet has been shown to result in a proinflammatory "obesity-linked" gene expression profile, whereas consumption of a mono-unsaturated fatty acid–rich diet caused a more anti-inflammatory profile (45).

Infectious origins

Just as evidence showed an infectious agent, *Helicobacter pylori*, to be an etiological agent for peptic ulcer disease, evolving data suggest that an infective etiology possibly exists for some obese phenotypes (1). A term associated with this postulated theory is "infectobesity," meaning obesity of infectious origin. Ten different microbes have been reported to cause obesity in various experimental models (26). Clearly, not every case of obesity is of infectious origin, but infection attributable to certain organisms should be included in the long list of potential etiological factors for obesity (95).

Be aware that production of obesity is not a characteristic of all animal or human pathogens and that certain infections may cause obesity without the obesogenic behavior of overeating or physical inactivity. Many of the animal viruses that cause obesity do so by damaging the CNS (97).

In the past two decades, adipogenic (fat-causing) pathogens have been reported; these pathogens include human and nonhuman viruses, prions, bacteria, and gut microflora (mentioned previously). Two pathogens of note are the avian adenovirus SMAM-1 and the human adenovirus 36 (Ad-36). SMAM-1 was the first virus to be implicated in human obesity.

- SMAM-1
  - An avian adenovirus from India.
  - Acts directly on adipocytes; causes fat deposition (adiposity) in chickens.
  - The only animal virus to date to show a serological association with human obesity (95,97).
  - Dhurandhar et al. (98) screened 52 obese humans for antibodies to SMAM-1 virus. Approximately 20% of the subjects had antibodies to SMAM-1. The antibody (+) subjects had significantly greater body weight compared with the antibody (–) group.
- Ad-36
  - First human adenovirus linked with obesity. Data show an association of Ad-36 antibodies with human obesity, but do not establish a causative relationship (95). May lead to increases in appetite by decreasing norepinephrine and leptin levels.
  - Has a direct effect on adipocytes to turn on the enzymes of fat accumulation (increases lipoprotein lipase) and accelerate the differentiation of preadipocytes to adipocytes through inhibition of leptin gene expression (99).
  - About 30% of obese adults and children and about 10% to 20% of nonobese people have been infected (100). Also causes obesity in chickens, mice, rats, and monkeys. In all animal models tested, Ad-36 infection did not significantly alter food intake.
  - In the United States, the prevalence of Ad-36 antibodies in adolescents aged 8 to 18 years was 15% overall, with 22% of the obese and 7% of the nonobese being seropositive. Of the seropositive children, 78% were obese and 4% were nonobese (101).
  - Subsequent to discovery of the linkage of Ad-36 with obesity, two additional human adenoviruses (of 50 known serotypes) have been associated with obesity and shown to affect adipocytes directly, Ad-5 and Ad-37 (97).
- Other suspected infectious agents promoting obesity
  - *Chlamydia pneumoniae*
    - The first bacterium reported to be associated with increased BMI in humans. At this time, the link remains somewhat uncertain (95).
  - *Selenomonas noxia*
  - *Helicobacter pylori*
  - Herpes simplex viruses 1 and 2
  - Gut microflora (microbiome)

BEHAVIORAL FACTORS

The final major category reviewed herein is that of behavioral factors. Factors such as dietary intake, daily energy expenditure, and physical inactivity can be modified to help reverse the global obesity trend. A healthy lifestyle can offset some of the genetic predisposition to obesity (102). Although large behavior changes are needed to produce and maintain reductions in body weight, small behavior changes may be sufficient to prevent excessive weight gain (16).

Remember that the three major categories discussed—global and community influences, personal characteristics, and behavioral factors—are interconnected. Each has an influence upon the others and always will.

In times past, obesity had been considered a "problem of the belly rather than of the brain." However, current thinking shows neurobiology and neurology play a prominent role. Adiposity can be initiated by pathological conditions of the brain and various signaling mechanisms, as we have indicated earlier. Obesity is mediated by learned patterns and may therefore be better understood by disciplines concerned with cognition and behavior (49).

We cannot attribute the obesity epidemic solely to our biology. We must also examine the role of our behavior patterns regarding diet and PA (or inactivity) as key pathways for how our social environment influences energy balance, overweight, and obesity. These primary factors are the source of day-to-day variations in energy balance, superimposed on top of our genetic fabric (77).

Dietary or nutrient intake

The first subcategory of behavioral factors is dietary or nutrient intake. The reason that this category is being addressed first is because it takes a lot of exercise to offset or undo very little extra "empty calorie" intake. Even small caloric excesses over expenditure as low as 100 cal per day cause obesity over time (47).

In the short term, humans eat a constant volume of food at meals, so that total energy intake increases with the energy density of the diet. Excess energy is efficiently stored in the body regardless of its source; however, excess energy from dietary fat is stored with a greater efficiency than excess energy from carbohydrates and proteins (77). Fat is energy dense (1 g = 9 cal [technically, kilocalories]) compared to carbohydrate and protein (1 g = 4 cal). However, debate remains as to whether these values, determined in a bomb calorimeter, hold true in vivo.

In September 2013, advice from the Swedish Council on Health and Technology Assessment came after a 2-year review of 16,000 scientific studies of diet. Among its conclusions was that the scientific evidence did not support a low (healthy)-fat diet. Instead, people should focus on reducing their intake of carbohydrates. The guideline advised that meat and fish rich in fat, along with nuts and olive oils, should form a large part of a healthy diet, and that the consumption of pasta, potatoes, and white bread should be reduced (103).

A somewhat different conclusion was reached regarding childhood obesity and fat intake in a separate review of various published papers. A large percentage of these studies found that, in general, obese compared to nonobese children consumed a higher percentage of energy from fats. Also, an increase in the percentage of fat intake was associated with higher BMIs (16).

There are definitely differences in body chemistry, hormonal response, and subsequent fat storage or use that depend upon the quantity and mixture of the food substrate. In regard to snacking, and given the high prevalence of snacking (average of three snacks per day on top of main meals in American children) (80), deleterious snacking is a major contributor to weight gain and poor nutrition (19).

Other factors associated with adiposity include the following:

- RATE of eating
  - Several epidemiological studies conducted among healthy participants have shown positive associations between eating quickly and obesity.
  - Decreased mastication in fast eaters and subsequent inactivation of neuronal histamine may be related to weight gain. Mastication-induced activation of histamine neurons suppresses physiological food intake.
  - A rapid eating style has also been shown to be associated with childhood obesity (104).

- TIME of eating
  - Importance of breakfast
    - Four prospective studies in which participants were followed for 3.7 to 10 years suggest a potential role of skipping breakfast in weight gain (105).
    - Eating breakfast regularly may protect against weight gain despite a higher total daily energy intake (33).
    - Subjects assigned to high caloric intake during breakfast lost significantly more weight than those assigned to high caloric intake during dinner (106).
    - A high-carbohydrate and -protein breakfast may prevent weight gain, possibly, in part, by changes in the circadian control of hunger and appetite (64).
  - Chrononutrition—meal timing to optimize circadian system reset
    - The timing of food intake itself may have a significant role in obesity. Feeding time affects body weight even under isocaloric conditions (51).
    - Food is one external synchronizer of our peripheral clocks. Unusual feeding time can produce a disruption of the circadian rhythmicity of many hormones involved in metabolism, such as insulin, glucagon, adiponectin, corticosterone, leptin, chemerin, lipocain, and visfatin.
    - When animals eat at the "wrong time," they become obese, although they apparently eat and expend the same amount of energy (106). A study in mice suggested that the temporal feeding pattern combined with nutrient quality reprograms the molecular mechanisms of energy metabolism and body weight regulation (107).
    - Although energy intake in the morning was not associated with obesity, those who consumed ≥33% of daily energy intake in the evening were twofold more likely to be obese than morning eaters (2). Eating more of the day's total energy intake at midday is associated with a lower risk of being overweight or obese.
    - The type of carbohydrate and the rate of absorption are important factors in the synchronizing effect.
    - Sodium, ethanol, and caffeine may alter circadian rhythms of several physiological functions (106).
    - Fat storage increases during the day and is the greatest after an evening meal (33). High-fat diets induce obesity and increase risk for metabolic diseases. However, time-restricted feeding with a high-fat diet without caloric reduction suppresses obesity and metabolic diseases (51).
    - A previous human study showed that caloric consumption after 8 p.m. was associated with increased BMI independently of sleep timing and duration (64).
- TYPE of intake
  - Liquids
    - We compensate very little in our subsequent food intake after we consume additional calories as a beverage. Higher consumption of SSBs was associated with a greater magnitude of weight gain.
    - US levels remain very high, with 400 kcal per day from beverages consumed by children and young adults and SSB intake remaining the highest component (108).
    - As for experimental studies, the evidence currently suggests that obesity risk may be lower when artificially sweetened beverages (ASBs) replace SSBs in the diet.
    - In a large pooled analysis of 120,877 adult women and men, in contrast to increases in SSBs intake, which were positively and robustly associated with weight gain, increases in ASBs intake appeared to be protective against weight gain over time in these cohorts (109).

- Solids with high GI, leading to tendency for insulin resistance and weight gain
  - Many processed grains (e.g., white bread) produce even higher glycemic responses than simple sugars.
  - Nicotinamide fortification may contribute to the increased GI of refined grains (14).
- Micronutrients
  - In humans, low-calcium consumers displayed reduced daily fat oxidation. Thus, a low calcium intake might promote fat partitioning toward storage rather than oxidation (110).
  - Excess vitamins may trigger obesity through multiple mechanisms, including increasing fat synthesis, causing insulin resistance, disturbing neurotransmitter metabolism, and inducing epigenetic changes.
  - It is known that niacin can stimulate appetite. Also ecological studies showed that there are strong correlations between US per capita consumption of B vitamins (B1, B2, and niacin) and the prevalence of obesity and diabetes.
  - Other vitamins, even those that have antioxidant function (e.g., vitamins C and E), when used in large doses can increase reactive oxygen species generation. Thus, high consumption of some vitamins may contribute to the development of obesity (14).

Below are a few of the known dietary and caloric causes contributing to overweight and obesity. Some of these causes have already been mentioned previously in this chapter.

- Dietary factors associated with a higher BMI
  - Dietary patterns of high energy density may lead to body weight increase in adults.
  - Some evidence suggests a certain level of association between high ethanol intake and weight gain.
  - Frequent intake of sugared beverages is associated with a higher BMI. A high intake of meat and processed meat products might increase weight gain and WC.
  - Offering larger portions conditions an increase in the individual's caloric intake.
  - The absence of supermarkets with fruit and vegetable availability and their location at greater distances (in particular from neighborhoods with low socioeconomic levels) are conditioning factors for a higher population mean BMI.
  - The habitual intake of fast food (more than once a week) might contribute to increased energy intake and to weight gain and obesity.
- Dietary factors associated with a lower BMI
  - Diets with higher content of complex carbohydrates (approximately ≥50% of the total energy intake) are associated with a lower BMI in healthy adults.
  - A high dietary fiber intake in the context of a diet rich in food of vegetable origin is associated with a better control of body weight in healthy adults.
  - A high intake of fruit and vegetables is associated with a lower long-term body weight increase in adults.
  - A high intake of whole grains is associated with a lower BMI.
  - Even results are inconsistent, the studies to date suggest a possible role of the "Mediterranean" diet in the prevention of overweight and obesity.
  - The existing evidence suggests that greater adherence to the Mediterranean diet might prevent increases in WC.
  - Vegetarian diets are associated, in healthy adults, with a lower BMI (16).

Decisions, such as what food to consume and at what quantities, may be explained by the interplay of competing processes. Choices of food intake are based not only on homeostatic criteria but also on hedonic criteria. The influence of hedonic criteria is evident when we take a closer look at fast-food establishments that tend to serve oversized portions; high energy density, highly processed, high fat content foods; and large amounts of refined starch and added sugars (111). Ingestion of a high-fat/high-sucrose diet increases gene expression of the opioid peptide dynorphin, which can have reinforcing properties on future intake (83).

Daily energy expenditure

The second facet of behavioral factors is daily energy expenditure and its subcomponents: PA, BMR, TEF, and nonexercise activity thermogenesis (NEAT) (49). Genetic influences appear to affect resting energy expenditure, TEF, and adaptive body fat changes to short-term overfeeding. Resting energy expenditure, which generally comprises 50% to 80% of daily energy expenditures, depends largely on body mass, especially fat-free mass, which is more metabolically active than fat tissue.

Since this chapter deals with etiologies of obesity, it does not fully elucidate the positive weight-reducing and maintenance benefits of exercise, but just mentions a few physiological facts regarding them. The prospective Norfolk study of 20,000 men and women showed PA to attenuate the genetic predisposition to common obesity by 40%. Similar findings showed higher levels of PA in adolescence can prevent the development of obesity in adulthood, and the genetic predisposition to weight gain can be counteracted by an active lifestyle (96). For example, for each 1 hour per day of brisk walking, there was a 24% reduction in the risk of becoming obese over a period of 6 years.

PA behavior is the largest modifiable component of energy expenditure and is assumed to be one of the major behavioral determinants affecting the dramatic increase in obesity over the past decades. The thermal effect of PA is the most variable daily component and can constitute from 15% to 30% of 24-hour energy expenditure (112).

In the average overweight person, the amount of energy expended in PA and exercise often is insufficient to counter the generally sedentary nature of the remainder of their lifestyle and the influence of excessive caloric consumption (79). For example, being seated rather than upright for an hour per day can result in approximately a 6-kg weight gain over the course of 1 year (≈0.5 kg per month). If this extra hour of sitting is coupled with television viewing, then there is the addition of exposure to food marketing, increased opportunity for snacking on high-energy foods and drinks, decreased opportunity for PA, and reinforcement of sedentary behavior (83).

As we consider the various subcomponents of daily energy expenditure, one of the biggest contributors is the BMR and its quasi-surrogate, the RMR. The BMR is the energy expenditure of laying still at rest, awake, in the overnight postabsorptive state. A true BMR is measured after awakening, but before arising from bed. The RMR is similarly defined, but is not necessarily measured before arising from bed. For most sedentary adult Americans, the RMR represents the major portion of energy expended during the day and may range from less than 1200 kcal per day to more than 3000 kcal per day. Coupling geography with genetics, basal BMRs are highest in people in "arctic" areas, intermediate in white Europeans, and lowest in African Americans (50).

Most of the BMRs (≈80%) are directly proportional to the amount of lean tissue mass, although age, sex (women have slightly lower BMRs than men), and fat mass also affect the BMR. Small changes in BMR occur during the menstrual cycle (luteal phase > follicular phase). There is also evidence that heritable or family factors do influence BMR, accounting for as much as 10% of the interindividual differences.

Not all components of lean tissue consume oxygen at the same rate. Visceral or splanchnic bed tissues account for approximately 25% of RMR, but a much smaller proportion of body weight. The brain, which is only a small percentage of body weight, accounts for almost 15% of RMR. Likewise, the heart ($\approx$7%) and kidneys ($\approx$5%–10%) account for greater portions of resting energy needs relative to their contribution to body mass. In contrast, resting muscle makes up 40% to 50% of lean tissue mass but accounts for only 25% of RMR. This contribution changes dramatically with exercise, at which time muscle can account for 80% to 90% of energy expenditure, especially during high-intensity exercise.

With an energy-restricted diet, significant reductions in BMR relative to the amount of fat-free mass occur. Reductions in the production of T3 from thyroxine are thought to contribute to this phenomenon. Likewise, during brief periods of overfeeding, it has been shown that RMR increases more than would be expected for the amount of lean tissue present. Most of the variability in RMR not explained by body size and composition is related to differences in SNS activity (113).

THERMIC EFFECT OF FOOD

TEF is another component of energy expenditure to be considered. The heritability of TEF is estimated to be about 30%. Approximately 10% of the energy content of food is expended in digestion, absorption, and metabolism of nutrients. There is a significant interindividual variability in this value, however, ranging from a low of approximately 5% to a high of 15% of meal calories that are "wasted" in the postprandial interval. Values for TEF from macronutrients average 5%–8% for carbohydrates, 2%–3% for fat, and 20%–30% for protein (114).

Both obligatory and facultative components of the TEF have been identified. The obligatory components reflect the energy costs of digestion, absorption, and storage of nutrients. Approximately 60%–70% of the thermic effect of meals is obligatory, and the remaining 30%–40% is facultative thermogenesis. The two factors thought to play a role in the facultative component of TEF are the postprandial insulin response and activation of the SNS. The TEF is somewhat lower in insulin-resistant obese humans.

NONEXERCISE ACTIVITY THERMOGENESIS

A fairly significant subcomponent of daily energy expenditure is NEAT. NEAT represents the calorie expense of performing all activities other than exercise. The range of observed NEAT under controlled (metabolic chamber) conditions has been from less than 100 to about 800 kcal per day. There is probably a much wider range in free-living individuals (49). Spontaneous activity-related energy expenditure represents about 30% of total energy expenditure and is a most variable component. The available evidence suggests that reduced activity-related energy expenditure is a potentially important contributor to the predisposition to obesity (115).

It has been shown that NEAT can increase in response to increased food intake in an unconscious manner. In fact, modulation of NEAT can be a significant factor that acts to stabilize weight despite variations in food intake. Low levels of NEAT have been reported to predict future weight gain in some populations, and there may be differences between lean and obese persons in the daily amount of NEAT, which could relate to differential tendencies to regulate weight (49). Some studies are linking genes and SNPs with quantity of NEAT exhibited.

At the beginning of the twentieth century, 90% of the population of the world was rural. However, over the last century, more than 2 billion agriculturalists have become city dwellers. In this transition, PA has declined. In particular, chair use has replaced ambulation so that obese individuals tend to sit approximately 2.5 hours per day more than their lean counterparts. Walking is the principal component of NEAT. Even at slow velocities, walking doubles energy expenditure.

Other components of NEAT, the activities of daily living, are somewhat difficult to measure. A plethora of labor-saving conveniences (e.g., drive-through food and banking, escalators, remote controls, e-mail, and on-line shopping) have been introduced into the modern environment. Each of these further reduces the energy humans must expend to get through the day. Little hard data exist to document how much change has actually occurred, although future studies may help shed light on this topic.

Physical inactivity

Finally, we discuss physical inactivity, a known contributor for acquiring and maintaining obesity (16). Many Americans get as few as 4000 to 5000 steps per day, whereas it may take as many as 15,000 to 17,000 steps per day to help those who have lost significant amounts of weight to maintain that lower weight. The relative risk of being overweight or obese (BMI $\geq$ 25 kg/m^2) was 12% higher in workers with mostly sitting occupations compared to workers with mostly standing occupations. This risk was independent of PA and reported leisure-time sitting. Epidemiologically, the relationship of physical inactivity to weight gain appears to be more consistent than the relationship of excess energy intake to weight gain (115).

Excessive sitting is associated with obesity and diabetes, independent of PA (17). A 28-year follow-up of 8182 Finnish twin pairs (discordant for PA) revealed that although the physically inactive (79.5 $\pm$ 18.4 kg) and active twins (72.9 $\pm$ 11.9 kg) had only small differences in body weight, the inactive twins had 170% more liver fat and 54% more intramuscular fat than the active twins. Thus, the value of PA (or harm of inactivity) should not be judged only by its effects on body weight (96).

Obesity sometimes tracks the sales of TVs, cars, and computers more closely than trends in energy and fat intake (17). "Calorie amnesia" and other forms of denial or inattentiveness make true honesty with oneself difficult when evaluating overconsumption and inactivity. For example, in a weight-discordant twin study, self-reported analyses could show no differences in energy intake or the amount of physical activity between the co-twins. However, using more objective measurement via doubly labeled water revealed a substantial reporting bias by the obese co-twins: the under-reporting of energy intake (3.2 $\pm$ 1.1 MJ per day) and over-reporting of physical activity (1.8 $\pm$ 0.8 MJ per day) in the obese twins equaled as much as one Big Mac hamburger with a 16-oz bottle of soft drink and almost 90 minutes of walking (3 mph), respectively (96).

More than half of the US adult population maintains an almost totally sedentary lifestyle. Perhaps it's time to stand up and be counted in a healthy movement to eat less processed and more whole and natural food, at breakfast and the right time of the day, chew our food slowly, limit snacking, drink from glass rather than plastic containers, watch our vitamin intake, move or stand even when we do not have to, get out of our TNZ from time to time, and get the proper amount of sleep for our age. Such a commitment should be something we can live with.

REFERENCES

1. Hamdy O, Uwaifo GI, Oral EA. eMedicine—Obesity. 2014. http://emedicine. medscape.com/article/123702-overview, accessed September 2, 2014.
2. Jou C. The biology and genetics of obesity—A century of inquiries. *N Engl J Med* 2014; 370(20): 1874–7.
3. Shift Obesity System Influence Diagram. http://www.shiftn.com/obesity/Full-Map. html?, accessed September 4, 2014.
4. World Health Organization. *Fact Sheet: Obesity and Overweight*. Fact Sheet 311. World Health Organization; 2012.
5. Gauthier KI, Krajicek MJ. Obesogenic environment: A concept analysis and pediatric perspective. *J Spec Pediatr Nurs* 2013; 18(3): 202–10.
6. Wilding J. Are the causes of obesity primarily environmental? Yes. *BMJ* 2012; 345: e5843.
7. Tillotson JE. America's obesity: Conflicting public policies, industrial economic development, and unintended human consequences. *Annu Rev Nutr* 2004; 24: 617–43.
8. Johnston BC, Kanters S, Bandayrel K, Wu P, Naji F, Siemieniuk RA, et al. Comparison of weight loss among named diet programs in overweight and obese adults: A meta-analysis. *JAMA* 2014; 312(9): 923–33.
9. Bazzano LA, Hu T, Reynolds K, Yao L, Bunol C, Liu Y, et al. Effects of low-carbohydrate and low-fat diets: A randomized trial. *Ann Intern Med* 2014; 161(5): 309–18.
10. Yale J, Levian C, Ruiz E, Yang X. The pathogenesis of obesity from a genomic and systems biology perspective. *Biol Med* 2014; 87(2): 113–26. eCollection 2014.
11. Malik VS, Schulze MB, Hu FB. Intake of sugar-sweetened beverages and weight gain: A systematic review. *Am J Clin Nutr* 2006; 84: 274–88.
12. Ouyang X, Cirillo P, Sautin Y, McCall S, Bruchette JL, Diehl AM, et al. Fructose consumption as a risk factor for non-alcoholic fatty liver disease. *J Hepatol* 2008; 48: 993–9.
13. Ludwig DS, Friedman MI. Increasing adiposity: Consequence or cause of overeating? *JAMA* 2014; 311(21): 2167–8. Erratum in: *JAMA* 2014; 311(21): 2168.
14. Zhou SS, Zhou Y. Excess vitamin intake: An unrecognized risk factor for obesity. *World J Diabetes* 2014; 5(1): 1–13.
15. Nackers LM, Appelhans BM. Food insecurity is linked to a food environment promoting obesity in households with children. *J Nutr Educ Behav* 2013; 45(6): 780–4.
16. Serra-Majem L, Bautista-Castaño I. Etiology of obesity: Two "key issues" and other emerging factors. *Nutr Hosp* 2013; 28 Suppl 5: 32–43.
17. Lear SA, Teo K, Gasevic D, Zhang X, Poirier PP, Rangarajan S, et al. The association between ownership of common household devices and obesity and diabetes in high, middle and low income countries. *Can Med Assoc J* 2014; 186(4): 258–66.
18. Kumanyika SK. Environmental influences on childhood obesity: Ethnic and cultural influences in context. *Physiol Behav* 2008; 94: 61–70.
19. Bellisle F. Meals and snacking, diet quality and energy balance. *Physiol Behav* 2014; 134: 38–43.
20. Airhihenbuwa CO, Kumanyika S, Agurs TD, Lowe A, Saunders D, Morssink CB. Cultural aspects of African American eating patterns. *Ethn Health* 1996; 1: 245–60.
21. Fernández-Amesto F. *Near a Thousand Tables—A History of Food*. New York: Free Press; 2002.
22. Wright SM, Aronne LJ. Causes of obesity. *Abdom Imaging* 2012; 37(5): 730–2.

23. Jerome NW, Kandel RF, Pelto GH, eds. *Nutritional Anthropology: Contemporary Approaches to Diet and Culture*. Pleasantville, NY: Redgrave Publishing; 1980.

24. Kimbro RT, Brooks-Gunn J, McLanahan S. Racial and ethnic differentials in overweight and obesity among 3-year-old children. *Am J Public Health* 2007; 97: 298–305.

25. Ceballos N, Czyzewska M. Body image in Hispanic/Latino vs. European American adolescents: Implications for treatment and prevention of obesity in underserved populations. *J Health Care Poor Underserved* 2010; 21: 823–38.

26. McAllister EJ, Dhurandhar NV, Keith SW, Aronne LJ, Barger J, Baskin M, et al. Ten putative contributors to the obesity epidemic. *Crit Rev Food Sci Nutr* 2009; 49(10): 868–913.

27. Rojas J, Aguirre M, Velasco M, Bermúdez V. Obesity genetics: A monopoly game of genes. *Am J Ther* 2013; 20(4): 399–413.

28. Beauchamp GK, Mennella JA. Early flavor learning and its impact on later feeding behavior. *J Pediatr Gastroenterol Nutr* 2009; 48: S25–30.

29. Townsend E, Pitchford NJ. Baby knows best? The impact of weaning style on food preferences and body mass index in early childhood in a case–controlled sample. *BMJ Open* 2012; 2: e000298.

30. Levitsky DA, Youn T. The more food young adults are served, the more they overeat. *J Nutr* 2004; 134: 2546–9.

31. Howarth NC, Huang TT, Roberts SB, Lin BH, McCrory MA. Eating patterns and dietary composition in relation to BMI in younger and older adults. *Int J Obes* 2007; 31: 675–84.

32. van der Heijden AA, Hu FB, Rimm EB, van Dam RM. A prospective study of breakfast consumption and weight gain among U.S. men. *Obesity (Silver Spring)* 2007; 15(10): 2463–9.

33. Kahleova H, Belinova L, Malinska H, Oliyarnyk O, Trnovska J, Skop V, et al. Eating two larger meals a day (breakfast and lunch) is more effective than six smaller meals in a reduced-energy regimen for patients with type II diabetes: A randomized crossover study. *Diabetologia* 2014; 57(8): 1552–60.

34. Kaiser Foundation Report, 2010. Generation M²: Media in the Lives of 8- to 18-Year-Olds. http://kaiserfamilyfoundation.wordpress.com/uncategorized/report/generation-m2-media-in-the-lives-of-8-to-18-year-olds/, accessed September 4, 2014.

35. Church TS, Thomas DM, Tudor-Locke C, Katzmarzyk PT, Earnest CP, Rodarte RQ, et al. Trends over five decades in US occupation-related physical activity and their associations with obesity. *PLoS One* 2011; 6: e19657.

36. Frank LD, Engelke PO, Schmid TL. *Health and Community Design: The Impact of the Built Environment on Physical Activity*. Washington, DC: Island Press; 2003.

37. Pruchno R, Wilson-Genderson M, Gupta AK. Neighborhood food environment and obesity in community-dwelling older adults: Individual and neighborhood effects. *Am J Public Health* 2014; 104(5): 924–9.

38. Maddock J. The relationship between obesity and the prevalence of fast food restaurants: State-level analysis. *Am J Health Promot* 2004; 19: 137–43.

39. Casey R, Oppert J-M, Weber C, Charreire H, Salze P, Badariotti D, et al. Determinants of childhood obesity: What can we learn from built environment studies? *Food Qual Prefer* 2011; 31: 164–72. doi: 10.1016/j.foodqual.2011.06.003.

40. Cleland V, Crawford D, Baur LA, Hume C, Timperio A, Salmon J. A prospective examination of children's time spent outdoors, objectively measured physical activity and overweight. *Int J Obes* 2008; 32: 1685–93.

41. Bassett DR Jr, Pucher J, Buehler R, Thompson DL, Crouter SE. Walking, cycling, and obesity rates in Europe, North America, and Australia. *J Phys Act Health* 2008; 5: 795–814.
42. National Center for Safe Routes to School. Trends in walking and bicycling to school report. 2013. http://www.saferoutesinfo.org/data-central/national-progress/federal-reports, accessed September 2, 2014.
43. Lillycrop KA, Burdge GC. Epigenetic changes in early life and future risk of obesity. *Int J Obes (Lond)* 2011; 35(1): 72–83.
44. O'Rourke RW. Metabolic thrift and the genetic basis of human obesity. *Ann Surg* 2014; 259(4): 642–8.
45. St-Onge MP. The role of sleep duration in the regulation of energy balance: Effects on energy intakes and expenditure. *J Clin Sleep Med* 2013; 9(1): 73–80.
46. Ordovás Muñoz JM. Predictors of obesity: The "power" of the omics. *Nutr Hosp* 2013; 28 Suppl 5: 63–71.
47. Redinger RN. The prevalence and etiology of nongenetic obesity and associated disorders. *South Med J* 2008; 101(4): 395–9.
48. Oken E, Levitan EB, Gillman MW. Maternal smoking during pregnancy and child overweight: Systematic review and metaanalysis. *Int J Obes (Lond)* 2008; 32: 201–10.
49. Jensen MD. Obesity. In: Goldman L, Schafer A, eds. *Cecil Textbook of Medicine*, 24th ed. Philadelphia, PA: Saunders Elsevier; 2012, pp. 1409–17.
50. Sellayah D, Cagampang FR, Cox RD. On the evolutionary origins of obesity: A new hypothesis. *Endocrinology* 2014; 155(5): 1573–88.
51. Oike H, Oishi K, Kobori M. Nutrients, clock genes, and chrononutrition. *Curr Nutr Rep* 2014; 3: 204–12. eCollection 2014.
52. Bayon V, Leger D, Gomez-Merino D, Vecchierini MF, Chennaoui M. Sleep debt and obesity. *Ann Med* 2014; 46(5): 264–72.
53. Janesick AS, Schug TT, Heindel JJ, Blumberg B. Environmental chemicals and obesity. In: Bray G, Bouchard C, eds. *Handbook of Obesity: Epidemiology, Etiology, and Physiopathology*, 3rd ed., Vol. 1, Chap 43. Boca Raton, FL: CRC Press; 2014, pp. 471–87.
54. Kelishadi R, Poursafa P, Jamshidi F. Role of environmental chemicals in obesity: A systematic review on the current evidence. *J Environ Public Health.* 2013; 2013: 896789, 8 p. doi: 10.1155/2013/896789.
55. Thayer KA, Heindel JJ, Bucher JR, Gallo MA. Role of environmental chemicals in diabetes and obesity: A national toxicology program workshop review. *Environ Health Perspect* 2012; 120: 779–89.
56. Karoutsou E, Polymeris A. Environmental endocrine disruptors and obesity. *Endocr Regul* 2012; 46(1): 37–46.
57. Tontonoz P, Spiegelman BM. Fat and beyond: The diverse biology of PPARgamma. *Annu Rev Biochem* 2008; 77: 289–312.
58. Hofstetter A, Schutz Y, Jéquier E, Wahren J. Increased 24-hour energy expenditure in cigarette smokers. *N Engl J Med* 1986; 314: 79–82.
59. Clair C, Chiolero A, Faeh D, Cornuz J, Marques-Vidal P, Paccaud F, et al. Dose-dependent positive association between cigarette smoking, abdominal obesity and body fat: Cross-sectional data from a population-based survey. *BMC Public Health* 2011; 11: 23.
60. Annalisa N, Alessio T, Claudette TD, Erald V, Antonino de L, Nicola DD. Gut microbioma population: An indicator really sensible to any change in age, diet, metabolic syndrome, and life-style. *Mediators Inflamm* 2014; 2014: 901308.

61. Moreno-Indias I, Cardona F, Tinahones FJ, Queipo-Ortuño MI. Impact of the gut microbiota on the development of obesity and type 2 diabetes mellitus. *Front Microbiol* 2014; 5: 190. eCollection 2014.

62. Muccioli GG, Naslain D, Bäckhed F, Reigstad CS, Lambert DM, Delzenne NM, et al. The endocannabinoid system links gut microbiota to adipogenesis. *Mol Syst Biol* 2010; 6: 392.

63. Lee JH, Reed DR, Price RA. Familial risk ratios for extreme obesity: Implications for mapping human obesity genes. *Int J Obes Relat Metab Disord* 1997; 21: 935–40.

64. Garaulet M, Gómez-Abellán P, Alburquerque-Béjar JJ, Lee YC, Ordovás JM, Scheer FA. Timing of food intake predicts weight loss effectiveness. *Int J Obes (Lond)* 2013; 37(4): 604–11. Erratum in: *Int J Obes (Lond)* 2013; 37(4): 624.

65. Garaulet M, Gómez-Abellán P. Chronobiology and obesity. *Nutr Hosp* 2013; 28 Suppl 5: 114–20.

66. Lee YS. Genetics of nonsyndromic obesity. *Curr Opin Pediatr* 2013; 25(6): 666–73.

67. Integratomics TIME. Human obesity—Chromosomal gene map. 2014. http://www. integratomics-time.com/fat_deposition/genomic_view/human, accessed August 31, 2014.

68. Carroll L, Voisey J, van Daal A. Mouse models of obesity. *Clin Dermatol* 2004; 22(4): 345–9.

69. Yu W, Gwinn M, Clyne M, Yesupriya A, Khoury MJ. A navigator for human genome epidemiology. *Nat Genet* 2008; 40(2): 124–5.

70. Shriner D, Coulibaly I, Ankra-Badu G, Bay TM, Allison DB. Genetic contributions to the development of obesity. In: Akabas S, Lederman S, Moore B, eds. *Textbook of Obesity: Biological, Psychological, and Cultural Influences.* West Sussex, UK: Wiley-Blackwell; 2012, pp. 79–86.

71. Lindgren CM, McCarthy MI. Mechanisms of disease: Genetic insights into the etiology of type 2 diabetes and obesity. *Nat Clin Pract Endocrinol Metab* 2008; 4(3): 156–63.

72. Ichihara S, Yamada Y. Genetic factors for human obesity. *Cell Mol Life Sci* 2008; 65(7–8): 1086–98.

73. Pérusse L, Chagnon YC, Bouchard C. Etiology of massive obesity: Role of genetic factors. *World J Surg* 1998; 22(9): 907–12.

74. Papoutsakis C, Dedoussis GV. Gene–diet interactions in childhood obesity: Paucity of evidence as the epidemic of childhood obesity continues to rise. *Per Med* 2007; 4(2): 133–46.

75. Xia Q, Grant SF. The genetics of human obesity. *Ann N Y Acad Sci* 2013; 1281: 178–90.

76. Gorkin DU, Ren B. Genetics: Closing the distance on obesity culprits. *Nature* 2014; 507(7492): 309–10.

77. Hill JO. Understanding and addressing the epidemic of obesity: An energy balance perspective. *Endocr Rev* 2006; 27(7): 750–61.

78. Adair LS. Child and adolescent obesity: Epidemiology and developmental perspectives. *Physiol Behav* 2008; 94(1): 8–16.

79. Racette SB, Deusinger SS, Deusinger RH. Obesity: Overview of prevalence, etiology, and treatment. *Phys Ther* 2003; 83(3): 276–88.

80. Fernández JR, Casazza K, Divers J, López-Alarcón M. Disruptions in energy balance: Does nature overcome nurture? *Physiol Behav* 2008; 94(1): 105–12.

81. Karatsoreos IN, Thaler JP, Borgland SL, Champagne FA, Hurd YL, Hill MN. Food for thought: Hormonal, experiential, and neural influences on feeding and obesity. *J Neurosci* 2013; 33(45): 17610–16.

82. Zimmermann-Belsing T, Feldt-Rasmussen U. Obesity: The new worldwide epidemic threat to general health and our complete lack of effective treatment. *Endocrinology* 2004; 145(4): 1501–2.
83. Knecht S, Ellger T, Levine JA. Obesity in neurobiology. *Prog Neurobiol* 2008; 84(1): 85–103.
84. Kelesidis T, Kelesidis I, Chou S, Mantzoros CS. Narrative review: The role of leptin in human physiology: Emerging clinical applications. *Ann Intern Med* 2010; 152(2): 93–100.
85. Kalra SP. Central leptin insufficiency syndrome: An interactive etiology for obesity, metabolic and neural diseases and for designing new therapeutic interventions. *Peptides* 2008; 29(1): 127–38.
86. Miegueu P, St Pierre D, Broglio F, Cianflone K. Effect of desacyl ghrelin, obestatin and related peptides on triglyceride storage, metabolism and GHSR signaling in 3T3-L1 adipocytes. *J Cell Biochem* 2011; 112: 704–14.
87. Cottrell EC, Ozanne SE. Early life programming of obesity and metabolic disease. *Physiol Behav* 2008; 94(1): 17–28.
88. Milewicz A, Jedrzejuk D. Climacteric obesity: From genesis to clinic. *Gynecol Endocrinol* 2006; 22(1): 18–24.
89. Yamada T, Katagiri H. Avenues of communication between the brain and tissues/organs involved in energy homeostasis. *Endocr J* 2007; 54(4): 497–505.
90. López-Guimerà G, Dashti HS, Smith CE, Sánchez-Carracedo D, Ordovas JM, Garaulet M. CLOCK 3111 T/C SNP interacts with emotional eating behavior for weight-loss in a Mediterranean population. *PLoS One* 2014; 9(6): e99152.
91. Thorgeirsson TE, Gudbjartsson DF, Sulem P, Besenbacher S, Styrkarsdottir U, Thorleifsson G, et al. A common biological basis of obesity and nicotine addiction. *Transl Psychiatry* 2013; 3: e308.
92. Foss B, Dyrstad SM. Stress in obesity: Cause or consequence? *Med Hypotheses* 2011; 77(1): 7–10.
93. Allison KC, Grilo CM, Masheb RM, Stunkard AJ. High self-reported rates of neglect and emotional abuse, by persons with binge eating disorder and night eating syndrome. *Behav Res Ther* 2007; 45: 2874–83.
94. Bailer BA, Bradley LE, Allison KC. Obesity and related eating disorders. In: Bray G, Bouchard C, eds. *Handbook of Obesity: Epidemiology, Etiology, and Physiopathology*, 3rd ed., Vol. 1, Chap 29. Boca Raton, FL: CRC Press; 2014, pp. 327–38.
95. Pasarica M, Dhurandhar NV. Infectobesity: Obesity of infectious origin. *Adv Food Nutr Res* 2007; 52: 61–102.
96. Naukkarinen J, Rissanen A, Kaprio J, Pietiläinen KH. Causes and consequences of obesity: The contribution of recent twin studies. *Int J Obes (Lond)* 2012; 36(8): 1017–24.
97. Atkinson RL. Viruses as an etiology of obesity. *Mayo Clin Proc* 2007; 82(10): 1192–8.
98. Dhurandhar NV, Kulkarni PR, Ajinkya SM, Sherikar AA, Atkinson RL. Association of adenovirus infection with human obesity. *Obes Res* 1997; 5(5): 464–9.
99. Hur SJ, Kim DH, Chun SC, Lee SK. Effect of adenovirus and influenza virus infection on obesity. *Life Sci* 2013; 93(16): 531–5.
100. Atkinson RL. Current status of the field of obesity. *Trends Endocrinol Metab* 2014; 25(6): 283–4.
101. Dhurandhar NV, Dhurandhar EJ, Atkinson RL. Viral infections and adiposity. In: Bray G, Bouchard C, eds. *Handbook of Obesity: Epidemiology, Etiology, and Physiopathology*, 3rd ed., Vol. 1, Chap 27. Boca Raton, FL: CRC Press; 2014, pp. 303–13.

102. Li S, Zhao JH, Luan J, Ekelund U, Luben RN, Khaw KT. Physical activity attenuates the genetic predisposition to obesity in 20,000 men and women from EPIC-Norfolk prospective population study. *PLoS Med* 2010; 7(8): e1000332.
103. Hansen A. Swedish health advisory body says too much carbohydrate, not fat, leads to obesity. *BMJ* 2013; 347: f6873.
104. Ohkuma T, Fujii H, Iwase M, Kikuchi Y, Ogata S, Idewaki Y, et al. Impact of eating rate on obesity and cardiovascular risk factors according to glucose tolerance status: The Fukuoka Diabetes Registry and the Hisayama Study. *Diabetologia* 2013; 56(1): 70–7.
105. McCrory MA. Meal skipping and variables related to energy balance in adults: A brief review, with emphasis on the breakfast meal. *Physiol Behav* 2014; 134: 51–4.
106. Garaulet M, Gómez-Abellán P. Timing of food intake and obesity: A novel association. *Physiol Behav* 2014; 134: 44–50.
107. Hatori M, Vollmers C, Zarrinpar A, DiTacchio L, Bushong EA, Gill S, et al. Time-restricted feeding without reducing caloric intake prevents metabolic diseases in mice fed a high-fat diet. *Cell Metab* 2012; 15(6): 848–60.
108. Popkin BM. Patterns of beverage use across the lifecycle. *Physiol Behav* 2010; 100: 4–9.
109. Pereira MA. Diet beverages and the risk of obesity, diabetes, and cardiovascular disease: A review of the evidence. *Nutr Rev* 2013; 71(7): 433–40.
110. Melanson EL, Sharp TA, Schneider J, Donahoo WT, Grunwald GK, Hill JO. Relation between calcium intake and fat oxidation in adult humans. *Int J Obes Relat Metab Disord* 2003; 27: 196–203.
111. Garcia G, Sunil TS, Hinojosa P. The fast food and obesity link: Consumption patterns and severity of obesity. *Obes Surg* 2012; 22(5): 810–18.
112. Levine JA. Non-exercise activity thermogenesis. *Proc Nutr Soc* 2003; 62: 667–79.
113. Toth MJ, Poehlman ET. Sympathetic nervous system activity and resting metabolic rate in vegetarians. *Metabolism* 1994; 43: 621–5.
114. Tappy L. Thermic effect of food and sympathetic nervous system activity in humans. *Reprod Nutr Dev* 1996; 36(4): 391–7.
115. Weinsier RL, Hunter GR, Heini AF, Goran MI, Sell SM. The etiology of obesity: Relative contribution of metabolic factors, diet, and physical activity. *Am J Med* 1998; 105(2): 145–50.

3

Health hazards of obesity

G. MICHAEL STEELMAN

Even if obesity were only a cosmetic problem, it would still be of significance in our society. Obesity is a disease with considerable social stigma (1–6), and obese individuals are subject to derision, discrimination, and prejudice, even from health care professionals (7–18).

But obesity is, in fact, one of our nation's biggest (no pun intended) health care problems. Although there is some controversy about the number, it has been estimated that over 300,000 deaths per year in America are attributable to obesity (19,20), making it the second most frequent preventable cause of death (after tobacco use). It is linked to cardiovascular disease (CVD), diabetes mellitus (DM), and various types of cancer, as well as many other health problems (21).

This chapter reviews basic information on some of the health hazards and comorbidities associated with obesity.

OBESITY AND INFLAMMATION

While the primary function of adipose tissue is to store energy as triglycerides during periods of energy excess and release free fatty acids during periods of energy need, it also has far more important functions than merely serving as a fuel tank. Adipocytes produce a significant number of substances which have autocrine, paracrine, and/or endocrine activity (22). Thus, obesity can be considered a proinflammatory condition.

Many of the morbidities associated with obesity are mediated through a low-grade "metabolic inflammation," including the development of insulin resistance (23–26). Although white adipose tissue is the main site mediating inflammation, muscle and liver may also demonstrate mild inflammatory responses caused by obesity (27).

Interestingly, adipose tissue secretes both proinflammatory and anti-inflammatory substances. Anti-inflammatory substances are preferentially secreted by the adipose tissue in lean individuals (e.g., adiponectin, interleukins [IL]-4, -10, and -13, IL-1 receptor antagonist, and apelin), whereas in obese individuals, it secretes proinflammatory cytokines including tumor necrosis factor (TNF)-α, IL-6, leptin, visfatin, resistin, angiotensin II, and plasminogen activator inhibitor 1 (25). Table 3.1 provides more information about many of these compounds (22). It is hoped that future research in this area will help identify targets for effective pharmacological therapy to reduce the health consequences of obesity.

DIABETES MELLITUS TYPE 2

According to the American Diabetes Association, an estimated 25.8 million Americans have been diagnosed with diabetes and an additional 7 million have undiagnosed diabetes (28). Furthermore, they report that 79 million more have prediabetes. The medical and social costs of diabetes are significant even in normal weight individuals. There is an even greater impact in those who are also obese (29). It has been projected that the number of Americans living with diabetes will nearly double by 2034, resulting in medical costs of approximately $336 billion (30).

The etiology of DM2 includes the development of insulin resistance, and/or pancreatic beta cell dysfunction. One suggested pathway for the development of the disease is that insulin resistance is the primary abnormality and that beta cell dysfunction arises later as the pancreatic cells "burn out" in response to the increased demand placed on them as they attempt to maintain normoglycemia in the state of increasing insulin resistance (31). Thus, in the initial stages of the disease, normal blood glucose levels are maintained by an increased supply of insulin.

Obesity contributes significantly to the development of insulin resistance. Eighty to ninety-five percent of patients with DM2 are obese, and most often demonstrate the android (apple-shaped) morphology, with an elevated waist-to-hip ratio (32,33).

Visceral fat when compared with subcutaneous fat produces more compounds that are associated with the development of insulin resistance; for example, angiotensin, IL-6, and plasminogen activator inhibitor 1 (34,35). It also releases less adiponectin, an insulin-sensitizing compound. Visceral adiposity is associated with increased deposition of triglyceride in liver and skeletal muscle and with subsequent insulin resistance in these tissues. It has been postulated that triglyceride or metabolic byproducts may produce insulin resistance through the impairment of mitochondrial function (36).

In high-risk overweight individuals, the progression to frank diabetes can be abated with weight loss; weight loss, as little as 5% to 10%, can bring about glycemic control and lessen attendant morbidity (37,38). More drastic weight loss may, at times, eliminate diabetes altogether (39,40).

Medications for diabetes often cause weight gain, especially insulin, sulfonylurea drugs, and thiazolidinediones. Metformin and incretin mimetics, like exenatide, are considered weight neutral and are also less likely to cause hypoglycemia.

Table 3.1 Adipokines increased in obesity, and/or diabetes

Adipokine	Distribution	Function	Increased in obesity
Leptin	Secreted predominantly by WAT, and to a lesser degree in hypothalamus, gastric epithelium, placenta, and gonads	Regulates energy intake, expenditure, and feeding behavior; also regulates storage of fat and insulin in signaling	Increased in mouse models of obesity; increased in human obesity and correlated with BMI and decreased with weight loss
Resistin	In rodents, secreted by adipocytes; in humans, secreted predominantly by circulating macrophages and monocytes, and to a lesser degree by WAT	Implicated in glucose metabolism in the regulation of neoglucogenesis and insulin resistance in rodents; more proinflammatory role in humans	Increased circulating concentrations in mouse models of obesity; increased in human obesity and correlated with insulin resistance in diabetic patients
Interferon α	Expressed by macrophages and adipocytes (visceral WAT > subcutaneous WAT)	Affects insulin and glucose metabolism; provokes insulin resistance and stimulates lipolysis	Increased in mouse models of obesity; increased in human obesity and correlated with BMI
IL-6	One-third of total circulating levels are expressed predominantly by adipocytes; also expressed in macrophages, skeletal muscle, endothelial cells, and fibroblasts	Controversial role in the development of insulin resistance; affects glucose metabolism	Increased circulating levels in human subjects and correlated with adiposity and reduced with weight loss; increased in plasma of T2D patients
IL-7	Secreted by stromal and vascular endothelial cells	Homeostatic immune cytokine; also regulates body weight, adipose tissue mass and function, and insulin signaling	Increased in morbidly obese subjects
IL-8	Secreted by adipocytes (visceral WAT > subcutaneous WAT) and macrophages	Neutrophil chemotaxis	Increased in obese subjects and related to fat mass and tumor necrosis factor α levels
IL-1	Secreted mainly by adipocytes and macrophages	Role in macrophages chemotaxis and thermogenesis	Increased in obese mice; increased in human obesity and predictive of T2D

(Continued)

Table 3.1 (*Continued*) Adipokines increased in obesity, and/or diabetes

Adipokine	Distribution	Function	Increased in obesity
Retinol-binding protein 4	Secreted by adipocytes, macrophages, and hepatocytes	Affects insulin sensitivity, hepatic glucose output, and muscle insulin signaling	Increased circulating levels in obese subjects and correlated with BMI and insulin resistance
Monocyte chemotactic protein 1	Secreted by adipose tissue	Affects insulin sensitivity and increases macrophage recruitment in adipose tissue and inflammation	Increased in mouse models of obesity; increased in T2D subjects
Plasminogen activator inhibitor 1	Expressed by WAT	Potent inhibitor of fibrinolytic pathway	Increased in human obesity and T2D subjects
CXC-chemokine ligand 5	Secreted by macrophages within the stromal vascular fraction	Interferes with insulin signaling in muscle	Circulating levels are higher in obese, insulin-resistant individuals than in obese, insulin-sensitive individuals and decreased after a 4-week period on low-calorie diet
Visfatin	Expressed in liver, muscle, WAT, bone marrow, and lymphocytes	Role in insulin sensitivity, insulin secretion, and inflammatory properties	Increased in obesity and correlates with visceral adiposity in humans
Chemerin	In rodents and humans, expressed in placenta and WAT	Regulates adipocyte development and metabolic function	Increased circulating levels in obese and T2D patients and correlated with body fat, glucose, and lipid metabolism
Vaspin	Secreted by WAT, hypothalamus, pancreatic islets, and skin	Improves insulin sensitivity	Increased in obesity and T2D patients

Source: Adapted from Makki K, Froguel P, Wolowczuk I. *ISRN Inflamm* 2013; 2013: 139–239.
Note: BMI, body mass index; IL, interleukin; T2D, type 2 diabetes; WAT, white adipose tissue.

CARDIOVASCULAR DISEASE

Obesity has been identified as an independent risk factor for CVD, the definition of which includes coronary heart disease (CHD), myocardial infarction (MI), congestive heart failure (CHF), hypertension, atrial fibrillation, and stroke (41,42). The Framingham Heart Study showed obesity to increase the age-adjusted relative risk (RR) for CVD to 1.46 and 1.64 in men and women, respectively, and an even higher age-adjusted risk for hypertension (2.21 in men and 2.75 in women) (43). In a follow-up study (44), the risk for CVD in normal weight, nondiabetic women and men were 54.8% and 78.6%, respectively, compared with 78.8% and 86.9% in obese, diabetic women and men, respectively. European studies (45,46) have shown such associations as well, and abdominal obesity has been recognized as a risk factor for CVD worldwide (47,48).

Obesity is associated with numerous structural and functional changes in the cardiovascular system, even in the absence of frank CVD. Some of these changes are presented in Table 3.2.

Obese individuals often experience *venous insufficiency* in the lower extremities. Pedal edema may be associated with several factors, including elevated ventricular filling pressure despite elevation of cardiac output (49,50), high-volume lymphatic overload, increased intravascular volume, decreased mobility (leading to less pumping action in the calf and leg muscles), and increased venous valvular incompetence.

Obesity increases the risk for CHF (51–55). Each incremental increase of BMI by 1 unit has been estimated to increase the risk for CHF by 5% for men and 7% for women (53). Paradoxically, once CHF is present, patients with higher BMI have a lower risk for hospitalization and death than patients with a healthy BMI (56–61). This phenomenon has been called the "obesity paradox" and is discussed later in the chapter along with its association with several other conditions.

Hypertension is strongly associated with obesity (62,63). Its prevalence is about 6 times more frequent in the obese, with a majority of people with hypertension being overweight (64). A 10 kg higher weight is associated with a 3.0 mm higher systolic and a 2.3 mm higher diastolic blood pressure, with estimated increases of 12% risk for CVD and 24% risk for stroke (65).

An increase in BMI from <25 to >30 kg/m^2 is associated with an increased prevalence of hypertension from 15% to 40% (66). A prospective study of about 30,000 normotensive men

Table 3.2 Cardiovascular system manifestations associated with obesity

↑	Total blood volume
↑	Cardiac output
↑	Stroke volume
↑	(±) Heart rate
↑	LV filling and pressure (especially during exercise)
↑	Left atrial hypertrophy
↑	LV hypertrophy (especially eccentric type)
↑	LV diastolic dysfunction
↑	Adipositas cordis (fatty heart)
↑	PR interval, QRS interval, QTc
↑	↓ QRS voltage
↑	ST depression and other ST-T abnormalities
↑	False-positive inferior MI on electrocardiogram

Note: LV, left ventricular; MI, myocardial infarction.

and women (67) showed that an increase in BMI compared with baseline was associated with a 1.4-fold increase in the risk for hypertension.

Weight loss in obese patients is associated with a reduction in blood pressure. In 50% or more of individuals, blood pressure decreases an average of 1 to 4 mmHg systolic and 1 to 2 mmHg diastolic per kilogram of weight reduction (68–70).

The *sudden cardiac mortality* rate in obese men and women has been estimated to be about 40 times higher than the rate in a matching nonobese population. This association is not newly found; Hippocrates is said to have stated, "Sudden death is more common in those who are naturally fat than in the lean" (71). Alterations in electrical activity of the heart may predispose the obese patient to various arrhythmias (72), especially in light of the structural changes often present in the heart of the severely obese individual. A 10% increase in weight decreases the parasympathetic tone and increases the heart rate, whereas the heart rate decreases on weight reduction (73). Heart rate variability, the fluctuation of heart rate around the mean heart rate, is associated with increased cardiac mortality (74–76) and improves with weight loss (77).

Atherosclerosis and *CHD* are also associated with obesity. Postmortem examination of young people who died from homicide, suicide, or accidental injuries revealed that the extent of fatty streaks and advanced lesions in the abdominal aorta and right coronary artery were associated with obesity and with the size of the abdominal panniculus (78–81).

Several studies (43,82–84) that have reported follow-up data of 20 years or more have well documented that obesity is an independent predictor of clinical CHD. Central fat distribution appears to be a greater factor for atherosclerosis than general fat distribution (85).

While obesity increases the risk of MI, reminiscent of the previous discussion regarding CHF, there is an inverse relationship between BMI and mortality in patients after an acute MI (86,87).

There is a correlation between obesity and the incidence of *stroke* (88–96). For every unit increase of BMI, there is a corresponding increase in the incidence of ischemic stroke by 4% and of hemorrhagic stroke by 6%. This relationship appears to be independent of the effect of hypertension, dyslipidemia, or diabetes (97). It is thought that the link may be related to the prothrombotic and proinflammatory changes that are associated with excess adiposity (98,99).

Metabolic syndrome (MetS), first described by Reaven (100) and associated with an increased risk of mortality from CVD (101), is a combination of several associated cardiovascular risk factors, including abdominal obesity, hypertension, elevated fasting glucose, increased triglycerides, and low high-density lipoprotein levels. One set of diagnostic criteria is outlined in Table 3.3. Weight reduction, even as little as 8 kg, has been shown to lower the prevalence of MetS significantly (102,103).

Weight reduction in obese patients can improve or prevent many obesity-related risk factors. Some of the benefits of weight loss on the cardiovascular system are listed in Table 3.4. However, treatment of the obese patient with CVD is not without risks. The use of very low

Table 3.3 Cardiovascular system manifestations associated with weight loss

↓	Total blood volume
↓	Cardiac output
↓	Stroke volume
↓	(±) Heart rate
↓	LV filling and pressure (especially during exercise)
↓	LV diastolic dysfunction
↓	PR interval, QRS interval, QT interval corrected

Note: LV, left ventricular.

Table 3.4 Metabolic syndrome

Diagnostic criteria (3 out of 5) of the following	
Abdominal obesity (waist circumference)	≥40 in. in men
	≥35 in. in women
Triglycerides	≥150 mg/dL
High-density lipoprotein	≤40 mg/dL for men
	≤50 mg/dL for women
Blood pressure	≥130/80 mmHg
Fasting glucose	≥100 mg/dL

calorie diets, liquid protein diets, and bariatric surgery has been associated with prolonged QT and QTc intervals (104–106). Nutritionally deficient diets may lead to increased predisposition to arrhythmias. Anorectic medications can potentially increase heart rate or blood pressure and are contraindicated in the face of unstable CVD (107). The use of such modalities is best left to those with special interest and training in their use in patients with CVD.

OBESITY AND CHRONIC RENAL DISEASE

There has been a steady increase in the incidence of chronic renal disease (CRD) that appears to parallel the increase in the rates of obesity, overweight, obese, and BMI (108). While hypertension, diabetes, dyslipidemia, atherosclerosis, and inflammation are linked causally to CRD, there is also evidence that renal dysfunction may be associated with obesity independent of diabetes and hypertension (109).

Hsu et al. (110) retrospectively analyzed more than 300,000 subjects who had been followed for ≤15 years and found that the adjusted RR for end-stage renal disease increased incrementally with increasing BMI. This relationship existed even after adjusting for blood pressure, diabetes, smoking, age, cholesterol levels, proteinuria, serum creatinine, and history of MI.

Burton et al. (111) demonstrated reduced estimated glomerular filtration rates (GFRs) and increased CRD in association with increasing BMI and waist circumference in a study of more than 6000 nondiabetic participants. Abdominal obesity (defined as a waist circumference >102 cm in men or >88 cm in women) was associated with a higher risk of renal dysfunction even after adjusting for elevated blood pressure, glucose, or lipids or for BMI in those with hypertension.

Excessive weight gain leads to increased renal tubular sodium reabsorption, which is followed by a compensatory renal vasodilation and increased GFR (109,112,113). This is then followed by a gradual decrease in GFR, as obesity-associated hypertension and diabetes lead to renal injury and nephron loss.

Obese humans often develop proteinuria, sometimes at levels in the nephrotic range. This can be followed by progressive worsening of kidney function, even in the absence of hypertension of diabetes (114). A review of almost 7000 autopsies revealed that the most common renal lesions seen in obese individuals were focal and segmental glomerulosclerosis and glomerulomegaly (115).

Ectopic obesity is the deposition of lipids into nonadipose tissue, including the kidney. It has been postulated that this can lead to the accumulation of toxic metabolites, which in turn may lead to mitochondrial dysfunction, endoplasmic reticulum stress, apoptosis, and subsequent injury and renal dysfunction (109).

Obese subjects have increased sympathetic nervous system (SNS) activation (112,113). Blood pressure is reduced to a greater extent by adrenergic receptor blockade in obese patients compared with lean patients (116). The mechanisms of renal SNS activation in obesity are not completely known, but several factors have been suggested, such as hyperleptinemia, angiotensin II, hyperinsulinemia, impaired baroreflex sensitivity, and physical compression of the kidneys by fat. For an in-depth analysis, refer to Hall et al. (109).

As mentioned earlier in association with certain other conditions, there is a paradoxical lowering of mortality rate in obese patients on dialysis or with end-stage renal disease (117–119). Intentional weight loss, whether by surgical or nonsurgical methods, has been demonstrated to improve renal dysfunction (120–122).

Concern is often expressed that the use of so-called high-protein diets may cause or worsen renal injury. Most of the diets advocated by trained bariatric specialists do not supply an amount of protein that is high in an *absolute* sense but rather an amount of protein that is high *relative* to the other macronutrients. An analysis of the effects of isocaloric diets categorized as low carbohydrate (CHO) (4% CHO, 35% protein, 61% fat) or high carbohydrate (46% CHO, 24% protein, 30% fat) in 68 subjects with abdominal obesity revealed that at 1-year follow-up, there were no changes in serum creatinine or estimated GFR associated with the use of either diet (123).

CANCER

Numerous studies have shown a correlation between obesity and the risk of developing or dying from cancer (124–128). The Million Women Study (126) showed a significant increase in obese individuals in the incidence of cancer (at 5.4 years) and of cancer mortality (at 7 years). This increase was true for all cancers combined and for leukemia, multiple myeloma, non-Hodgkin's lymphoma, and cancer of the endometrium, esophagus, kidney, breast (in postmenopausal women), and colon and rectum (in premenopausal women). A prospective study (125) in the United States involving 900,000 subjects (cancer free at baseline) for more than 15 years showed those with a BMI >39.9 had a 50% to 60% increase in overall cancer mortality and, specifically, had higher death rates from cancer of the colon and rectum, gallbladder, liver, pancreas, kidney, esophagus, and multiple myeloma and non-Hodgkin's lymphoma.

Studies have shown an increase in the incidence and mortality rate of prostate cancer in association with obesity (127). Furthermore, the risk of high-grade, nonmetastatic prostate cancer has been shown to be reduced as a result of weight reduction (127).

OSTEOARTHRITIS

Osteoarthritis (OA) is a common problem that leads to decreased mobility, lost productivity, chronic pain, and disability. Obesity has been shown to increase the risk of OA, especially in the knee and hip (129). OA of the knee has been shown to reduce ambulatory capacity, exercise capacity, and quality of life (130–134).

In the Rotterdam Study (129), the progression of OA of the knee over a 6.5-year period was found to be more than three times more likely in patients with a BMI >27 kg/m^2. Data from the Framingham Heart Study (135) showed that the risk of developing knee OA over a 10-year period in a group of elderly individuals without disease at baseline increased by 1.6 for each 5-unit increase in BMI.

Weight loss has been shown to significantly reduce the signs and symptoms of OA and to improve functional capacity and quality of life in afflicted obese patients (136–141). A randomized study of 87 elderly adults with symptomatic OA of the knee showed those randomized to the weight loss intervention group lost 8.7% body weight (compared with no loss in the placebo group), and they had significant improvement in their functional status. A meta-analysis (136) of four trials (454 total patients) showed that even a modest weight loss (5%) was associated with lessened physical disability.

The possibility of lessened pain and improved functional capacity and quality of life, may serve as a strong motivating factor to encourage weight reduction in appropriate patients.

NONALCOHOLIC FATTY LIVER DISEASE

Nonalcoholic fatty liver disease (NAFLD), associated with obesity, hypertension, and dyslipidemia, affects 15% to 30% of the general population and up to 70% of patients with DM2 (142). It is a spectrum of disorders that ranges from steatosis and nonalcoholic steatohepatitis to, ultimately, cirrhosis and hepatocellular carcinoma (143). Studies (144,145) have shown that obesity is associated with NAFLD significantly and independently.

In one multivariate study (143), an increased BMI (>26.9) was shown to be the primary variable associated with NAFLD (odds ratio [OR] = 6.2). Another report (146) showed the prevalence of NAFLD in a group of Israeli people to be more common in men (38%) than in women (21%) and independently associated with obesity (OR = 2.9). A BMI >30 and the lack of physical fitness were shown to be significantly and independently associated with NAFLD in a group of nonsmoking, healthy men (145). Fortunately, weight loss may be beneficial for reducing the risk of NAFLD in obese patients (147).

INSOMNIA AND OBSTRUCTIVE SLEEP APNEA

Obesity and impaired metabolic functions have been shown to be associated with short sleep duration (148), impaired sleep quality (149), and irregular sleep–wake patterns (150). Table 3.5 lists some of the obesity-associated conditions affected by sleep disturbances (151).

It is beyond the scope of this chapter to address all the connections between insomnia and its role in the etiology and management of obesity in detail. Schmid et al. (151) provide a good review of this topic.

More attention is warranted for obstructive sleep apnea (OSA), a specific sleep disorder and cause of insomnia associated with obesity. OSA occurs in 2% to 3% of middle-aged females and in 4% to 5% of middle-aged males, but its prevalence is >30% in obese patients and 50%

Table 3.5 Obesity-associated conditions affected by sleep disturbances

Prevalence of metabolic syndrome
Increased body weight and obesity
Type 2 diabetes
Dyslipidemia
Hypertension
Mortality
Appetite and food intake (hormonal and central)

Source: Adapted from Schmid SM, Hallschmid M, Schultes B. *Lancet* 2015; 3(1): 52–62.

to 98% in morbidly obese patients (152–154). Obesity is the most important risk factor for the development of OSA, and the RR in obese patients is high (RR = 10) (155). Complications associated with OSA include pulmonary hypertension, right heart failure, stroke, hypertension, and cardiac arrhythmias (21).

One prospective study (153) showed a 32% increase in the apnea–hypopnea index and a sixfold increase in the odds of developing significant sleep-disordered breathing in association with a 10% weight gain during the study. Another study showed those with a 10-kg weight increase had an associated 2.5- to 5-fold increase in the risk of developing >15 respiratory events per hour (154).

Weight loss has been shown (156) to produce significant reduction in symptoms of OSA, including apnea, snoring, and daytime sleepiness.

GALLBLADDER DISEASE

An alliterative characterization of those at higher risk for gallbladder disease is that they are fat, aged 40, female, fertile, and flatulent. Gallbladder disease is a common cause of hospitalization for women and significantly adds to overall health care costs (157).

A study of more than 1 million English and Scottish women showed a strong association between gallbladder disease and obesity (157). After adjusting the data to account for other factors such as age and socioeconomic status, subjects having a higher BMI were more likely to be admitted for gallbladder disease and to have longer hospital stays than their thinner counterparts. Twenty-five percent of hospital days for gallbladder disease were attributed to obesity.

The risk of gallbladder disease is also increased in men who are obese. In the Health Professions Follow-Up Study of men originally free of gallbladder disease (158), those with a BMI >28.5 kg/m^2 had a 2.5 times greater risk of having gallstones. Both overweight and obesity were associated with a significant increase in the risk (OR = 1.86 and 3.38, respectively) of developing symptomatic gallstones in a study of Swedish twins (159).

MENTAL HEALTH ISSUES

The National Epidemiologic Survey on Alcohol and Related Conditions (160) showed that BMI was significantly associated with mood, anxiety, and personality disorders. The lifetime prevalence of major depressive disorder (MDD), specifically, was increased 1.5- to 2-fold for obese individuals compared with normal weight subjects. The OR for a psychiatric disorder was similarly elevated in the study group.

The 2006 Behavioral Risk Factor Surveillance System (161) included data on more than 200,000 individuals. It showed that the prevalence of moderate-to-severe MDD increased from 6.5% to 25.9%, with an increase in BMI from 25 to 35 kg/m^2. Similarly, the prevalence of obesity increased from 25.4% among those without MDD to 57.8% in those with moderate-to-severe MDD.

The nature of the relationship between MDD and obesity is unclear and may be multifactorial. Obese individuals are subject to ridicule, rejection, and other forms of bias and negative stereotyping in our society. Many psychotropic medications are associated with weight gain. Food, especially high-carbohydrate and high-fat items, is often used for comfort in times of emotional distress.

Weight loss may improve depression in many individuals. Some patients will benefit from a change in their psychotropic medications to alternatives that are more weight neutral. There has been a suggestion that an anorectic agent, such as phentermine or diethylpropion, may help alleviate the symptoms of depression (162). The clinician must work carefully with people who use their weight or food consumption as an important emotional defense mechanism (e.g., abuse victims). A nonjudgmental, compassionate physician functions as an extremely valuable part of a potentially life-changing pursuit of the obese patient, particularly in those patients whose weight is creating, or worsening, major social or emotional challenges.

THE OBESITY PARADOX

It appears that obesity offers some protection from mortality in patients with a variety of serious conditions, including MI, CHF, stroke, cancer, diabetes, and other debilitating diseases (56,117,119,163–167). There are several explanations for this seeming protection.

Patients who are more obese may present earlier in the course of their disease compared with their less obese counterparts. The obese patient with mild CHF, for example, may present with more shortness of breath because of the additive effects of CHF and obesity-related respiratory difficulties.

Another possibility is that the lean individual with a cachexia-producing disease has less fat stores to obtain energy and thus enters a severe catabolic state sooner, losing critical protein stores in the process.

It has also been suggested that the obesity paradox may simply be the result of statistical and methodological problems associated with epidemiological studies (167–169). Obese patients should not use this paradox to avoid a healthier lifestyle and attain a better body composition. This remains an area of controversy and, until it becomes more clear, common sense would suggest that "an ounce of prevention is worth a pound of cure."

METABOLICALLY HEALTHY OBESE PATIENTS: IS THERE SUCH A THING?

Similar to the concept of an obesity paradox, there has also been discussion of a subset of obese patients who do not display the typical metabolic disease markers associated with the disease. They have been referred to as the metabolically healthy obese (MHO) as opposed to the metabolically unhealthy phenotype. Additional phenotypes include the metabolically healthy normal weight (MHNW) and metabolically abnormal normal weight (MANW).

One recent report estimated that 10% to 25% of obese individuals fit the MHO phenotype, whereas 5% to 6% of people with normal BMI have metabolic syndrome and thus fall in the MANW subset (170). Appleton et al. (171) reported that those in the MHO subset were not more likely to develop CVD or stroke compared with those in the MHNW subset over a 5- to 10-year time frame, but that 10-year fatal CVD risk was higher in MANW subjects than those in the MHO subset.

Kramer et al. (172) undertook a meta-analysis of 12 studies to further clarify the issue. Using only studies with a follow-up period of 10 years or more, the MHO group had increased CVD and mortality risk compared with the MHNW group. Breaking down results based on BMI categories, they found a stepwise increase in blood pressure, waist circumference, and insulin resistance from normal weight to overweight to obesity.

Thus, there may not be such an entity as MHO if one takes the long-term (>10-year) view. Studies that evaluate over shorter terms may misinterpret those with subtle changes. Excess weight, even in the short term, has been associated with chronic inflammation (173,174), left ventricular changes (175,176), impaired vasoreactivity (175), and increased carotid artery thickness and coronary calcification (177,178). In addition, studies based *solely* on

BMI may include individuals who are in the MANW subset and are "contaminating" the control group.

Kramer et al. (172) sum it up in their statement: "Metabolically healthy obese individuals are at increased risk for death and CV events over the long term compared with metabolically healthy normal weight persons suggesting that (obesity) is not a benign condition even in the absence of metabolic abnormalities."

FINAL THOUGHTS

Obesity is a medical condition with numerous comorbidities and deserves to be approached as a serious health threat. It has reached epidemic proportions and is continuing to increase in prevalence. Recent estimates place obesity-related health expenditures at $147 billion (179). The days of simply handing the patient a preprinted 1000-calorie diet plan with the admonition to "push away from the table" have passed. Overweight patients deserve competent, compassionate, and comprehensive treatment by medical personnel who are willing to take the time and have the patience to see them through a long-term treatment regimen.

REFERENCES

1. Allon N. The stigma of overweight in everyday life. In: Wolman BB, DeBerry S (eds). *Psychological Aspects of Overweight: A Handbook*. New York: Van Nostrand Reinhold; 1982, pp. 130–174.
2. Weiner B. *Judgements of Responsibility: A Theory of Social Conduct*. New York: Guilford; 1955.
3. Pingitore R, Dugoni BL, Tindale RS, et al. Bias against overweight job applicants in a simulated employment interview. *J Appl Psychol* 1994; 79: 909–917.
4. Roehling MV. Weight-based discrimination in employment: Psychological and legal aspects. *Pers Psychol* 1999; 52: 969–1016.
5. Canning H, Mayer J. Obesity: An influence on high school performance? *Am J Clin Nutr* 1967; 20: 352–354.
6. Hebl MR, Heatherton TF. The stigma of obesity: The differences are black and white. *Pers Soc Psychol Bull* 1997; 24: 417–526.
7. Hebl MR, Xu J. Weighing the care: Physician's reactions to the size of a patient. *Int J Obes* 2001; 25: 1246–1252.
8. Harvey EL, Hill AJ. Health professionals' views of overweight people and smokers. *Int J Obes* 2001; 25: 1253–1261.
9. Maddox GL, Back K, Liederman V. Overweight as social deviance and disability. *J Health Soc Behav* 1968; 9: 287–298.
10. Breytspraak LM, McGee J, Conger JC, et al. Sensitizing medical students to impression formation processes in the patient interview. *J Med Educ* 1977; 52: 47–54.
11. Blumberg P, Mellis LP. Medical students' attitudes toward the obese and morbidly obese. *Int J Eat Disord* 1985; 4: 169–175.
12. Price JH, Desmond SM, Krol RA, et al. Family practice physicians beliefs, attitudes and practices regarding obesity. *Am J Prev Med* 1987; 3: 339–345.
13. Bagley CR, Conklin DN, Isherwood RT, et al. Attitudes of nurses toward obesity and obese patients. *Percept Mot Skills* 1989; 68: 954.
14. Peternelj-Taylor CA. The effects of patient weight and sex on nurses' perceptions: A proposed model of nurse withdrawal. *J Adv Nurs* 1989; 14: 744–754.

15. Oberrieder H, Walker R, Monroe D, et al. Attitude of dietetics students and registered dietitians toward obesity. *J Am Diet Assoc* 1995; 95: 914–916.
16. Young LM, Powelll B. The effects of obesity on the clinical judgments of mental health professionals. *J Health Soc Behav* 1985; 26: 233–246.
17. Ferrante JM, Piasecki AK, Ohman-Strickland PA, et al. Family physicians' practices and attitudes regarding care of extremely obese patients. *Obesity* 2009; 17: 1710–1716.
18. Kaminsky J, Gadaleta D. A study of discrimination within the medical community as viewed by obese patients. *Obes Surg* 2002; 12: 14–18.
19. Mokdad AH, Marks JS, Stroup DF, et al. Actual causes of death in the United States, 2000. *JAMA* 2004; 291: 1238–1245.
20. Masters R, Reither EN, Powers D, et al. The impact of obesity on US mortality levels: The importance of age and cohort factors in population estimates. *Am J Public Health* 2013; 103(10): 1895–1901.
21. Pi-Sunyer X. The medical risks of obesity. *Postgrad Med* 2009; 121(6): 21–33.
22. Makki K, Froguel P, Wolowczuk I. Adipose tissue in obesity-related inflammation and insulin resistance: Cells, cytokines, and chemokines. *ISRN Inflamm* 2013; 2013: 139239.
23. Gregor MF, Hotamisligil GS. Inflammatory mechanisms in obesity. *Ann Rev Immun* 2011; 29: 415–445.
24. Hotamisligil GS. Inflammation and metabolic disorders. *Nature* 2006; 444(7121): 860–867.
25. Ouchi N, Parker JL, Lugus JJ, et al. Adipokines in inflammation and metabolic disease. *Nat Rev Immun* 2011; 11(2): 85–97.
26. Shoelson SE, Lee J, Goldfine AB. Inflammation and insulin resistance. *J Clin Invest* 2006; 16(7): 1793–1801.
27. Odegaard JI, Chawla A. Pleiotropic actions of insulin resistance and inflammation in metabolic homeostasis. *Science* 2013; 339: 172–177.
28. American Diabetes Association. Fast facts: Data and statistics about diabetes. 2014. http://professional.diabetes.org/admin/UserFiles/0%20Sean/FastFacts%20March%20 2013.pdf, accessed October 22, 2015.
29. Sullivan PW, Ghushchyan V, Ben-Joseph RH. The effect of obesity and cardiometa-bolic risk factors on expenditures and productivity in the Unites States. *Obesity (Silver Spring)* 2008; 16: 2155–2162.
30. Huang ES, Basu A, O'Grady M, et al. Projecting the future diabetes population size and related costs for the U.S. *Diabetes Care* 2009; 32(12): 2225–2229.
31. Weir GC, Laybutt DR, Kaneto H, et al. Beta-cell adaption and decompensation during the progression of diabetes. *Diabetes* 2001; 50(Suppl 1): S154–S159.
32. Astrup A. Healthy lifestyles in Europe: Prevention of obesity and type II diabetes by diet and physical activity. *Public Health Nutr* 2001; 4(2B): 499–515.
33. Perrini S, Leonardini A, Laviola L, et al. Biological specificity of visceral adipose tissue and therapeutic intervention. *Arch Physiol Biochem* 2008; 114: 277–286.
34. Mafong D, Henry RR. Pathophysiology and complications of type 2 diabetes. *Pract Diabetol* 2009; 6: 13–26.
35. Hevener AL, Febbraio MA, Stock Conference Working Group. The 2009 stock con-ference report: Inflammation, obesity, and metabolic disease. *Obes Rev* 2010; 11(9): 635–644. doi: http://dx/doi.org/10.1111/j.1467-789X.2009.00691.x.
36. Abdul-Ghani MA, DeFronzo RA. Mitochondrial dysfunction, insulin resistance, and type 2 diabetes mellitus. *Curr Diab Rep* 2008; 8: 173–178.
37. Knowler WC, Barrett-Conner E, Fowler SE, et al. Reduction in the incidence of type 2 diabetes with lifestyle intervention or metformin. *N Engl J Med* 2002; 346: 393–403.

38. Wadden TA, Berkowitz RI, Womble LG, et al. Randomized trial of lifestyle modification and pharmacotherapy for obesity. *N Engl J Med* 2005; 353: 2111–2120.
39. Dixon JB, Obrien PE. Health outcomes of severely obese type 2 diabetic subjects 1 year after laparoscopic adjustable gastric banding. *Diabetes Care* 2002; 25: 358–363.
40. Buchwald H, Estok R, Fahrback K, et al. Weight and type 2 diabetes after bariatric surgery: Systematic review and meta-analysis. *Am J Med* 2009; 1222: 248–256.
41. Must A, Spadano J, Coakley EH, et al. The disease burden associated with overweight and obesity. *JAMA* 1999; 282(16): 1523–1529.
42. Klein S, Burke LE, Bray GA, et al. Clinical implications of obesity with specific focus on cardiovascular disease: A statement for professionals from the American Heart Association Council on Nutrition, Physical Activity, and Metabolism: Endorsed by the American College of Cardiology Foundation. *Circulation* 2004; 110(8): 2952–2967.
43. Wilson PW, D'Agostina RB, Sullivan L, et al. Overweight and obesity as determinants of cardiovascular risk: The Framingham experience. *Arch Intern Med* 2002; 162(16): 1867–1872.
44. Fox CS, Pencina MJ, Wilson PW, et al. Lifetime risk of cardiovascular disease among individuals with and without diabetes stratified by obesity status in the Framingham Heart Study. *Diabetes Care* 2008; 31(8): 1582–1584.
45. Balkau B, Deanfield JE, Despres JP, et al. International Day for the Evaluation of Abdominal Obesity (IDEA): A study of waist circumference, cardiovascular disease, and diabetes mellitus in 168,000 primary care patients in 63 countries. *Circulation* 2007; 116(7): 1942–1951.
46. Wannamethee SG, Shaper AG, Walker M. Overweight and obesity and weight change in middle aged men: Impact on cardiovascular disease and diabetes. *J Epidemiol Community Health* 2005; 59(2): 134–139.
47. Poierier P, Eckel RH. Obesity and cardiovascular disease. *Curr Atheroscler Rep* 2002; 4: 448–453.
48. Poirier P, Eckel RH. The heart and obesity. In: Fuster V, Alexander RS, King S, et al. (eds). *Hurst's The Heart*. New York: McGraw-Hill; 2000, pp. 2289–2303.
49. deDivitiis O, Fazio S, Petitto M, et al. Obesity and cardiac function. *Circulation* 1981; 4: 447–482.
50. Nakajima T, Fujioka S, Tokunaga K, et al. Correlation of intra-abdominal fat accumulation and left ventricular performance in obesity. *Am J Cardiol* 1989; 64: 369–373.
51. Kortelainen ML. Myocardial infarction and coronary pathology in severely obese people examined at autopsy. *Int J Obes Relat Metab Disord* 2002; 26: 73–79.
52. He J, Ogden LOG, Bazzano LA, et al. Risk factors for congestive heart failure in US men and women: NHANES I epidemiologic follow-up study. *Arch Intern Med* 2001; 161: 996–1002.
53. Kenchaiah S, Evans JC, Levy D, et al. Obesity and the risk of heart failure. *N Engl J Med* 2002; 347: 305–313.
54. Chen YT, Vaccarino V, Williams CS, et al. Risk factors for heart failure in the elderly: A prospective community-based study. *Am J Med* 1999; 10: 605–612.
55. Wilhelmsen L, Rosengren A, Eriksson H, et al. Heart failure in the general population of men: Morbidity, risk factors and prognosis. *J Intern Med* 2001; 249: 253–261.
56. Horwich TB, Fonarow GC, Hamilton MA, et al. The relationship between obesity and mortality in patients with heart failure. *J Am Coll Cardiol* 2001; 38: 780–795.

57. Osman AF, Mehra MR, Lavie CH, et al. The incremental prognostic importance of body fat adjusted peak oxygen consumption in chronic heart failure. *J Am Coll Cardiol* 2000; 36: 2126–2131.
58. Lissin LW, Gauri AJ, Froelicher VF, et al. The prognostic value of body mass index and standard exercise testing in male veterans with congestive heart failure. *J Card Fail* 2002; 8: 206–215.
59. Davos CH, Doehner W, Rauchhaus M, et al. Body mass and survival in patients with chronic heart failure without cachexia: The importance of obesity. *J Card Fail* 2003; 9: 29–55.
60. Lavie CJ, Osman AF, Milani RV, et al. Body composition and prognosis in chronic systolic heart failure: The obesity paradox. *Am J Cardiol* 2003; 91: 891–894.
61. Mosterd A, Cost B, Hoes AW, et al. The prognosis of heart failure in the general population: The Rotterdam study. *Eur Heart J* 2001; 22: 1318–1327.
62. Johnson AL, Cornini JC, Cassel JC, et al. Influences of race, sex and weight on blood pressure behavior in young adults. *Am J Cardiol* 1975; 35: 523–530.
63. Voors AW, Webber LS, Frerichs RR, et al. Body height and body mass as determinants of basal blood pressure in children: The Bogalusa Heart Study. *Am J Epidemiol* 1977; 106: 101–108.
64. Stamler R, Stamler J, Riedlinger WF, et al. Weight and blood pressure: Findings in hypertension screening of 1 million Americans. *JAMA* 1978; 240: 1607–1610.
65. National Institutes of Health. Clinical guidelines on the identification, evaluation, and treatment of overweight and obesity in adults: The evidence report. *Obes Res* 1998; 6(Suppl 2): 51S–209S.
66. Brown CD, Higgins M, Donato KA, et al. Body mass index and the prevalence of hypertension and dyslipidemia. *Obes Res* 2000; 8: 605–619.
67. Dreyvold WB, Midthjell K, Nilsen J. Change in body mass index and its impact on blood pressure: A prospective population study. *Int J Obes (Lond)* 2005; 29(6): 650–655.
68. Schotte DE, Stunkard AJ. The effects of weight reduction on blood pressure in 301 obese patients. *Arch Intern Med* 1990; 150: 1701–1704.
69. Novi RF, Porta M, Lamberto M, et al. Reductions of body weight and blood pressure in obese hypertensive patients treated by diet. A retrospective study. *Panminerva Med* 1989; 31: 13–15.
70. Staessen J, Fagard R, Amery A. The relationship between body weight and blood pressures. *J Hum Hypertens* 1988; 2: 207–217.
71. Lavie CJ, Milani RV, Ventura HO. Obesity and cardiovascular disease: Risk factor, paradox, and impact of weight loss. *J Am Coll Cardiol* 2009; 53(21): 1925–1932.
72. Poirier P, Giles TD, Bray GA, et al. Obesity and cardiovascular disease: Pathophysiology, evaluation, and effect of weight loss; an update of the 1997 American Heart Association Scientific Statement on Obesity and Heart Disease from the Obesity Committee of the Council on Nutrition, Physical Activity, and Metabolism. *Circ J Am Heart Assoc* 2006; 113: 898–918.
73. Hirsch J, Leibel RL, Mackintosh R, et al. Heart rate variability as a measure of autonomic function during weight change in humans. *Am J Physiol* 1991; 261: R1418–R1423.
74. Kannel WB, Kannel C, Paffenbarger RS Jr, et al. Heart rate and cardiovascular mortality: The Framingham study. *Am Heart J* 1987; 113: 1489–1494.

75. Seccareccia F, Pannozzo F, Dima F, et al. Malattie Cardiovascolari Aterosclerotiche Istituto Superiore di Sanita Project. Heart rate as a predictor of mortality: The MATISS project. *Am J Public Health* 2001; 91: 1258–1263.

76. La Rovere MT, Bigger JT Jr, Marcus FI, et al. Baroreflex sensitivity and heart-rate variability in prediction of total cardiac mortality after myocardial infarction. ATRAMI (Autonomic Tone and Reflexes After Myocardial Infarction) Investigators. *Lancet* 1998; 351: 478–484.

77. Poirier P, Hernandez TL, Weil KM, et al. Impact of diet-induced weight loss on the cardiac autonomic nervous system in severe obesity. *Obes Res* 2003; 11: 1040–1047.

78. McGill HC Jr, McMahan CA, Herderick EE, et al. Origin of atherosclerosis in childhood and adolescence. *Am J Clin Nutr* 2000; 72: 1307S–1315S.

79. Berenson GS. Bogalusa Heart Study: A long-term community study of a rural biracial (black/white) population. *Am J Med Sci* 2001; 322: 267–274.

80. Enos WF, Holmes RH, Beyer J. Coronary disease among United States soldiers killed in action in Korea. *JAMA* 1953; 152: 1090–1093.

81. McGill HC Jr, McMahan CA, Malcom GT, et al. Relation of glycohemoglobin and adiposity to atherosclerosis in youth. Pathobiological Determinants of Atherosclerosis in Youth (PDAY) Research Group. *Arterioscler Thromb Vasc Biol* 1995; 15: 431–440.

82. Rabkin SW, Mathewson FA, Hsu PH. Relation of body weight to development of ischemic heart disease in a cohort of young North American men after a 26 year observation period: The Manitoba Study. *Am J Cardiol* 1977; 39: 452–458.

83. Hubert HB, Feinleib M, McNamara PM, et al. Obesity as an independent risk factor for cardiovascular disease: A 26-year follow-up of participants in the Framingham Heart Study. *Circulation* 1983; 67: 968–977.

84. Manson JE, Colditz GA, Stampfer MJ, et al. A prospective study of obesity and risk of coronary heart disease in women. *N Engl J Med* 1990; 322: 882–889.

85. Fontaine KR, Redden DT, Wang C, et al. Years of life lost due to obesity. *JAMA* 2003; 289: 187–193.

86. Dagenais GR, Yi Q, Mann JF, et al. Prognostic impact of body weight and abdominal obesity in women and men with cardiovascular disease. *Am Heart J* 2005; 149: 54–60.

87. Kragelund C, Hassager C, Hildebrandt P, et al. Impact of obesity on long-term prognosis following acute myocardial infarction. *Int J Cardiol* 2005; 98: 123–131.

88. Abbott RD, Behrens GR, Sharp DS, et al. Body mass index and thromboembolic stroke in nonsmoking men in older middle age: The Honolulu Heart Program. *Stroke* 1994; 25: 2370–2376.

89. Rhoads GG, Kagan A. The relation of coronary disease, stroke, and mortality to weight in youth and in middle age. *Lancet* 1983; 1: 492–495.

90. Shinton R, Shipley M, Rose G. Overweight and stroke in the Whitehall study. *J Epidemiol Community Health* 1991; 45: 138–142.

91. Rexrode KM, Hennekens CH, Willett WC, et al. A prospective study of body mass index, weight change, and risk of stroke in women. *JAMA* 1997; 227: 1539–1545.

92. Lapidus L, Bengtsson C, Larsson B, et al. Distribution of adipose tissue and risk of cardiovascular disease and death: A 12 year follow up of participants in the population study of women in Gothenburg, Sweden. *BMJ (Clin Res Ed)* 1984; 289: 1257–1261.

93. Folsom AR, Prineas RJ, Kaye SA, et al. Incidence of hypertension and stroke in relation to body fat distribution and other risk factors in older women. *Stroke* 1990; 21: 701–706.

94. Terry RB, Page WF, Haskell WL. Waist/hip ratio, body mass index and premature cardiovascular disease mortality in US Army veterans during a twenty-three year follow-up study. *Int J Obes Relat Metab Disord* 1992; 16: 417–423.

95. Walker SP, Rimm EB, Ascherio A, et al. Body size and fat distribution as predictors of stroke among US men. *Am J Epidemiol* 1996; 144: 1143–1150.

96. Pyorala M, Miettinen H, Lasko M, et al. Hyperinsulinemia and the risk of stroke in healthy middle-aged men: The 22-year follow-up results of the Helsinki Policemen Study. *Stroke* 1998; 29: 1860–1866.

97. Kurth T, Gaziano JM, Berger K, et al. Body mass index and the risk of stroke in men. *Arch Intern Med* 2002; 162: 2557–2562.

98. Rost NS, Wolf PA, Kase CS, et al. Plasma concentration of C-reactive protein and risk of ischemic stroke and transient ischemic attack: The Framingham study. *Stroke* 2001; 32: 2575–2579.

99. Sriram K, Benkovic SA, Miller DB, et al. Obesity exacerbates chemically induced neurodegeneration. *Neuroscience* 2002; 115: 1335–1346.

100. Reaven GH. Role of insulin in human disease. *Diabetes* 1988; 37: 1595–1607.

101. Gao W, DECODE Study Group. Does the constellation of risk factors with and without abdominal adiposity associate with different cardiovascular mortality risk? *Int J Obes* 2008; 32(5): 757–762.

102. Ilanne-Parikka P, Eriksson JG, Lindstrom J, et al. Effect of lifestyle intervention on the occurrence of metabolic syndrome and its components in the Finnish Diabetes Prevention Study. *Diabetes Care* 2008; 31(4): 805–807.

103. Phelan S, Wadden TA, Berkowitz RI, et al. Impact of weight loss on the metabolic syndrome. *Int J Obes* 2007; 31: 1442–1448.

104. Sours HE, Frattali VP, Brand CD, et al. Sudden death associated with very low calorie weight reduction regimens. *Am J Clin Nutr* 1981; 34: 453–461.

105. Isner JM, Sours HE, Pari AL, et al. Sudden unexpected death in avid dieters using the liquid-protein-modified-fast diet. Observations in 17 patients and the role of the prolonged QT interval. *Circulation* 1979; 60: 1401–1412.

106. Drenick EJ, Fisler JS. Sudden cardiac arrest in morbidly obese surgical patients unexplained after autopsy. *Am J Surg* 1988; 155: 720–726.

107. Shape Up America!, American Obesity Association. *Guidance for Treatment of Adult Obesity*. Bethesda, MD: Shape Up America!; 1996.

108. Hall JE, Henegar JR, Dwyer TM, et al. Is obesity a major cause of chronic renal disease? *Adv Ren Replace Ther* 2004; 11(1): 41–54.

109. Hall ME, do Carmo JM, da Silva AA, et al. Obesity, hypertension, and chronic kidney disease. *Int J Nephrol Renal Dis* 2014; 7: 75–88.

110. Hsu CY, McCulloch CE, Iribarren C, et al. Body mass index and risk for end-stage renal disease. *Ann Intern Med* 2006; 144(1): 21–28.

111. Burton JO, Gray LJ, Webb DR, et al. Association of anthropometric obesity measures with chronic kidney disease risk in a non-diabetic patient population. *Nephrol Dial Transplant* 2012; 27(5): 1860–1866.

112. Hall JE, Crook ED, Jones DW, et al. Mechanisms of obesity-associated cardiovascular and renal disease. *Am J Med Sci* 2002; 324(3): 127–137.

113. Hall JE, da Silva AA, do Carmo JM, et al. Obesity-induced hypertension: Role of sympathetic nervous system, leptin, and melanocortins. *J Biol Chem* 2010; 285(23): 17271–17276.

114. Morales E, Valero MA, Leon M, et al. Beneficial effects of weight loss in overweight patients with chronic proteinuric nephropathies. *Am J Kidney Dis* 2003; 41(2): 319–327.

115. Kambham N, Markowitz GS, Valeri AM, et al. Obesity-related glomerulopathy: An emerging epidemic. *Kidney Int* 2001; 59(4): 1498–1509.

116. Wofford MR, Anderson DC, Brown CA, et al. Antihypertensive effect of alpha- and beta-adrenergic blockade in obese and lean hypertensive subjects. *Am J Hypertens* 2001; 14(7 Pt 1): 694–698.

117. Lowrie EG, Lew NL. Death risk in hemodialysis patients: The predictive value of commonly measured variables and an evaluation of death rate differences between facilities. *Am J Kidney Dis* 1990; 15(5): 458–482.

118. Schuster DP, Teodorescu M, Mikami D, et al. Effect of bariatric surgery on normal and abnormal renal function. *Surg Obes Relat Dis* 2011; 7(4): 459–464.

119. Molnar MZ, Streja E, Kovesdy CP, et al. Associations of body mass index and weight loss with mortality in transplant-waitlisted maintenance hemodialysis patients. *Am J Transplant* 2011; 11(4): 725–736.

120. Shen WW, Chen HM, Chen H, et al. Obesity-related glomerulopathy: Body mass index and proteinuria. *Clin J Am Soc Nephrol* 2010; 5(8): 1401–1409.

121. Fenske WK, Dubb S, Bueter M, et al. Effect of bariatric surgery-induced weight loss on renal and systemic inflammation and blood pressure: A 12-month prospective study. *Surg Obes Relat Dis* 2013; 9(4): 559–568.

122. Navaneethan SD, Yehnert H, Moustarah F, et al. Weight loss interventions in chronic kidney disease: A systematic review and meta-analysis. *Clin J Am Soc Nephrol* 2009; 4(10): 1565–1574.

123. Brinkworth GD, Buckley JD, Noakes M, et al. Renal function following long-term weight loss in individuals with abdominal obesity on a very-low-carbohydrate diet vs. high-carbohydrate diet. *J Am Diet Assoc* 2010; 110(4): 633–638.

124. Thygesen LC, Grenbaek M, Johansen C, et al. Prospective weight change and colon cancer risk in male US health professionals. *Int J Cancer* 2008; 123(5): 1160–1165.

125. Calle EE, Rodriguez C, Walker-Thurmond K, et al. Overweight, obesity, and mortality from cancer in a prospectively studied cohort of US adults. *N Engl J Med* 2003; 348(17): 1625–1638.

126. Reeves GK, Pirie K, Beral V, et al. Cancer incidence and mortality in relation to body mass index in the Million Women Study: Cohort study. *BMJ* 2007; 335(7630): 1134.

127. Wright ME, Chang SC, Schatzkin A, et al. Prospective study of adiposity and weight change in relation to prostate cancer incidence and mortality. *Cancer* 2007; 109(4): 675–684.

128. Rodriguez C, Freedland SJ, Deka A, et al. Body mass index, weight change, and risk of prostate cancer in the Cancer Prevention Study II Nutrition Cohort. *Cancer Epidemiol Biomarkers Prev* 2007; 16(1): 63–69.

129. Reijman M, Pols HA, Bergink AP, et al. Body mass index associated with onset and progression of osteoarthritis of the knee but not of the hip: The Rotterdam Study. *Ann Rheum Dis* 2007; 66(2): 158–162.

130. Creamer P, Lethbridge-Cejku M, Hochberg MC. Factors associated with functional impairment in symptomatic knee osteoarthritis. *Rheumatology* 2000; 39(5): 490–496.

131. Jinks C, Jordan K, Croft P. Disabling knee pain—Another consequence of obesity: Results from a prospective cohort study. *BMC Public Health* 2006; 6: 258.

132. Marks R. Obesity profiles with knee osteoarthritis: Correlation with pain, disability, disease progression. *Obesity (Silver Spring)* 2007; 15(7): 1867–1874.

133. Sutbeyaz ST, Sezer N. Koseoglu BF, et al. Influence of knee osteoarthritis on exercise capacity and quality of life in obese adults. *Obesity (Silver Spring)* 2007; 15(8): 2071–2076.

134. Tukker A, Visscher T, Picavet H. Overweight and health problems of lower extremities: Osteoarthritis, pain and disability. *Public Health Nutr* 2009; 12(3): 359–368.
135. Felson DT, Zhang Y, Hannan MT, et al. Risk factors for incident radiographic knee osteoarthritis in the elderly: The Framingham Study. *Arthritis Rheum* 1997; 40(4): 728–733.
136. Christensen R, Bartels EM, Astrip A, et al. Effect of weigh reduction in obese patients diagnosed with knee osteoarthritis: A systematic review and meta-analysis. *Ann Rheum Dis* 2007; 66(4): 433–439.
137. Fransen M. Dietary weight loss and exercise for obese adults with knee osteoarthritis: Modest weight loss targets, mild exercise, modest effects. *Arthritis Rheum* 2004; 50(5): 1366–1369.
138. Huang MH, Chen CH, Chen TW, et al. The effects of weight reduction on the rehabilitation of patients with knee osteoarthritis and obesity. *Arthritis Care Res* 2000; 13(6): 398–405.
139. Messier SP, Loeser RF, Miller GD, et al. Exercises and dietary weight loss in overweight and obese older adults with knee osteoarthritis: The arthritis, diet and activity promotion trial. *Arthritis Rheum* 2004; 50(5): 1501–1510.
140. Miller GD, Nicklas BJ, Davis C, et al. Intensive weight loss program improves physical function in older obese adults with knee osteoarthritis. *Obesity (Silver Spring)* 2006; 14(7): 1219–1230.
141. VanGool CH, Penninx BW, Kempen GI, et al. Effects of exercise adherence on physical function among overweight older adults with knee osteoarthritis. *Arthritis Rheum* 2005; 53(1): 24–32.
142. Targher G, Arcaro G. Non-alcoholic fatty liver disease and increased risk of cardiovascular disease. *Atherosclerosis* 2007; 191(2): 235–240.
143. Preiss D, Sattar N. Non-alcoholic fatty liver disease: An overview of prevalence, diagnosis, pathogenesis and treatment considerations. *Clin Sci (Lond)* 2008; 115(5): 141–150.
144. Riquelme A, Arrese M, Soza A, et al. Non-alcoholic fatty liver disease and its association with obesity, insulin resistance and increased serum levels of C-reactive protein in Hispanics. *Liver Int* 2009; 29(1): 82–88.
145. Church TS, Kuk JL, Ross R, et al. Association of cardiorespiratory fitness, body mass index, and waist circumference to nonalcoholic fatty liver disease. *Gastroenterology* 2006; 130(7): 2023–2030.
146. Zelber-Sagi S, Nitzan-Kaluski D, Halpert Z, et al. Prevalence of primary non-alcoholic fatty liver disease in a population-based study and its association with biochemical and anthropometric measures. *Liver Int* 2006; 26(7): 856–863.
147. Adams LA, Angulo P. Treatment of non-alcoholic fatty liver disease. *Postgrad Med J* 2006; 82(967): 315–322.
148. Hall MH, Muldoon MF, Jennings JR, et al. Self-reported sleep duration is associated with the metabolic syndrome in midlife adults. *Sleep* 2008; 31: 635–643.
149. Hun HC, Yang YC, Ou HY, et al. The association between self-reported sleep quality and overweight in a Chinese population. *Obesity (Silver Spring)* 2013; 21: 486–492.
150. Pan A, Schernhammer ES, Sun Q, et al. Rotating night shift work and risk of type 2 diabetes: Two prospective cohort studies in women. *PLoS Med* 2011; 8: e1001141.
151. Schmid SM, Hallschmid M, Schultes B. The metabolic burden of sleep loss. *Lancet* 2015; 3(1): 52–62. doi: http://dx/doi.org/10.1016/S2213-8587(14)70012-9.
152. Resta O, Foschino-Barbaro MP, Legari G, et al. Sleep-related breathing disorders, loud snoring and excessive daytime sleepiness in obese subjects. *Int J Obes Relat Metab Disord* 2001; 25(5): 669–675.

153. Peppard PE, Young T, Palta M, et al. Longitudinal study of moderate weight change and sleep-disordered breathing. *JAMA* 2000; 284(23): 3015–3021.
154. Newman AB, Foster G, Givelber R, et al. Progression and regression of sleep-disordered breathing with changes in weight: The Sleep Heart Health Study. *Arch Intern Med* 2005; 165(20): 2408–2413.
155. Pillar G, Shehadeh N. Abdominal fat and sleep apnea: The chicken or the egg? *Diabetes Care* 2008; 31(Suppl 2): S303–S309.
156. Grunstein RR, Stenlof K, Hedner JA, et al. Two year reduction in sleep apnea symptoms and associated diabetes incidence after weight loss in severe obesity. *Sleep* 2007; 30(6): 703–710.
157. Liu B, Balkwill A, Spencer E, et al. Relationship between body mass index and length of hospital stay for gallbladder disease. *J Public Health (Oxf)* 2008; 30(2): 161–166.
158. Tsai CJ, Leitzmann MF, Willett WC, et al. Prospective study of abdominal adiposity and gallstone disease in US men. *Am J Clin Nutr* 2004; 80(1): 38–44.
159. Katsika D, Tuvblad C, Einarsson C, et al. Body mass index, alcohol, tobacco and symptomatic gallstone disease: A Swedish twin study. *J Intern Med* 2007; 262(5): 581–587.
160. Petry NM, Barry D, Pietrzak RH, et al. Overweight and obesity are associated with psychiatric disorders: Results from the National Epidemiologic Survey on alcohol and related conditions. *Psychosom Med* 2008; 70(3): 288–297.
161. Strine TW, Mokdad AH, Dube SR, et al. The association of depression and anxiety with obesity and unhealthy behaviors among community dwelling US adults. *Gen Hosp Psychiatry* 2008; 30(2): 127–137.
162. Meldman MJ. Diet medications as useful antidepressants. *Am J Bariatric Med* 2009; 24(1): 234–235.
163. Kalantar-Zadeh K, Block G, Humphreys MH, et al. Reverse epidemiology and cardiovascular risk factors in maintenance dialysis patients. *Kidney Int* 2003; 63: 793–808.
164. Kalantar-Zadeh K, Block G, Horwich T, et al. Reverse epidemiology of conventional cardiovascular risk factors in patients with chronic heart failure. *J Am Coll Cardiol* 2004; 43(8): 1439–1444.
165. Leavey SF, McCullough K, Hecking E, et al. Body mass index and mortality in 'healthier' as compared with 'sicker' haemodialysis patients: Results from the Dialysis Outcomes and Practice Patterns Study (DOPPS). *Nephrol Dial Transplant* 2001; 16(12): 2386–2394.
166. Fung F, Sherrard DJ, Gillen DL, et al. Increased risk for cardiovascular mortality among malnourished end-stage renal disease patients. *Am J Kidney Dis* 2002; 40(2): 307–314.
167. Banack HR, Kaufman JS. The "obesity paradox" explained. *Epidemiology* 2013; 24(3): 461–462.
168. Lajous M, Bijon A, Fagherazzi G, et al. Body mass index, diabetes, and mortality in French women: Explaining away a "paradox." *Epidemiology* 2014; 25(1): 10–14.
169. Standl E, Erbach M, Schnell O. Defending the con side: Obesity paradox does not exist. *Diabetes Care* 2013; 36(Suppl 2): S282–S286.
170. Bluher M. The distinction of metabolically 'healthy' from 'unhealthy' obese individuals. *Curr Opin Lipidol* 2010; 21: 38–43.
171. Appleton SL, Seaborn CJ, Visvanathan R, et al. Diabetes and cardiovascular disease outcomes in the metabolically healthy obese phenotype: A cohort study. *Diabetes Care* 2013; 36: 2388–2394.
172. Kramer CK, Zinman B, Retnakaran R. Are metabolically healthy overweight and obesity benign conditions? *Ann Intern Med* 2013; 159(11): 758–769.

173. Wildman RP, Kaplan R, Manson JE, et al. Body size phenotypes and inflammation in the Women's Health Initiative Observational Study. *Obesity (Silver Spring)* 2011; 19: 1482–1491.
174. Marques-Vidal P, Velho S, Waterworth D, et al. The association between inflammatory biomarkers and metabolically healthy obesity depends on the definition used. *Eur J Clin Nutr* 2012; 66: 426–435.
175. Lind L, Siegbahn A, Ingelsson E, et al. A detailed cardiovascular characterization of obesity without the metabolic syndrome. *Arterioscler Thromb Vasc Biol* 2011; 31: e27–e34.
176. Park J, Kim SH, Cho GY, et al. Obesity phenotype and cardiovascular changes. *J Hypertens* 2011; 29: 1765–1772.
177. Stefan N, Kantartzis K, Machann J, et al. Identification and characterization of metabolically benign obesity in humans. *Arch Intern Med* 2008; 168: 1609–1616.
178. Khan UI, Wang D, Thurston RC, et al. Burden of subclinical cardiovascular disease in "metabolically benign" and "at-risk" overweight and obese women: The Study of Women's Health Across the Nation (SWAN). *Atherosclerosis* 2011; 217: 179–186.
179. Finkelstein EA, Trogdon JG, Cohen JW, et al. Annual medical spending attributable to obesity: Payer-and service-specific estimates. *Health Aff (Millwood)* 2009; 28(5): w822–w831.

4

Evaluation of the obese patient

G. MICHAEL STEELMAN AND JAMES T. COOPER*

* Deceased.

APPROACH TO THE PATIENT

The importance of how you interact with your patients who are obese cannot be emphasized enough. Your success or failure as a treating physician, or member of a treatment team, is often determined during the first encounter with the patient. The unspoken communication that you send to your patient can be stronger than the actual words that you speak. An unconscious shrug of your shoulders, a smile that is taken as a smirk, a look of disbelief, or any of dozens of gestures and expressions can turn the patient off. Such a response could happen in spite of your genuine desire to help the patient.

The first thing to understand about someone with a chronic obesity problem is that she (the female pronoun is used in this chapter exclusively, but all such text also applies to males) may be accustomed to failure and rejection. You may be the latest in a long line of doctors who have all failed to be of help, for one reason or another, in the management of this person's situation. When you are successful, you become the last and most effective therapist that she will need.

There is a widespread attitude among physicians that obesity is a self-induced condition that could be cured promptly if only each patient would exercise some self-control and just "push away from the table." Since alcoholism has been relatively destigmatized, obesity remains one of the only diseases that is perceived as a character weakness and an unwillingness to change and improve oneself.

Obesity is a disease that is difficult to treat successfully; therefore, doctors who cannot help their obese patients to become slim may turn to blaming the patient for the failure. They may unconsciously reject the patient, just as many physicians have difficulties dealing with the terminally ill. The doctor's professional sense of omnipotence and omniscience can be threatened. Many doctors will send an obese patient off with a diet sheet, a pat on the shoulder, and perhaps a month's supply of anorectic agents, along with the admonition to not come back "until you lose 10 pounds."

It is no wonder that the doctor who is successful in treating overweight patients soon has a crowded waiting room. Word soon gets out that this doctor, although not promising miracles, at least promises tolerance, understanding of the problem, and a sensible approach that has a better-than-even chance at success.

For the primary or secondary physician who is not involved in directly treating the obese patient, it remains important to seize an opportunity to direct the patient toward treatment (1,2). This direction can often be accomplished by following the 5 "A's":

- ASK for permission to discuss body weight and explore readiness to change
- ASSESS parameters such as weight, waist circumference, and body mass index (BMI) as are appropriate for your specialty
- ADVISE about the health risks, benefits of weight loss, and treatment options
- AGREE on realistic weight loss expectations and treatment objectives
- ARRANGE or ASSIST in identifying barriers and resources and in following up with appropriate plans and health care providers (e.g., an obesity medicine specialist)

THE BARIATRIC VISIT

The initial interview and history should be done in an atmosphere of understanding, respect, and kindness. The patient should not be patronized during this or any other visit to your office. Such belittling turns off the flow of information that is so vital to your success with her.

The sexual history and food contact history are somewhat neglected in other medical workups, but they could be quite productive when working with overweight patients. The food contact history does not have to be part of the initial workup; it can be compiled and evaluated by the use of diaries and food contact interviews as treatment proceeds.

Many patients are anxious when they first come to your office. Being in a strange office produces part of the anxiety, and part of the anxiety also is related to the fact that you are going to "take food away" from them. In this type of setting, it is best to be kind and patient with an obese patient. Even if you have to repeat or explain something several times because of anxiety-generated poor attention, be helpful and considerate of the patient's feelings.

A good way to get a lot of data quickly is to have the patient fill out the history form before the initial interview. Software is available so that the patient can complete the form in the Internet before the clinic visit. If the patient has any difficulty with reading or writing, you might have to have someone on your staff go through the questions with them. You can then take the completed form and review it with the patient. Make notes on the areas of the sheets where the answers were given, or on a separate place in the problem list that could be attached to the history. Many offices make use of yellow highlighter markers to point out the important positive responses in the body of the history. Notes in the doctor's handwriting may be in black, for further information on positive responses, and in red when medications and/or allergies are mentioned.

You can then summarize the history by listing problems that are active and important to management of the patient. Medications and their frequency of use are listed. Impressions of the patient's apparent strengths and weaknesses are important to note at each visit. These impressions may not always be correct, but several regular visits with the treatment team can often uncover most of the most pressing problems that need to be addressed before each patient can learn to deal with her eating problem.

The description of the history and physical examination on a beginning bariatric patient may seem familiar, but certain elements deserve special attention. Bariatrics, or medical weight control, could be considered a branch of internal medicine, family practice, or gynecology. The bariatrician is a physician and should still practice medicine, including an excellent history, physical, and laboratory workup, and proper follow-through. Anything less than excellent is not acceptable for this extremely neglected segment of the patient population, the obese. Of course, the history and physical procedures given here will need to be suited to your style of practice and to the patient's individual medical conditions.

THE HISTORY

The bariatric history has unique aspects that enable the bariatrician to identify underlying comorbidities and to develop an individualized treatment plan to optimize the patient's likelihood of success. The main purpose of the history is to understand what has happened in the past and what is happening to this patient now. Without this overall understanding, you can give all the diets that you want, and you will almost never produce lasting weight loss. Most practitioners use a standard medical history format (Table 4.1).

The first task is to understand what the individual's goals and needs are in a weight loss program. Many practitioners use open-ended questions for this task, or questions pertaining to desired weight, monthly weight loss goal, and clothing size (Table 4.2). If it appears that the weight loss goals are not realistic, then work to make the goals become realistic is needed.

Table 4.1 Example components of a bariatric history

Reason for consultation
Weight history
   Onset: child, teen, adult, perimenopausal
   Rate: rapid vs. slow
   Inciting factors: stress, marriage, divorce, illness, medication
Weight loss history (what has worked and what has not worked)
   Previous dietary approaches, medicine use, weight loss surgery
Dietary history
   Patterns of eating, eating triggers, problem foods, favorite foods
Activity/exercise assessment
   Current physical activity level, favorite activity, barriers to physical activity
Past medical history
Past surgical history
Medications and supplements
Allergies (food and medication)
Menstrual/obstetric history
Psychiatric history
Family medical history
   Presence of obesity, type 2 diabetes, hypertension, coronary artery disease,
   hyperlipidemia, thyroid disease, psychiatric illness (dysthymia, depression, addictions)
Social history
   Family and work environments, support of spouse and family, tobacco and alcohol use,
   sleep cycles, major life stressors, readiness to change, major motivators for weight loss
Review of systems

Table 4.2 Example questions for initial visit

Questions assessing knowledge of the weight loss process

Sometimes patients do not lose weight on their scale, but continue to shrink in size. Their clothes become looser as the size of the body gets smaller. Will it bother you if this happens to you?

What is the difference between the loss of fat and the temporary loss or gain of water?

How would it affect you if water retention caused your weight to go up on the scales?

How many calories does your body burn per day with your present level of activity?

How many calories per day will you need to maintain your new slim weight when you reach it?

Eating less than we burn in a day produces a calorie deficit. How much of a daily deficit would it take to lose 1 pound of fat per week?

How much of a calorie deficit to lose 2 pounds per week?

If you burned an extra 200 cal per day through exercise, how many extra pounds a month would you lose in addition to those pounds lost through dieting?

How many calories are in a pound of fat?

Questions about understanding adherence

If you are not as successful as you think you should be, but are not quite following the diet program as you should, would you be willing to continue the program and follow the routine more closely?

(Continued)

Table 4.2 (*Continued*) Example questions for initial visit

If nobody helps you, supports you, compliments you, or otherwise encourages you to continue your weight loss program, what would you do?

What tactics will you use if you have to do the whole thing alone?

Questions assessing goals and expectations

What do you expect from us in assisting you in your efforts to lose weight?

What will happen to you when you lose all your unwanted fat? Will life be different, and if so, how?

Will a new figure help you or hinder you in any way?

Do you have any fears connected with losing weight? What are they?

Questions assessing social support

Will your husband/wife/partner help, hinder, or be neutral while you are losing weight?

Do you now notice, or have you ever detected, any resentment in your spouse about your getting slimmer? How did you determine this? Please give examples of his or her negative behavior, if present.

Will your new lower weight keep you from doing something, or feeling a certain way? Please explain.

How much jealousy do you expect to see in those close to you when you lose all your unwanted pounds? How do you plan to handle it? (Gaining weight back to stop their complaints is not the correct answer.)

Questions assessing self-image

If someone compliments you now, how do you handle the compliment?

Will your new lower weight have any effect on your sexuality? If so, how will it affect you at home, or away from home?

Do you have any fears or misgivings about being more attractive to people other than your spouse or friends? How might it possibly affect your spouse?

Will your new lower weight cause people to respect you more, or make it easier for you to be promoted or advanced at work? Please explain.

Will those around you respect you more when you slim down? Please explain your answer.

Will you be able to function better or worse in your home, work, or social life when you reach your goal weight? Please explain.

If you do not reach your goal, what will it mean to you, and what will you do?

How do you plan to maintain your lower weight, once it is reached?

Will it be harder or easier for you to keep your weight off once you have started a maintenance program? How?

Questions screening for sleep apnea

Do you snore on most nights (more than three times per week)?

Do you (or have you been told that you) stop breathing while sleeping?

Do you wake suddenly during the night?

Do you suddenly wake up gasping for air?

Do you wake up in the morning feeling tired?

Do you wake up in the morning with a headache?

Special questions regarding the weight loss history and what has and has not worked are important to include. As bariatric surgery has been used for decades, some of your patients may even have already had some sort of surgical procedure for weight loss. Many malabsorptive procedures require ongoing nutritional and vitamin supplementation. Some sort of assessment of daily physical activity and exercise is needed.

The past medical history will often reveal common conditions that accompany obesity, such as prediabetes (glucose intolerance), hypertension, type 2 diabetes, metabolic syndrome, insulin resistance, nonalcoholic fatty liver disease, hyperlipidemia, hypothyroidism, and obstructive sleep apnea. The review of systems may disclose lack of energy, some degree of shortness of breath, joint pains, or snoring or spouse complaint of snoring. Sometimes there is a "positive review of systems" due to the multisystem effects of obesity.

It is important to state clearly that any information given to the clinic will be kept confidential and not shared with other doctors or insurance companies unless the patient specifically gives permission. This is also a good time to ask the patient to be candid and honest, as you are trying to work together toward the same goal of weight loss.

THE PHYSICAL EXAMINATION

In most disciplines of medical practice, the physical examination, or *laying on of hands*, can make or break the doctor–patient relationship. You can usually establish immediate rapport by meeting the patient prior to the physical examination and greeting her in a friendly manner. Most physicians have the patient fill out a history form and discuss the positive and significant answers with the patient prior to the physical. In my experience, it is better to go over the discussion of the history first with the patient fully clothed, and then do the physical after the patient changes into a gown. A careful look at the history will help you decide how you approach certain examinations during the physical. Obtaining a comprehensive history and review of systems shows your genuine interest and makes it easier to spot and identify early problems that may impede progress.

Keep in mind that specific findings on the physical exam may be reflective of any medical problem, although the obese patient has a greater likelihood of having diabetes, vascular disease, skin problems, cancer, cataracts, and other medical comorbidities of obesity. You should have the patient change into a gown and examine all body areas, just as you would on any patient on whom you perform a comprehensive examination. Your thoroughness will be rewarded by identifying problems in advance. Some practitioners use their clinical judgment to abbreviate some parts of the examination as necessary.

Be sure that there is ample light in the room and that the patient is not too hot or too cold. Many heavy patients are extremely sensitive to cold. Be sure to have appropriately sized gowns, and chairs that accommodate your patients (bariatric chairs, sofa, or chairs without arms). A blanket (for security or warmth) that the patient can get without getting off the table will be greatly appreciated. Proper instruments are those found in any standard exam room, and should include an ophthalmoscope, an otoscope, a gooseneck sinus illuminator, tongue blades, a stethoscope with a nonchill head, cotton balls, a dull safety pin, a reflex hammer, and a floor lamp with an aimable light beam.

The table should be wide enough and sturdy enough for an obese person. Some physicians have a table that sits on 4′ × 4′ legs, is 42″ wide and 72″ long, with heavy padding, and can hold patients who weigh more than 600 pounds. This design will have to be custom-made for your office, but it costs less than the standard table. This type of table can also double as an extra pediatric exam table for those who see children too.

Pertinent negatives are as important as positive findings, and show that each part of the physical has been performed. Documenting each item properly avoids confusion and may prevent overlooking important and possibly treatable items.

Skin

The complete dermal examination includes inspection of the axillae, the groin, and between the toes. The intertriginous areas under the breast, under the abdominal panniculus if present, and in the groin and buttocks area should be checked. These areas are often the site of maceration, discoloration, and infection that could point out a diabetic condition in its early stages.

Acanthosis nigricans is a velvety black-to-light brown maculopapular lesion commonly found in the axillae, groin, or the side or back of the neck. Acanthosis nigricans is associated with insulin resistance or type 2 diabetes mellitus, so its presence warrants testing for these conditions.

The scalp and hair can provide a great deal of information about the nutritional status of the patient, and can alert you to the presence of psoriasis, seborrhea, and general dryness or oiliness of the skin. Hypothyroidism can lead to thinning of the lateral third of the eyebrows and general skin changes of dryness and scaliness. The area behind the neck and on the upper surface and posterior of the pinna may have had a lot of sun exposure and these are good places to look for possible malignancies. Lesions and nevi on the palms of the hands and the soles of the feet should be looked for carefully. Acne may be a reflection of polycystic ovary syndrome or hypercortisolism. Hyperpigmentation can also occur with hypercortisolism.

The vascular flush area of the cheeks and the bridge of the nose should be carefully checked. Other similar areas are on the neck, the upper chest, the genital areas, and the flexor surface of the extremities. You may see vascular disturbances here that could tell you about systemic diseases, such as systemic lupus erythematosus.

Lipomas can be the cause of mechanical problems, and sebaceous cysts can sometimes be sources of infection. The nails can give valuable clues to systemic disease and should be checked on both the hands and the feet.

Eyes

A complete exam should include assessment of visual acuity, visual fields, and ocular movements, a check of the external eye and the lids, and a funduscopic examination. Particular care should be taken to observe for cataracts, eyeground changes, and the state of the macula and optic nerve head in each eye. Check the intraocular pressure with a tonometer, or estimate the pressure through gentle tactile pressure. If you do not actually get a pressure yourself, make sure the patient gets one on his or her next visit to an ophthalmologist. Pupillary light reflexes should be tested, as well as accommodation changes in the pupils. Vertical nystagmus may reflect low magnesium levels.

Nose and sinuses

The external shape of the nose may give clues to previous trauma. The mucous membranes should be checked for congestion, visible mucous (noting color if present), and possible erosions. A gooseneck light attachment to your otoscope battery handle will allow you to look deep inside the mouth and direct your beam of light accurately. In a totally dark examining room, it can be used to illuminate the frontal and maxillary sinuses. Place the head of the light above the infraorbital rim to see the maxillary sinuses and under the medial aspect of the supraorbital rim to see the frontal sinus areas. The hard palate and the forehead are observed to see whether the sinuses illuminate.

Ears and throat

The tongue should be checked for abnormalities of texture and color, as well as swelling and enlarged lymph nodes. A small hypopharynx is a risk factor for sleep apnea. Erosion of dental enamel and swollen parotid glands should raise the possibility of bulimia.

Neck

The thyroid, larynx, and lymph node chains should be visually inspected and palpated carefully. Goiters, nodules, and other thyroid pathology must be distinguished from a sometimes quite prominent pretracheal fat pad. A neck circumference of ≥17 in. in men and ≥16 in. in women increases the likelihood of the presence of obstructive sleep apnea. A buffalo-hump fat pad suggests hypercortisolism.

Chest

A careful examination of the entire chest with inspection, palpation, percussion, and auscultation is carried out. Many overweight patients have early congestive heart failure and hypertension. Expect a decrease in vital capacity and tidal volume in extreme obesity. An increase in respiratory rate may be seen to maintain minute ventilation if the tidal volume is decreased.

Heart

Evidence of arteriosclerotic heart disease, hypertensive heart disease, and congestive heart failure would be of special interest in the examination. You should be as thorough in a cardiac examination of an obese person as any other type of patient, even if it may be difficult to move the patient around to do a complete examination, and is sometimes difficult to hear heart tones.

Back

Examine the entire back, from the occipital area down to the coccyx. There may be a lot of back pain in this type of patient, requiring palpation and light percussion over the vertebral area. Pilonidal sinuses and cysts should be looked for, as well as old surgical scars in this lower spine area. Lightly percuss over the costophrenic angles where the kidneys are located.

Breasts

A breast examination in a massively obese female should be carried out. Careful and systematic exam may detect any abnormalities that are present. If there is the slightest doubt about possible abnormalities, mammography and/or ultrasound studies should be considered. Mammography should be performed on all obese women with a significant family history of breast cancer.

Abdomen

The abdomen of an overweight patient may have a large panniculus that overhangs the belly and pubic areas. It may be difficult or impossible to palpate the liver and spleen, but this should be attempted. Check for ascitic fluid and hernias. Do the usual inspection, palpation, percussion, and auscultation that you do on other types of patient. The following gauge for the size of the pannus has been suggested: Grade 1, pannus covers the pubic hairline but not the entire mons pubis; Grade 2, pannus covers the entire mons pubis; Grade 3, pannus extends to cover the upper thigh; Grade 4, pannus extends to the mid-thigh; and Grade 5, pannus extends to the knee and beyond.

Anus and rectum

It can be difficult to do a careful rectal examination on a lot of overweight men and women, but I find two positions are the most comfortable for them. The first position has the patient lying on his or her left side, facing away from the examiner. The patient takes the right hand and reaches around, lifting up his or her right buttock as much as possible. The examining finger is then well lubricated, and the external and internal exam takes place. The second position places the male patient in the lithotomy position. The examination is carried out in the same way as a usual examination, except that you must palpate upward instead of downward to feel for the prostate.

Pelvic examination

The pelvic examination a necessary part of every obese female patient's physical, unless another competent practitioner is following this patient closely. The anterior abdominal fat is often quite thick and difficult to examine through. The size and texture of the uterine body and the adnexal structures can be obscured to a great degree by this heavy layer of fat. A complete examination should include the vulvar areas and rectovaginal palpation.

Extremities

Checking the color, turgor, and musculature of the arms and legs often gives clues to other medical problems. Look for evidence of edema, passive congestion of the lower legs, pallor, cyanosis, clubbing, varicosities, and lymphedema. Many obese patients have poorly healing ulcers and scars on the lower legs, with atrophic and unhealthy skin that is thin, shiny, and has a great deal of darker pigmentation. Dry, cracking heels may be a result of diabetes, hypothyroidism, or essential fatty acid deficiency.

Check for range of motion of all the joints from the digits to the hips and shoulders. Look for signs of arthritic swelling, particularly in the proximal and distal interphalangeal joints. A fair number of patients may have early or advanced Dupuytren's contracture. Tophi may indicate a history of gout. The pulses in all four extremities should be palpated.

Neurologic exam

A complete neurologic exam includes tests for light touch, pain, proprioception, and heat and cold senses. All cranial nerves can be checked. The olfactory senses can be checked with perfume. Deep tendon reflexes are checked on all four extremities. Many doctors use the tips of their two fingers or the edge of the hand to elicit reflexes. The hand is less threatening to a patient than a hammer, and it is one less item to have to carry around to the hospital or keep in the examination room. The possibility of neuropathy from problems peculiar to obesity (e.g., diabetes) makes a thorough job important. Particularly look for decreased sensitivity and signs of neuropathy in the lower extremities. Abnormal reflexes exhibiting a decreased relaxation time may suggest hypothyroidism or undertreatment with thyroid replacement. Hyperactive reflexes may indicate hypomagnesemia.

Mental status

Observation of the mental status of the patient are valuable in the physical and evaluation process. Orientation as to time, place, and purpose of the visit can be easily obtained. Overly friendly or hostile patients may be manifesting an underlying anxiety and acting out in their usual way. Any possible resentment of authority is noted and possibly discussed on the follow-up visit as an addressable problem that could slow down the weight loss. Dementia or delirium should raise the possibility of nutritional deficiencies, especially in the case of an individual who has had a prior surgical malabsorptive procedure.

Most of the mental status evaluation is obtained from the questions answered (or not answered) on the history. Careful and patient questioning on the part of the therapist can yield a good rapport that permits coverage of some potentially serious problems in the patient's lifestyle, family, work situation, or other areas of her environment.

MEASUREMENTS

Special considerations concerning the evaluation of an obese patient are discussed in this section. They include proper blood pressure measurement techniques, estimation of the extent of the obesity problem in each patient, an electrocardiogram (ECG), and laboratory work to tailor treatment.

Blood pressure

It is important to use an appropriately sized blood pressure cuff. If the cuff is too small, the blood pressure values may be artificially elevated. The bladder length should wrap around more than two-thirds of the middle of the upper arm and the width should exceed the diameter of this point by 20%. An arm that is obviously above normal in size and circumference should be fitted with an adult thigh cuff to minimize distortions in measurement of the blood pressure.

Waist circumference

The waist circumference and waist-to-hip ratio (WHR) are easily obtained and usually reproducible. The waist is measured at the level of the umbilicus, without pulling the tape too tight. The hips are measured at the widest point. Divide the waist measurement by the hip measurement to get the WHR. A waist circumference greater than 40 in. in men or 35 in. in women or a WHR greater than 1.0 for men or 0.8 for women is a sign of central obesity (android type or apple shaped) and indicates a higher likelihood of insulin resistance, metabolic syndrome, and other comorbidities. A WHR less than those figures indicates the gynecoid type of obesity (pear shaped), which is less likely to be associated with the comorbidities.

The therapist who is just starting out might want to measure the patient using several methods before deciding which method or combination of methods to use. Remember to take a good look at the patients when they are disrobed. Note the relative presence or lack of muscle mass and degree of fatness visible. The WHR will give an indication if the body shape has central obesity (android, apple shaped) or lower body obesity (gynecoid, pear shaped).

SEVERITY OF OVERWEIGHT OR OBESITY

Obesity is defined as an excess of total body fat—not just excess weight. For example, there are differences between a sedentary accountant who weighs 235 pounds and a football player who weighs the same, even if their height is the same. Obviously, the less active accountant may have a greater percentage of the body composed of fat versus the football player, who would have a much heavier mass of muscle tissue.

The most widely used measurement of degree of fatness in the body is the BMI. A BMI of ≤24 is considered normal, 24–27 shows a modest degree of obesity, 27–30 is borderline significant obesity, and >30 is medically significant obesity. To calculate BMI, the weight in pounds is converted into kilograms (pounds × 0.454) and the height in inches is changed into meters (inches × 0.0254). BMI is then calculated by dividing the weight in kilograms by the square of the height in meters. BMI also can be calculated by the following formula: BMI = 703 (weight in pounds)/(height in inches) × (height in inches). Although imperfect, the BMI does correlate well with body fat, morbidity, and mortality.

An estimate of body composition (fat mass and fat-free mass) can be obtained using bioelectrical impedance (BIA). For this determination, a machine is used to introduce an imperceptible electrical current through the body and measure its conduction. The total body mass is divided into two compartments: nonconductive (fat mass) and conductive (fat-free mass: water, muscle, other tissues). Based on the amount of electrical impedance, the relative size of the different compartments can be determined. The advantages of BIA are that it is safe, rapid, easy to use, and inexpensive. Disadvantages are that it is affected by hydration status, fasting, and recent exercise, and there are some difficulties applying its use to athletes, children, and the elderly. Using percent body fat, obesity is defined as >25% body fat for men and >30% body fat for women.

A simple, though not always accurate, rule to estimate "normal" weight is this: women should weigh 100 pounds at 5 feet tall and an additional 5 pounds for each additional inch of height. For men, it is 106 pounds at 5 feet tall and an additional 6 pounds for each additional inch above. In both sexes, you can vary by 10%. If the frame size is small, you can subtract up to 10%, and if the frame size is larger, you add an additional 10%.

Skinfold thickness measurement is used at many centers, but it presents challenges to accuracy and reproducibility. A good caliper, such as the Lange caliper, is the most accurate. This type of precision caliper exerts the same amount of pressure at any point on its scale, thereby eliminating major errors in measuring skinfold thickness.

ELECTROCARDIOGRAM

After years of reading ECGs from obese patients, what is remarkable to me is the relative lack of electrical pathology seen, even on massively obese patients. The most common abnormality I observe is incomplete right bundle branch block. There are a typical number of asymptomatic premature ventricular contractions, nonspecific ST segment changes, and U waves (usually associated with injudicious use of diuretics), both with and without significant T wave flattening or inversion. It is rare to see any great amount of distinguishable left ventricular hypertrophy on the tracing, even with radiographic evidence of the condition. Prolonged QT interval is sometimes seen, often as a sign of electrolyte imbalance, such as hypokalemia, hypomagnesemia, or hypocalcemia.

It is best to carefully do all 12 leads, plus any extra leads that are thought necessary. Care should be taken in placing the electrodes on the chest, particularly in light of the mechanical difficulties when the breasts are extremely large and overlay or obscure the points where the precordial leads are placed.

The exam table, such as that recommended earlier, should be wide enough to hold the largest patient you might see. It is unprofessional for a doctor or technician to attempt to do an ECG if the patient's arms, legs, buttocks, back, and shoulders are hanging off both sides of the table. This instability produces a nightmare of artifacts and prevents an accurate and usable tracing in many cases. Where suction cups are not used to make contact on the limb leads, it might be good to have long enough bands, or large enough clamps, to fit around the wrists and ankles of the patient.

Common indications for an ECG include coronary risk factors, diabetes mellitus, hypertension, coronary artery disease, family history of cardiovascular disease, diuretic use, and consideration of anorectic medication use. Additional cardiovascular evaluations and risk estimates may be required, depending on the degree of obesity of the patient and other factors.

LABORATORY EVALUATION

Laboratory tests are performed to identify metabolic problems and to tailor therapy. A fasting period of at least 10 hours prior to the drawing of the initial blood work is needed for accuracy in lipid measurements. A usual profile consists of a complete blood count, thyroid profile, and a chemical profile that includes triglycerides, cholesterol, high-density lipoprotein, and several other tests. Clean-voided, midstream urine is obtained when fasting blood is drawn. If a fasting glucose of ≥100 is detected, you may want to subsequently obtain an oral glucose tolerance test of at least 2-hour duration, with determinations at 30, 60, 90, and 120 minutes after ingestion of the test meal. Fasting insulin levels should be obtained if insulin resistance is suspected. The results of every test performed should be discussed with the patient, even if all the tests are within the normal range.

PROBLEM-ORIENTED SUMMARY

All the history, physical, laboratory, and other data (Table 4.3) obtained are put into a problem list, and a differential diagnosis is created. For example, is there a possibility of a hormonal cause of obesity that requires further testing? This type of problem-oriented medical record is assembled and should be updated on each visit. Medication of a chronic or acute nature is documented on a separate sheet inside the front cover of the medical chart. In our office, the medications are written in red ink for more rapid spotting. When a medication is discontinued or changed, a note is made to that effect (e.g., insulin discontinued and metformin 500 mg daily begun on 10-01-09). The problem-oriented summary becomes the foundation for a more thorough follow-up system for this patient. The time taken to systematically set up such a system pays dividends later in more efficient management of the patient. Although the details of the workup will vary from patient to patient, the completeness of your evaluation marks you as a caring and competent physician and helps you build valuable rapport with your patient.

Table 4.3 Example components of a bariatric physical and laboratory examination

Vital signs: height (first visit), weight, BMI, blood pressure, pulse, respiration

Measurements: waist circumference, hip circumference, waist-to-hip ratio, neck circumference

General appearance: (consider frontal and side photographs) apple shaped or pear shaped

HEENT: facial plethora, large neck, size of hypopharynx, teeth and gums for mastication

Heart: distant heart sounds, S3 gallop

Lungs: hypoventilation, wheezing

Abdomen: incisional scars from appendectomy, cholecystectomy

Skin: acanthosis nigricans, psoriasis, eczema, acne

Extremities: edema, varicosities, ecchymoses

Neurologic: muscle weakness, hyperreflexia (hypomagnesemia), hyporeflexia (hypothyroidism)

Optional: breast exam, genitorectal exam

Blood tests: complete blood count, chemistries, kidney function, liver function, fasting glucose, fasting lipid profile for cardiometabolic risk

ECG: QT interval

Body composition: bioimpedance, infrared conductance, skinfold thickness

REFERENCES

1. Vallis M, Piccinini-Vallis H, Sharma AM, et al. Clinical review: Modified 5 As: Minimal intervention for obesity counseling in primary care. *Can Fam Physician* 2013; 59: 27–31.
2. Alexander SC, Cox ME, Boling Turer CL, et al. Do the five A's work when physicians counsel about weight loss? *Fam Med* 2011; 43: 179–184.

BIBLIOGRAPHY

Bickley LS. ed. *Bates' Guide to Physical Examination and History Taking.* 10th ed. New York: Lippincott Williams & Wilkins; 2008.

Dubin D. *Rapid Interpretation of EKG's.* 6th ed. Tampa, FL: Cover Publishing; 2000.

Orient JM. *Sapira's Art and Science of Bedside Diagnosis.* New York: Lippincott Williams & Wilkins; 2009.

Ross EJ, Linch DC. Cushing's syndrome—Killing disease: Discriminatory value of signs and symptoms aiding early diagnosis. *Lancet* 1982; 2: 646–649.

Simel DL, Rennie D. *The Rational Clinical Examination: Evidence-Based Clinical Diagnosis.* New York: McGraw-Hill; 2009.

5

Dietary treatment of overweight and obesity

ERIC C. WESTMAN, MARY C. VERNON, AND JAMES A. WORTMAN

INTRODUCTION

Overweight and obesity are high-priority areas for primary care practitioners because they are associated with many medical consequences, such as diabetes mellitus and hypertension. Unfortunately, obesity can also be frustrating for the practitioner for lack of training in effective therapies. We started using low-carbohydrate diets for the treatment of obesity and found that they could be just as effective as medication therapy (1). Over the past 10 years, numerous randomized, controlled trials have shown that low-carbohydrate diets lead to weight loss and cardiometabolic risk factor improvements (2–5).

The underlying principle of dietary treatment of overweight and obesity is to create a negative energy balance by reducing energy intake. Reducing energy intake can be achieved by explicitly controlling energy intake (calorie restriction), or by controlling carbohydrate intake (carbohydrate restriction). Carbohydrate restriction works by reducing the appetite, probably as a consequence of nutritional ketosis (6–8). Nutritional ketosis occurs when carbohydrate consumption is less than approximately 50 g per day, and the body uses fatty acids and ketone bodies as its major metabolic fuels (9,10). When carbohydrate consumption is high, fatty acids and glucose are the major metabolic fuels. This metabolic change from using glucose to using ketones has to occur to some extent for any method of adipose tissue loss to be effective, because lipolysis leads to an increase in ketone body production. One of the major hormonal changes that occurs is a reduction in serum insulin levels to approximately basal levels. The alteration of the insulin/glucagon ratio leads to a reduction in glycolytic/lipogenic activity and an enhancement of fatty acid/ketone use. Herein, we describe several methods that take advantage of nutritional ketosis and discuss how to implement this type of diet in a medical outpatient practice.

WHAT IS HEALTHY NUTRITION DURING WEIGHT LOSS?

Before a discussion of optimal diets for weight loss, a discussion of what nutrient inputs are needed for the body's proper structure and function is appropriate. A balanced diet is one that meets all of the minimal requirements for essential nutrients, including amino acids, fatty acids, vitamins, minerals, and vitamin-like substances (Table 5.1) (11). Although minimal requirements are set by governmental advisors for the general population to prevent nutritional deficiencies, the nutritional requirements during weight loss are different from the nutritional needs of the otherwise healthy individual. An optimal diet during weight loss provides all of the nutrients in a way that maintains optimal health, which may include

Table 5.1 Essential human nutrients

- Vitamins: A, B1 (thiamine), B2 (riboflavin), B3 (niacin), B5 (pantothenic acid), B6 (pyridoxine), B7 (biotin), B9 (folic acid), B12 (cyanocobalamin), C (ascorbic acid), D, E, K
- Minerals: calcium, phosphorus, magnesium, iron
- Trace minerals: zinc, copper, manganese, iodine, selenium, molybdenum, chromium
- Electrolytes: sodium, potassium, chloride
- Amino acids: histidine, isoleucine, leucine, lysine, methionine, phenylalanine, threonine, tryptophan, valine
- Essential fatty acids: linoleic, α-linolenic

Source: Adapted from Makki K, et al. *ISRN Inflamm* 2013; 2013: 139239.

changes in body composition, during the adipose tissue loss process. Because carbohydrates are simply a source of energy, if energy needs are otherwise met, there is no dietary need for carbohydrate intake. Because dietary protein is used for structure (muscle, bone connective tissue) and provides more than just an energy source, this macronutrient is indispensable. Likewise, essential fatty acids are required for optimal health. It is very important to keep in mind that there may be differences in requirements based upon individual variation.

Water

Water has so many uses in the body and is so essential for human life that it must be consumed daily for optimal function. A few of the important functions that water performs are dissolving nutrients to make them accessible to cells, assisting in moving nutrients through cells, keeping mucous membranes moist, lubricating joints, evaporating for body temperature regulation, and removing waste from the body. For most people, the daily water losses are about 6 cups (1.5 L) of urine, 2 cups (0.5 L) of sweat, and 1 cup (0.25 L) from breathing. In sum, about 9 cups (2.25 L) is required for most people each day, but the body has many regulatory systems to allow for a wide variation in water intake. Interestingly, about 20% of the water is obtained from the water in food and metabolic processes. For practical purposes, the general recommendation to "drink when you are thirsty" will suffice during the weight loss process.

Protein

Protein is the major structural component of the human body. Dietary protein is the source of amino acids to provide the building blocks to make proteins, and when used for energy, burned in a bomb calorimeter, contains 4 kcal/g. Protein is required in the human diet because there are nine essential amino acids that the body cannot manufacture by itself ("essential" means that the body is unable to synthesize the nutrient). Although maintenance dietary protein needs are estimated to be from 0.7 to 1.0 mg/kg/day, 1.2 to 1.5 g/kg lean body weight of dietary protein is needed for preservation of lean body mass and physical performance during weight loss (12). Picking the value of 1.5 g/kg/day, for adults with reference weights ranging from 60 to 80 kg, this translates into total daily protein intakes between 90 and 120 g/day. When expressed in the context of total daily energy expenditures of 2000 to 3000 kcal/day, about 15% of an individual's daily energy expenditure (or intake if the diet is eucaloric) needs to be provided as protein. During weight loss, especially if strenuous exercise is a component of the process, more dietary protein may be advantageous.

Fat

Fat is a major component of cell structure and hormones, and it is the body's primary source of energy, containing 9 kcal/g when burned in a bomb calorimeter. Fat is required in the human diet because there are two essential fatty acids. A tolerable upper limit intake level is not set for total fat because there is no known level of fat at which an adverse effect occurs. Dietary fat may enhance fatty acid oxidation; thus, high-fat diets may be desirable to achieve the goal of dietary treatment of the obese individual. The optimal type of fat to eat during weight loss is not known, although recent evidence indicates that in the absence of carbohydrate intake ($\leq$20 g/24 hours) high-fat diets lead to lower levels of bloodstream saturates than in those eating a low-fat diet (13,14).

Carbohydrate

Carbohydrates are a source of energy containing 4 kcal/g when burned in a bomb calorimeter. Some single carbohydrates (monosaccharides) are used in physiological compounds such as glycoproteins and mucopolysaccharides. Although some dietary carbohydrates contain vitamins and minerals, there is no requirement for carbohydrate in the human diet because metabolic pathways exist within the body to produce carbohydrate from dietary protein and fat. Dietary and endogenously created carbohydrate is stored as glycogen or converted to and stored as fat.

Source of energy

To achieve lipolysis and increased fat oxidation in the dietary treatment of the obese individual, an important goal is to maximize fat as the major fuel source—fat from the diet and from adipose tissue stores. Carbohydrate then becomes a fuel source of much less importance because ketones can substitute for glucose in most tissues. Because carbohydrate used as a fuel is linked with lipogenesis, lipolysis and fat mobilization are reduced when carbohydrate is a dominant fuel source. For optimal lipolysis and adipose tissue mobilization, keeping carbohydrate as an energy source to a minimum is preferable.

Vitamins and minerals

Essential dietary vitamins and minerals are required in small amounts and occur naturally in a variety of foods. Functions of vitamins include hormonal signaling, mediators of cell signaling, regulators of cell and tissue growth and differentiation, precursors for enzymes, catalysts and coenyzmes, antioxidant activity, and substrates in metabolism. Vitamins and minerals are now available in inexpensive pill and liquid form. A multivitamin is recommended during weight loss.

NUTRITIONAL KETOSIS AS DIET THERAPY FOR OBESITY

The rationale of the dietary treatment of the obese individual is to alter the hormonal milieu to direct the body's metabolism away from fat storage (lipogenesis) and toward fat mobilization and oxidation. Using carbohydrate as the body's main fuel is metabolically linked to lipogenesis (Figure 5.1). Nutritional ketosis is useful for treating obesity and many similar conditions (Table 5.2). Body systems can be directed toward fat oxidation in many ways, for example, through carbohydrate restriction or caloric restriction since caloric restriction is usually achieved at least, in part, by carbohydrate restriction. Nutritional ketosis is a metabolic state in which fat and ketones are the major fuel sources to generate ATP while glycolysis is minimized (Figure 5.2). Although often misconstrued as harmful or unhealthy, nutritional ketosis is not known to cause any short- or long-term adverse consequences. In fact, many indigenous populations living on very-low–carbohydrate diets were likely in chronic nutritional ketosis. Nutritional ketosis causes a relatively low level of serum ketone elevation and is not associated with a reduction in pH or significant metabolic acidosis (15). Frequently, nutritional ketosis is confused with diabetic ketoacidosis—the metabolic state during which the absence of insulin leads to very high levels of ketones along with elevated blood glucose, dehydration, and a low blood pH.

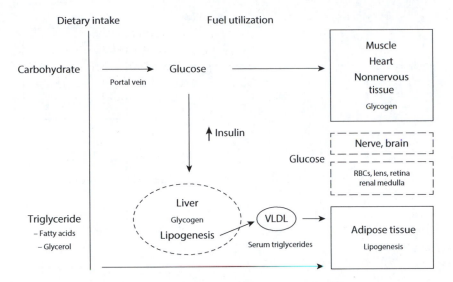

Figure 5.1 Glycolysis is linked to lipogenesis absorptive (postprandial) state. Boxes with solid line borders indicate glucose uptake is insulin dependent.

Table 5.2 Indications for medical nutritional program

- Overweight or obesity (body mass index >27 kg/m²)
- Type 2 diabetes mellitus
- Metabolic syndrome
- Hyperlipidemia
- Polycystic ovarian syndrome
- Nonalcoholic fatty liver disease
- Gluten hypersensitivity (celiac disease)
- Seizure disorder refractory to medication
- Obesity-related consequences: sleep apnea, hyperinsulinemia, hypertension, asthma, gastroesophageal reflux disorder, irritable bowel syndrome

   When an individual is adapted to nutritional ketosis, fatty acids and ketones become the major energy sources. Fatty acids are an excellent fuel source and can be used for energy by most tissues, including cardiac and skeletal muscle. Ketone bodies (β-hydroxybutyrate and acetoacetate) contain 4 kcal/g (when burned in a bomb calorimeter) and can be used by all cells, except those that do not have mitochondrial fat oxidation enzymes (erythrocytes, cornea, lens, retina, distal axons) or sufficient oxygen to support oxidative metabolism (renal medulla). During nutritional ketosis, it is estimated that the daily glucose need can be as low as 30 g per day because fatty acids and ketones are available for muscle and central nervous system use (6). Glucose becomes less important as a fuel source, with ketones substituting for glucose in most tissues that would otherwise use glucose. Glucose is manufactured through gluconeogenesis in both the liver and kidneys. Although the liver is the major gluconeogenic organ, capable of producing up to approximately 240 g of glucose per day when insulin levels are low, the kidneys may produce up to 20% of daily glucose needs (16). Precursors for gluconeogenesis come mainly from amino acids in the diet.

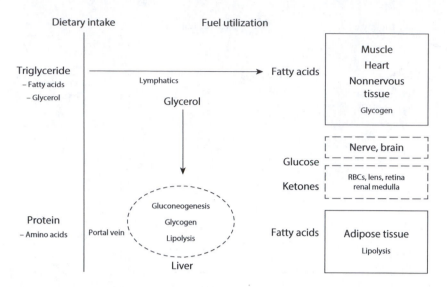

Figure 5.2 Fat oxidation is linked to lipolysis. Boxes with solid line borders indicate glucose uptake is insulin dependent.

As ketosis is desirable during weight loss, some individuals use urinary acetoacetate, blood β-hydroxybutyrate, and breath acetone monitoring to verify dietary adherence and the presence of the lipolytic state, colloquially known as "being in ketosis." However, there can be significant person-to-person variability in urinary ketone response even when subjects eat uniform diets. Diabetes can also reduce the likelihood of urinary acetoacetate. Most studies of the low-carbohydrate ketogenic diet (LCKD) have observed that the level of ketosis (urine and blood levels) decreases with time. It is unclear whether this effect is a result of increased efficiency at using ketone bodies for energy or a decrease in the production of ketone bodies over time (presumably from adding carbohydrates back into the diet). However, this effect was also observed in one inpatient study that closely controlled carbohydrate intake at 21 g over 2 weeks and measured urine ketones daily.

Nutritional ketosis enhances adipose tissue loss in several ways. First, a reduction in insulin facilitates lipolysis at the adipose tissue via hormone-sensitive lipase. Reduced insulin also leads to inhibition of metabolic pathways of lipogenesis (fat production) in many sites throughout the body (17–19). A diet that causes nutritional ketosis can also be regarded as a diet that lowers serum insulin.

Nutritional ketosis and sodium regulation

During nutritional ketosis, the conventional advice to limit sodium in the diet does not apply. It is actually important to provide 2 to 3 g of dietary sodium during nutritional ketosis, for patients who do not have salt-sensitive conditions. The reason for an increased intake of dietary sodium is that the prior higher levels of serum insulin promote sodium and water retention and, after dietary changes that decrease serum insulin, there is an increase in renal sodium excretion (20,21). This is one of the factors leading to the diuresis that occurs during the first few weeks of nutritional ketosis. Urinary ketone bodies can also act as an osmotic diuretic, and glycogen loss leads to water loss because water is stored with glycogen to keep the glycogen in aqueous form (3 g of water is stored with every 1 g of glycogen). Presumably, when the glycogen is used, the water is released, and if insulin is low, this water also becomes part of the initial diuresis.

Nutritional ketosis has many similarities to the metabolic state of zero nutritional intake (starvation) (9). The main similarities are that with zero or greatly reduced intake of exogenous carbohydrate, there is a shift from the use of fatty acids and glucose as fuel toward the use of fatty acids and ketones. During starvation, however, endogenous sources of protein are used for energy, resulting in significant loss of muscle mass. Conversely, under conditions of nutritional ketosis, if sufficient exogenous protein is eaten a very-low–carbohydrate diet can preserve lean body mass even during loss of adipose mass (17). Unlike starvation, glucose levels are sustained despite the lack of carbohydrate intake under low-carbohydrate conditions. So, the important differences between starvation and nutritional ketosis are that during nutritional ketosis, serum glucose levels are maintained and breakdown of endogenous protein (muscle mass) is minimized.

METHODS FOR ATTAINING NUTRITIONAL KETOSIS

Prior to any medical nutritional program, a complete history, physical, and laboratory evaluation are recommended (Table 5.3).

Carbohydrate restriction

Dietary carbohydrate is the primary insulin secretagogue. Because pancreatic insulin secretion is stimulated by the glucose/amino acid ratio in the portal vein and in response to an increase

Table 5.3 Medical evaluation prior to a medical nutritional program

- Complete medical history
- Physical examination (including waist measurement, blood pressure, pulse, and body composition measurement if available)
- Complete blood count, serum chemistries, fasting serum lipid profile, or lipid subfraction test
- Serum thyroid function tests (triiodothyronine, thyroxine, thyroid-stimulating hormone)
- Electrocardiogram if heart disease present or high risk for heart disease
- Glycosylated hemoglobin, high-sensitivity C-reactive protein, c-peptide
- Vitamin D
- Hormonal evaluation tailored to patient, including sex steroid status: testosterone, estrogen, progesterone; luteinizing hormone/follicle-stimulating hormone (consider if a.m. cortisol or dehydroepiandrosterone sulfate needed).
- Pelvic sonogram or hepatic sonogram to evaluate polycystic ovarian syndrome or nonalcoholic steatohepatitis, cholelithiasis
- 24-hour urine for creatinine clearance and quantitative urinary albumin or other measure such as creatinine/albumin
- 3- to 5-hour glucose tolerance test with insulin levels at each blood draw
  - No need for a glucose tolerance test in known diabetics
  - c-Peptide may indicate hyperinsulinemia and the presence of endogenous insulin production

in blood glucose, a powerful way to lower insulin levels is to reduce dietary carbohydrate. When the dietary intake of carbohydrate is reduced to less than 50 g per day, most individuals excrete ketones in the urine, leading to the descriptive name of ketogenic diet. Several popular diets have used the recommendation of very low levels of carbohydrate (<20 g per day) in the early stages of the diet to enhance lipolysis. The presence of urinary acetoacetate or increase in blood β-hydroxybutyrate or breath acetone may be indicators of an increase in fat oxidation. Several research groups have referred to this approach as a very-low–carbohydrate ketogenic diet (VLCKD), or LCKD (9). When dietary carbohydrate is low (20 g per day), insulin secretion remains low—close to basal levels—and fat burning (lipolysis) and protein burning (gluconeo-genesis) occur as glucagon levels rise. A low-carbohydrate diet is one that contains 50 to 150 g per day and is not typically associated with nutritional ketosis. When dietary carbohydrate is present in sufficient amounts for stimulating insulin secretion, fat storage will occur. This storage may even be true in situations where total energy intake is limited, resulting in fat storage and lean tissue breakdown. The dietary carbohydrate signals fat deposition, while the need for gluconeo-genesis in energy-limited diets results in lean tissue use. In general, the low-carbohydrate diet will raise high-density lipoprotein (HDL) cholesterol; lower triglycerides; and have little effect on low-density lipoprotein (LDL) cholesterol. The average weight loss over 6 to 12 months in clinical trials ranged from 5.1 to 12.2 kg, although in private clinical settings larger amounts of weight loss have been reported. Examples of popular carbohydrate-restricted programs include the Atkins Diet, the South Beach Diet, and the Protein Power Plan.

Calorie restriction

In calorie-restricted diets, calories are explicitly limited and instruction is given to either count calories or to follow a diet protocol that is low in calories. Calorie- and fat-reduced diets and balanced deficit diets generally do not achieve nutritional ketosis because they contain sufficient carbohydrate to prevent ketogenesis. Whereas calorie-restricted diets will lead to weight loss, they do not lead to the same pattern of cardiometabolic risk reduction or lean tissue sparing as low-carbohydrate diets. In general, the 30% fat calorie-restricted diet will lower LDL cholesterol, modestly impact triglycerides, and modestly raise HDL cholesterol. The average weight loss in clinical trials over 6 to 12 months ranged from 1.5 to 6.4 kg. Examples of popular calorie-restricted diet programs include Weight Watchers, Jenny Craig, and Nutrisystem.

Combination of calorie restriction and carbohydrate restriction (VLCD)

A very-low-calorie diet (VLCD), also referred to as supplemented fasting, is a diet that pro-vide between 300 and 800 kcal per day. VLCDs provide enough protein to meaningfully reduce lean tissue wasting and supply essential minerals and vitamins along with varying amounts of carbohydrates and fats. There are two general classes of VLCD: one class con-sists of common foods with dietary supplements of minerals and vitamins and the other class consists of a defined formula providing all nutrients as beverages, soups, and bars, or a combination, taken three to five times per day. The food-based VLCD consists mostly of lean meat, fish, and poultry, whereas the formula VLCD usually requires the addition of carbo-hydrate as sugar or modified starch to enhance palatability. The food-based VLCD provides a modest dose of fat inherent in the food choices, whereas fat is not always provided in the defined formula diets.

Upon initiation of a VLCD, through the natriuresis of fasting (insulin reduction) and the mobilization of liver and muscle glycogen, with its associated intracellular water release, up to 10 lb of total weight loss in the first week is possible. Along with the water loss, the adipose tissue loss may total 2 to 3 lb, plus 1 or 2 lb of lean body mass as the body adapts to nutritional ketosis. By the end of the second week of a VLCD, the patient's fluid and electrolyte status stabilizes and, given adequate protein and minerals, the loss of lean body mass is minimized. Then, the average weekly weight loss ranges from 1.5 lb per week for the shorter person with little activity to 3 lb per week for a taller and more active person. The total weight loss achievable with a VLCD varies greatly depending on many factors, such as initial weight, the degree of support provided to the patient, and the duration of diet use. The average weight loss in clinical trials over a 50-week period ranged from 6.2 to 19.9 kg (22).

Side effects

After instruction in a medical nutritional program, follow-up monitoring is recommended (Table 5.4). There are two groups of side effects based on whether they occur early or late in the process, and monitoring is recommended (Table 5.5). VLCDs (400–800 kcal per day) probably have a higher incidence of side effects than carbohydrate restriction using food (1200–1500 kcal per day) due to the lower caloric intake. During adaptation to carbohydrate restriction and nutritional ketosis, the most common side effects are weakness, fatigue, and lightheadedness. Although there is a modest reduction in peak aerobic performance in the first week or two of a VLCD, orthostatic symptoms occurring during normal daily activities are the result of the combination of diet-induced natriuresis and an inadequate sodium intake. These symptoms can be prevented by the addition of 2 to 3 g per day of sodium (taken as bouillon or broth for example) in all patients not requiring continued diuretic medication, along with attention to adequate dietary potassium.

After the first few weeks of adaptation to carbohydrate restriction, the most common side effects are constipation and muscle cramps. The constipation may result, in part, from the lower fiber content of dietary intake, but it is also exacerbated by dehydration. If increasing fluid intake to a minimum of 2 L per day does not resolve the constipation, then 1 teaspoon of milk of magnesia at bedtime, bouillon supplementation, or a carbohydrate-free fiber supplement can be used. Muscle cramps can occur either early or late in treatment, and they are more common in people with a history of diuretic medication use or prior heavy ethanol consumption.

Table 5.4 Follow-up medical evaluation

- Focused history (symptoms, hunger level) and physical exam (heart, lungs, waist, peripheral edema)
- Vital signs (blood pressure, pulse)
- Serum chemistry panel (electrolytes, renal function, liver function)
- Fasting serum lipid profile
- Serum thyroid function tests (triiodothyronine, thyroxine, thyroid-stimulating hormone)
- Glycosylated hemoglobin, c-peptide, high-sensitivity C-reactive protein, fasting and random serum glucose
- If muscle cramps, then check serum K^+, Mg^+, and supplement with magnesium
- Repeat of any previously abnormal values

Table 5.5 Medication management

Insulin
- Calculate the total number of units used per day.
- If the total daily dose of insulin is <20 units, stop the insulin on the morning (or night before if long acting) that the diet is started.
- Reduce the number of units of insulin by 50% on the first day of the diet. When the blood glucoses go below 150 mg/dL, decrease the total daily amount of insulin by one-third to one-half. Repeat until the insulin dose is below 10 units and then discontinue insulin.
- Instruct the patient to not take insulin if the blood glucose is <100 mg/dL.
- Instruct the patient to call if the blood glucose is >250 mg/dL, or if the blood glucose is <100 mg/dL.

Oral and injectable hypoglycemic medications
- Stop all oral or injectable hypoglycemic medication except metformin the day the diet is started.
- Continue metformin until the fasting blood glucose is <100 mg/dL.
- Instruct the patient to call if the blood glucose is >250 mg/dL (16 mmol/L), to see if any additional intervention is required.

Diuretics
- If the patient is normoglycemic, it is ok to stop the diuretic as soon as the patient has urinary ketones (usually sometime within the first week).
- If the patient has elevated blood glucoses, observe blood pressure. If blood pressure begins to drop, consider tapering diuretic first. If patient has edema, taper as tolerated by blood pressure and edema, allowing a few days for equilibration of edema.
- Once the patient is off the diuretic and free of edema, begin two bouillon servings daily to treat orthostatic symptoms, fatigue, and headache.

Other antihypertensives
- When the patient is no longer taking the diuretic, begin to taper the beta blocker as tolerated as long as normal blood pressure is maintained.
- When the patient is off the diuretic and beta blocker, consider tapering the angiotensin II receptor blocker or angiotensin-converting enzyme if blood pressure is low, the patient has evidence or symptoms of orthostatic hypotension, the blood glucose is normal, and proteinuria is absent.

In almost all cases, the muscle cramps respond promptly to supplementation with 1 teaspoon of milk of magnesia at bedtime or 200 mEq per day of slow-release magnesium chloride, suggesting prior depletion of this essential mineral as the root cause.

In patients with a history of gout, an attack of this acute arthritis can be induced during the adaptation period. The mechanism for this effect of ketogenic diets is the competition between β-hydroxybutyrate and uric acid for excretion in the renal tubule. This process induces a transient rise in serum uric acid in the first few weeks of a VLCD, during which time those patients prone to gout are at risk of an attack. With the subsequent adaptation to nutritional ketosis, however, the renal handling of uric acid returns to normal and the risk of an acute attack subsides. This can be managed by prophylaxis with allopurinol in selected patients with a history of gout, or by treatment of the acute event with a nonsteroidal anti-inflammatory drug (NSAID) or colchicine. Chronic nutritional ketosis may actually prevent gout because metabolic syndrome is one of the predisposing factors for gout, and nutritional ketosis improves all of the components of metabolic syndrome.

During the weight loss process, mobilization of adipose cell cholesterol results in increases in both serum cholesterol and increased biliary excretion of cholesterol (23). Cholestasis is best prevented by >20 g of fat per day in the nutritional intake. Given the typical individual net oxidation of 150 to 200 g per day of body fat, this modest dietary fat intake does not significantly impact the rate of weight loss. In addition, patients deemed high risk because of prior history of or existing gallstones can be treated prophylactically with ursodeoxycholic acid. Later onset side effects can include dry skin, hair loss, and loss of normal menstrual cycles in women, or resumption of normal menstrual cycles in amenorrheic women. Hair loss is telogen effluvium and is treated symptomatically or by reassurance of its self-limited nature. Some practitioners have reported that fatty acid (omega 3) supplementation decreases the telogen effluvium.

Excessive weight loss

After the first week, weight loss exceeding an average of 1.5 kg per week is a medical concern and warrants evaluation of potential inappropriate diuretic use or nonadherence to the prescribed diet. Patients need to understand that speeding weight loss by not consuming the prescribed nutrients sacrifices lean body mass and function, possibly increasing the risk of fluid and electrolyte imbalance and lean tissue loss.

FLUIDS AND ELECTROLYTES

The water loss associated with nutritional ketosis has been called the natriuresis of fasting and was for many years only thought to be a result of the osmotic effects of ketones in the distal tubule. Another likely mechanism for an increase in sodium excretion is the increase in the phospholipid arachidonic acid (ARA). Because ARA is the precursor of prostaglandin E2 (PGE2), an increase in ARA leads to an increase in PGE2. An increase in PGE2 causes an excretion of sodium, leading to water loss. If uncompensated sodium loss occurs, sodium depletion elicits aldosterone secretion, which then increases potassium excretion. This process may lead to hypokalemia and its attendant risks of muscle wasting and cardiac arrhythmias.

An examination of populations that lived on very little dietary carbohydrate may provide insight into the healthiest long-term use of a diet low in carbohydrate. The Inuit people of the Arctic lived much of the year on coastal ice (which is partially desalinated seawater), and much of their food consisted of soup made with meat in a broth from this brackish source of water. When they went inland to hunt, they traditionally added caribou blood (also a rich source of sodium) to their soup. With these empirically derived techniques, the Inuit culture had adapted the available resources to optimize their intakes of both sodium and potassium. When meat is baked, roasted, broiled, or when it is boiled but the broth discarded, potassium initially present in the meat is lost, making it more difficult to maintain potassium balance in the absence of fruit and vegetable intake. Using bouillon as a sodium supplement, the optimal amount of daily sodium intake of 3 to 5 g can be ensured. If dietary potassium supplementation is appropriate, "lite salt" may be used as well.

TREATMENT OF THE MAJOR CONSEQUENCES OF OBESITY

The major consequences of obesity that generally improve with weight loss treatment are diabetes mellitus; metabolic syndrome, which includes hypertension and hypertriglyceridemia; and gastroesophageal reflux disorder (GERD). The management of obesity in patients who are medicated for these comorbidities is more complicated because of the need to monitor and reduce or eliminate medications.

Diabetes mellitus

Carbohydrate restriction can have a potent effect on glycemic control of diabetes mellitus initially and can, in many cases, result in remission of type 2 diabetes. Although large-scale clinical trials regarding carbohydrate restriction are lacking, there are a growing number of small clinical trials and case series showing that the low-carbohydrate diet has a potent effect on type 2 diabetes mellitus and obesity (24–29). Among patients with type 1 diabetes, carbohydrate restriction generally leads to a reduction in the daily insulin dose requirement and may lead to a reduction in hypoglycemic events.

Metabolic syndrome

Successful adipose tissue loss will improve the components of the metabolic syndrome. The ATP III definition of metabolic syndrome includes any three or more of the following: (a) waist circumference: >102 cm in men, >88 cm in women; (b) serum triglycerides: >150 mg/dL; (c) HDL cholesterol: <40 mg/dL in men, <50 mg/dL in women; (d) blood pressure: >130/85 mm Hg; and (e) serum glucose: >110 mg/dL. Carbohydrate-restricted diets have a greater effect on improving these aspects of the metabolic syndrome than fat-restricted diets (19).

Gastroesophageal reflux disorder

Practitioners using carbohydrate-restricted diets have noted the resolution of heartburn symptoms in their patients for some time. This observation has been supported by recent research: first in a case series of five individuals noting improvement of their heartburn symptoms, and then in a subsequent, more detailed study (30). In the second study, eight obese individuals with GERD were instructed to follow a diet containing less than 20 g per day (31). One day prior to the initiation of the diet, participants completed the GERD Symptom Assessment Scale—distress subscale (GSAS-ds), a GERD-specific questionnaire, and underwent dual-channel 24-hour pH probe testing. After removal of the pH probe, participants initiated the diet. Three to 6 days later, a second pH probe was performed and the GSAS-ds was administered again. Outcomes included changes in GSAS-ds scores, percentage of total time with a pH <4 in the distal esophagus, and the Johnson–DeMeester score (a score based upon the pH probe measurements). All individuals showed an improvement in the severity of their symptoms, with the mean GSAS-ds score decreasing from 1.28 prior to the diet to 0.72 afterward ($P = 0.0004$). Participants had a significant decrease in the Johnson–DeMeester score (mean of 34.7 before the diet vs. 14.0 afterward, $P = 0.023$). Participants also exhibited a significant decrease in the percentage of time with a pH <4 (5.1 before the diet vs. 2.5 afterward, $P = 0.022$). Austin et al. (31) concluded that the initiation of a very-low–carbohydrate diet in obese patients with GERD significantly reduces distal esophageal acid exposure and improves the symptoms of GERD. Further research is needed to identify mechanisms.

Irritable bowel syndrome

After anecdotal reports of improvement in irritable bowel syndrome (IBS) symptoms after consuming low-carb diets, a prospective study was performed to determine whether this observation was robust (32). Patients with moderate-to-severe diarrhea-predominant IBS were provided a 2-week standard diet, then 4 weeks of a very-low–carbohydrate diet (20 g per day). A responder in symptoms was defined as having adequate relief of gastrointestinal symptoms for 2 or more weeks during the low-carbohydrate phase. Of the 17 participants enrolled, 13 completed the study and all 13 were responders. Seventy-seven percent reported adequate relief for all 4 weeks of the low-carbohydrate diet phase. The frequency of stools decreased and the consistency of the stool improved from diarrheal-to-normal form. Pain scores and quality-of-life measures also significantly improved. Austin et al. (32) concluded that a very-low–carbohydrate diet can provide adequate relief of IBS.

Clinical considerations

If your patient is otherwise healthy, and not taking diabetes or hypertensive medication, it is possible that all you need to do is to recommend or give permission to your patient to follow a low-carbohydrate popular diet book. Most of these books combine dietary advice with supportive and motivational writing to instruct individuals in lifestyle modification. At a minimum, check underlying organ function by using blood tests at baseline. Even this type of patient often has improved outcomes with physician support and monitoring.

If your patient is taking medication, then closer evaluation and follow-up are recommended after instruction. Many clinical practices have their patients return for a follow-up visit after 1 week of diet change to monitor self-reported adherence and to check adherence by using urinary ketones and food diaries. If your patient is taking diabetic or antihypertensive medication, then frequent medical monitoring is necessary for medication adjustment. Follow-up clinic visits may be scheduled at 1- to 2-week intervals, or more frequently if needed.

Patients taking medications for certain conditions require more attention, as many medications will need to be adjusted or discontinued due to the potent effect of nutritional ketosis. Common medications that may result in iatrogenic problems if doses are not adjusted include diuretics, antihypertensives, and hypoglycemics (both oral and injectable hypoglycemics). Thus, hypoglycemics and antihypertensives may require rapid tapering (days to weeks) to avoid hypoglycemia and hypotension (Table 5.5). Patient self-monitoring can be done using simple worksheets for patients to monitor their own food intake, glucose levels, or blood pressures can be very helpful during this initial phase, when medication adjustment is required. If the patient is taking vitamin K antagonists for anticoagulation, then more frequent monitoring may be needed if there has been a change in intake of leafy greens or other foods containing vitamin K.

Some medications create problems with the treatment of obesity because they inhibit lipolysis or increase appetite. Niacin and beta blockers block lipolysis via lipoprotein lipase and a reduction in sympathetic activity, respectively. Psychiatric medications, especially antipsychotic medications, and subcutaneous insulin injections are common offenders.

Hypertension

For patients taking antihypertensive medications, wean diuretics as soon as the patient measures positive for urinary ketones, as the natriuresis of ketosis will cause diuresis. If symptoms of dizziness, lightheadedness, or orthostatic hypotension occur, other antihypertensive medications should also be reduced with continued monitoring of the blood pressure. Supplementation with bouillon may be helpful to reduce symptoms during the first few weeks. (Drinking 1 g of sodium in the form of bouillon can improve symptomatic hypotension within a few minutes.) Check serum electrolytes, including calcium and magnesium, and replace deficits if salt supplementation does not relieve these symptoms. Even if serum magnesium is normal, a trial of magnesium supplementation may ameliorate fatigue and cramping.

Blood pressure monitoring at home or at the clinic is required because a reduction in blood pressure frequently occurs soon after the initiation of the diet. Taper or discontinue the antihypertensives if home or clinic blood pressures are less than 110 mmHg systolic. If the systolic blood pressure is 130 mmHg or below or diastolic is 70 mmHg or below, consider initiating taper. Due to their effect on weight loss, decrease beta blockers first, followed by calcium channel blockers, and then angiotensin-converting enzyme (ACE) inhibitor or angiotensin II receptor blocker (ARB). Until microalbuminuria is resolved, a low dose of renal protective medication may be continued if the patient does not become hypotensive. In diabetic patients, continue a low dose ACE or ARB until blood glucoses are normal and urinary microalbumin is normal. Consider the use of prophylactic potassium citrate if there is a history of kidney stones.

Most patients with hypertension have been told to *restrict* their sodium intake in the past, and they will probably continue to restrict sodium out of habit even after instruction to not be concerned about the sodium. It is very important during carbohydrate restriction to have adequate sodium intake to counteract the natriuresis that occurs because of the cessation of the insulin-induced sodium retention that accompany high-carbohydrate diets.

Type 2 diabetes mellitus

ORAL HYPOGLYCEMICS

For patients taking oral hypoglycemic medications, stop all oral hypoglycemic agents except metformin on the day that the diet begins. Patients with diabetes should monitor home glucoses once (fasting a.m. value will be the highest of the day) or twice daily. Because these meals do not raise the blood glucose, it no longer matters if the home glucoses are before or after meals. Because short-term hyperglycemia poses less immediate risk than hypoglycemia, the glucoses are allowed to go up to 200 to 250 mg/dL during the weight loss process. Restart oral hypoglycemic of choice if the blood glucose is >250 mg/dL after the first 3 days. If a downward trend in serum glucose is noted, continue to observe the patient without reintroducing the medication. Individuals with untreated type 2 diabetes should have fasting blood glucose values near normal within a few weeks of nutritional ketosis if they have intact insulin secretion. Metformin can be discontinued when the blood glucoses remain <100 mg/dL.

INJECTABLE HYPOGLYCEMICS

Because injectable hypoglycemics (insulin or exenatide) introduce the risk of severe hypoglycemia, it is recommended to discontinue these medications as quickly as tolerated. For patients with type 2 diabetes taking insulin, if the daily insulin use is less than 20 units per day, discontinue the insulin on the first day of the lifestyle change. In other patients, reduce the insulin or other injectable hypoglycemic by 50% at diet initiation. (Again, short-term hyperglycemia poses less immediate risk than hypoglycemia.) Patients should self-monitor their glucose level several times a day and record the results for reporting to their health care provider. When the fasting glucose is less than 200 mg/dL, decrease the insulin or exenatide dose by another 50%. Consider changing to short-acting insulin preparations because longer acting preparations do not allow flexible dosing when serum glucose levels are falling rapidly. Insulin is then discontinued when the daily dose is 10 to 20 units, depending upon the individual's response.

CAUTION: Some individuals may have a dramatic reduction in blood glucoses with the initiation of *nutritional ketosis* and *may* become hypoglycemic if the injectable hypoglycemic agent is not reduced or discontinued rapidly.

Hyperglycemic individuals may not demonstrate urinary ketones as quickly as normoglycemic individuals. As a result, the absence of urinary ketones does not accurately reflect adherence among patients with diabetes. When treating hyperglycemic patients, even if the preprandial glucose levels are similar to baseline, the next measurement of glycosylated hemoglobin (HgbA1c) will probably be lower than before because there are no large postprandial rises in glucose on the LCKD.

OTHER MEDICAL CONDITIONS

Other medical conditions that require consideration include congestive heart failure, gout, hyperchylomicronemia (triglycerides >1000 mg/dL), or history of calcium oxalate renal stones. Patients with heart failure may need to limit sodium and water consumption. Patients with a history of gout may be placed on prophylactic allopurinol prior to initiation or a prescription for colchicine or NSAID may be provided as well for the patient to initiate if needed. Patients with a history of calcium oxalate renal stones may reduce the risk of subsequent stones by taking potassium citrate supplements. GERD medications may be eliminated on a trial basis at any time—resume if the GERD recurs. After significant weight loss, continuous positive airway pressure therapy for sleep apnea may be discontinued if upon retesting, apnea and hypoxia are resolved. Some practitioners repeat a sleep study to document resolution of the sleep apnea. Although we have observed many patients with severe hypertriglyceridemia (>6500 mg/dL) improve with a low-carbohydrate diet, the current diet recommendation for these patients is a low-fat diet, due to the possibility of worsening hyperchylomicronemia. A high-fat diet in the presence of chylomicronemia may lead to pancreatitis (33). If the hypertriglyceridemia is chylomicron in origin, then a low-carbohydrate, high-fat diet is contraindicated. Test for this by asking your laboratory to measure for the presence of chylomicrons if the fasting serum triglycerides are >500 mg/dL. Careful clinical monitoring will show rapid decreases in serum triglycerides if the elevation is due to hyperinsulinemia. Triglyceride values will begin to decrease in a few days. Areas of the body that have a substantial loss of weight may require plastic surgery for removal of the stretched skin.

INSTRUCTIONS ON WHEN TO CALL THE CLINIC

Although some mild symptoms of fatigue may occur during the keto-adaptation phase, if your patients are taking medications, these symptoms can also occur due to overmedication by antihypertensive or hypoglycemic (Table 5.6). Instruct your patient to call the clinic if he or she experienced symptoms such as dizziness, lightheadedness, or muscle cramping. Home monitoring of glucose and/or blood pressure is recommended. Home glucose monitoring is highly recommended if the patient is taking insulin or taking multiple hypoglycemic agents. If fatigue or muscle cramping occurs, recommend one bouillon cube dissolved in hot water every 4 hours as needed. If symptoms persist, then bring the patient back to the clinic for measurement of serum electrolytes. Potassium or magnesium supplementation can be added if serum measurements are abnormally low. Because potassium and magnesium are intracellular electrolytes, serum levels are a poor indicator of total body depletion. For example, a history of muscle cramps and hyperreflexia on physical exam is highly suggestive

Table 5.6 Causes of dizziness during the first 2 weeks

Low blood pressure due to overmedication: reduce medication

Low blood glucose due to overmedication: reduce medication

Fluid shifts from diuresis: discontinue diuretic, add or increase bouillon (salt)

Other common illnesses: treat as indicated

Troubleshooting

- First take a diet history and then take a routine medical history.
- Is the patient strictly following the allowed foods? Are adequate salad greens and nonstarchy vegetables being consumed?
- Too much sucralose, NutraSweet, or alcohols may cause diarrhea.
- Overmedication or undermedication?
- Non–diet-related events can occur, such as adverse effects of medications.

of magnesium deficiency. As a preventive treatment for muscle cramping and constipation, a slow-release magnesium preparation like Slow-Mag or 1 teaspoon of milk of magnesia at bedtime is helpful. For patients who are taking insulin or other injectable hypoglycemic agents, we instruct patients to call the doctor on call when the glucoses go below 100 mg/dL.

HOSPITAL MANAGEMENT OF A PATIENT IN NUTRITIONAL KETOSIS

Many hospitals do not have a standard low-carbohydrate selection, even though foods that are low carbohydrate are available at the hospital. Choosing to not eat the carbs on the plate is an option. Stating that there is an allergy to wheat, milk, and fruit may lead to a discussion of personal dietary selections.

In regard to intravenous therapy during hospitalization, if the hospital has a pharmacy capable of making total parenteral nutrition (TPN), use 3% amino acids, 30 mEq of sodium, 20 mEq of potassium, 15 mM phosphorus, and 20 mEq of magnesium and run 2 L per day by peripheral vein after the first few liters of normal saline. If a customized TPN prescription is not available, use normal saline (without glucose or dextrose). Since about half of the water becomes intracellular, this can lead to hypernatremia after a few liters. Serum electrolytes, magnesium, and phosphorus should be measured daily. Oral fluid resuscitation should use bouillon and sugar-free gelatin. Small amounts of sugar substitutes or sugar-free beverages may be used for palatability.

REFERENCES

1. Vernon MC, Mavropoulos J, Transue M, et al. Clinical experience of a carbohydrate restricted diet: Effect on diabetes mellitus. *Metab Syndr Relat Disord* 2003; 1: 233–237.
2. Johnston BC, Kanters S, Bandayrel K, et al. Comparison of weight loss among named diet programs in overweight and obese adults. A meta-analysis. *JAMA* 2014; 312(9): 923–933.
3. Naude CE, Schoonees A, Senekal M, et al. Low carbohydrate versus isoenergetic balanced diets for reducing weight and cardiovascular risk: A systematic review and meta-analysis. *PLoS One* 2014; 9(7): e100652.

4. Bueno NB, de Melo IS, de Oliviera SL, et al. Very-low-carbohydrate ketogenic diet v. low-fat diet for long-term weight loss: A meta-analysis of randomised controlled trials. *Br J Nutr* 2013; 110(7): 1178–1187.

5. Nordmann AJ, Nordmann A, Briel M, et al. Effects of low-carbohydrate vs low-fat diets on weight loss and cardiovascular risk factors: A meta-analysis of randomized controlled trials. *Arch Intern Med* 2006; 166(3): 285–293.

6. Phinney SD, Horton ES, Sims EAH, Hanson JS, Danforth E Jr., LaGrange BM. Capacity for moderate exercise in obese subjects after adaptation to a hypocaloric, ketogenic diet. *J Clin Invest* 1980; 66: 1151–1161.

7. Phinney SD, Bistrian BR, Evans WJ, Gervino E, Blackburn GL. The human metabolic response to chronic ketosis without caloric restriction: Preservation of submaximal exercise capability with reduced carbohydrate oxidation. *Metabolism* 1983; 32: 769–776.

8. Phinney SD, Bistrian BR, Evans WJ, Gervino E, Blackburn GL. The human metabolic response to chronic ketosis without caloric restriction: Physical and biochemical adaptation. *Metabolism* 1983; 32: 757–768.

9. Westman EC, Feinman RD, Mavropoulos JC, et al. Low-carbohydrate nutrition and metabolism. *Am J Clin Nutr* 2007; 86(2): 276–284.

10. Westman EC, Mavropoulos J, Yancy WS, et al. A review of low-carbohydrate ketogenic diets. *Curr Atheroscler Rep* 2003; 5(6): 476–483.

11. Makki K, Froguel P, Wolowczuk I. Adipose tissue in obesity-related inflammation and insulin resistance: Cells, cytokines, and chemokines. *ISRN Inflamm* 2013; 2013: 139239.

12. Layman DK. Dietary guidelines should reflect new understandings about adult protein needs. *Nutr Metab (Lond)* 2009; 6: 12.

13. Forsythe CE, Phinney SD, Fernandez ML, et al. Comparison of low fat and low carbohydrate diets on circulating fatty acid composition and markers of inflammation. *Lipids* 2008; 43(1): 65–77.

14. Forsythe CE, Phinney SD, Feinman RD, et al. Limited effect of dietary saturated fat on plasma saturated fat in the context of a low carbohydrate diet. *Lipids* 2010; 45(10): 947–962. doi: 10.1007/s11745-010-3467-3.

15. Yancy WS Jr., Olsen MK, Dudley T, et al. Acid-base analysis of individuals following two weight loss diets. *Eur J Clin Nutr* 2007; 61(12): 1416–1422.

16. Harber MP, Schenk S, Barkan AL, Horowitz JF. Alterations in carbohydrate metabolism in response to short-term dietary carbohydrate restriction. *Am J Physiol Endocrinol Metab* 2005; 289: E306–E312.

17. Volek JS, Sharman MJ, Love DM, et al. Body composition and hormonal responses to a carbohydrate-restricted diet. *Metabolism* 2002; 51: 864–870.

18. Sharman MJ, Kraemer WJ, Love DM, et al. A ketogenic diet favorably affects serum biomarkers for cardiovascular disease in normal-weight men. *J Nutr* 2002; 132: 1879–1885.

19. Volek JS, Fernandez ML, Feinman RD, Phinney SD. Dietary carbohydrate restriction induces a unique metabolic state positively affecting atherogenic dyslipidemia, fatty acid partitioning, and metabolic syndrome. *Prog Lipid Res* 2008; 47: 307–318.

20. Horita S, Seki G, Yamada H, et al. Insulin resistance, obesity, hypertension, and renal sodium transport. *Int J Hypertens* 2011; 2011: 391762. doi: 10.4061/2011/391762.

21. DeFronzo RA, Cooke CR, Andres R. The effect of insulin on renal handling of sodium, potassium, calcium, and phosphate in man. *J Clin Invest* 1975; 55(4): 845–855.

22. Tsai AG, Wadden TA. The evolution of very-low-calorie diets: An update and meta-analysis. *Obesity* 2006; 14: 1283–1293.
23. Phinney SD, Tang AB, Waggoner CR, et al. The transient hypercholesterolemia of major weight loss. *Am J Clin Nutr* 1991; 53(6): 1404–1410.
24. O'Neill DF, Westman EC, Bernstein RK. The effects of a low-carbohydrate regimen on glycemic control and serum lipids in diabetes mellitus. *Metab Syndr Relat Disord* 2003; 1: 291–298.
25. Yancy WS Jr., Vernon MC, Westman EC. A pilot trial of a low-carbohydrate, ketogenic diet in patients with type 2 diabetes. *Metab Syndr Relat Disord* 2003; 1: 239–243.
26. Westman EC, Yancy WS Jr., Mavropoulos JC, Marquart M, McDuffie JR. The effect of a low-carbohydrate, ketogenic diet versus a low-glycemic index diet on glycemic control in type 2 diabetes mellitus. *Nutr Metab (Lond)* 2008; 5: 36.
27. Saslow LR, Kim S, Daubenmier JJ, et al. A randomized pilot trial of a moderate carbohydrate diet compared to a very low carbohydrate diet in overweight or obese individuals with type 2 diabetes mellitus or prediabetes. *PLoS One* 2014; 9(4): e91027.
28. Tay J, Luscombe-Marsh ND, Thompson CH, et al. A very-low carbohydrate, low saturated fat diet for type 2 diabetes management: A randomized trial. *Diabetes Care* 2014; 37(11): 2909–2918.
29. Yamada Y, Uchida J, Izumi H, et al. A non-calorie-restricted low-carbohydrate diet is effective as an alternative therapy for patients with type 2 diabetes. *Intern Med* 2014; 53(1): 13–19.
30. Yancy WS Jr., Provencale D, Westman EC. Improvement of gastroesophageal reflux disease after initiation of a low-carbohydrate diet: Five brief case reports. *Altern Ther Health Med* 2001; 7: 120–122.
31. Austin GL, Thiny MT, Westman EC, Yancy WS Jr., Shaheen NJ. A very low carbohydrate diet improves gastroesophageal reflux and its symptoms: A pilot study. *Dig Dis Sci* 2006; 51: 1307–1312.
32. Austin GL, Dalton DB, Hu Y, et al. A very-low-carbohydrate diet improves symptoms and quality of life in diarrhea-predominant irritable bowel syndrome. *Clin Gastroenterol Hepatol* 2009; 7: 706–708.
33. Buse GJ, Riley KD, Dress CM, Neumaster TD. Patient with gemfibrozil-controlled hypertriglyceridemia that developed acute pancreatitis after starting ketogenic diet. *Curr Surg* 2004; 61(2): 224–226.

6

The role of physical activity in the treatment of overweight and obesity

DEBORAH BADE HORN

INTRODUCTION

Obesity in America had been increasing throughout the end of the twentieth and beginning of the twenty-first century, and only recently is there consistent evidence that the epidemic problem may be stabilizing, at least in terms of prevalence. Using National Health and Nutrition Examination Survey data, The National Center for Health Statistics brief (1) found that the prevalence of obesity was not significantly different in 2011 to 2012 than it was in 2009 to 2010.

Using an alternate dataset—the Behavioral Risk Factor Surveillance System (BRFSS)—The State of Obesity: Better Policies for a Healthier America report (formerly known as the F as in Fat report series) now states that obesity rates increased in only six states compared to previous years, but did not decrease in a single state (2). Thus, the report concluded that a slowing of the epidemic of obesity is occurring. Both reports identify an obesity prevalence of 35%. If the obesity epidemic is indeed leveling off, it may be partially the result of increased physical activity. Physical activity levels in the United States have improved slightly over the past two decades. However, with the addition of updated physical activity guidelines in 2008 and 2009, the ability to compare earlier statistics to those collected more recently is diminished. The most recent statistics using updated guidelines demonstrate that only about 20% of US adults are meeting both the aerobic and muscle-strengthening components of the physical activity recommendations (3). Because physical activity can affect caloric expenditure and therefore energy balance, it plays an important role in a comprehensive approach to weight management, obesity treatment, and the obesity epidemic.

The Centers for Disease Control and Prevention (CDC) evaluates physical activity participation in America through the BRFSS survey via state health departments. The survey is a self-reported telephone survey and thus is subject to recall and social-desirability bias. After the release of the updated 2008 Physical Activity Guidelines for Americans by the US Department of Health and Human Services (HHS), the CDC reanalyzed BRFSS data from 2007 to determine the number of Americans sufficiently active to achieve health benefits. The CDC analysis found that 64.5% of surveyed participants were meeting the new guidelines as defined by the HHS. Interestingly, when the same responses were applied to the Healthy People 2010 recommendations, only 48.8% of respondents were meeting recommended guidelines. The CDC attributes the difference to two factors: (1) the updated HHS guidelines allow for an accumulation of physical activity over the entire week, as opposed to the previously prescribed number of minutes per day and a prescribed number of days per week; and (2) the updated guidelines offer an option of variable intensities that can be combined together to meet the requirements. When the analyzed data were reduced to participants with obesity over the age of 18, only 57% met the HHS guidelines. Similarly, when this subset was applied to the Healthy People 2010 recommendations, only 41% of individuals with obesity were meeting the guidelines (4).

In addition, the current HHS guidelines indicate that the amount of physical activity required to achieve health benefit and reduced risk of disease may be much less than the amount of exercise needed to affect change in weight or prevent weight gain and regain (5). Unfortunately, as reported above, individuals affected by overweight and obesity are less likely to meet even the minimum recommendations for physical activity. Finally, research is discovering that the physical activity required to affect weight change or weight maintenance may be highly variable from individual to individual (6,7).

This chapter reviews the concept of physical activity; the multiple sets of guidelines available for consideration; and the role that physical activity can play in preventing weight gain, achieving weight loss, and sustaining long-term weight maintenance after significant weight loss. Included is a practical approach to physical activity in individuals who struggle with overweight and obesity from exercise prescription to special needs in the bariatric population. Although public health experts, scientists, and clinicians agree that physical activity plays a key role in weight management, the recommended message to the patient is not always consistent and therefore can be confusing. The goal of this chapter is to review the current guidelines and tools and to assist clinicians as they initiate a dialogue regarding daily physical activity with their overweight and obese patients (Table 6.1).

Table 6.1 Example exercise prescription

	Frequency	Intensity	Time	Type
Cardio				
Strength				
Muscular endurance				
Flexibility				

PHYSICAL ACTIVITY VERSUS EXERCISE

Although the two terms are often used interchangeably, physical activity and exercise are not synonymous. Physical activity is a larger umbrella term that can include exercise and all other nonrest activities; it is defined as "movement produced by skeletal muscle and that results in energy expenditure" (8). Total energy expenditure (EE) is composed of resting energy expenditure (REE), the thermic effect of meals (TEM), and energy expenditure from physical activity (EEPA): EE = REE + TEM + EEPA (9). EEPA is EE from all physical activity accumulated throughout the day. Examples of EE from physical activity include walking from the car to the office, swimming, exercise class, walking the dog, household chores, gardening, and playing with one's children. Some researchers choose to categorize physical activity into three major areas: transportational, occupational, and leisure-time activities.

Exercise is more specific. It is a subset of physical activity or EEPA. Exercise is "planned, structured, and repetitive and has a final or an intermediate objective, the improvement or maintenance of physical fitness" (8). Examples can include jogging, rowing, cycling, lunchtime exercise class, yoga, or dance class. In the preceding categories, it would fall under leisure-time activities.

Most of the current literature on physical activity, obesity, and weight modification is reported as exercise. Research subjects are commonly asked to complete a specific physical activity, for a prescribed amount of time, with the goal to measure some aspect of improved health outcomes. Researchers choose prescribed or predetermined exercise intentionally because it is difficult to quantify, and/or instruct individuals to increase their overall daily physical activity, when activities and intensities could vary widely between study participants and dilute the potential results. As physical activity and obesity treatment research evolves, increasing the component of physical activity that is built into otherwise fixed daily responsibilities may provide an opportunity to achieve recommended levels of physical activity without dedicating as much isolated time specifically to exercise (see also Novel approaches section). Smaller amounts of "exercise" could potentially provide the cardiorespiratory benefits needed, whereas larger bouts of nonexercise physical activity may be able to contribute significantly to EE and maintenance of a healthier weight and body composition.

PHYSICAL ACTIVITY AND PREVENTING INITIAL WEIGHT GAIN: TRUE PRIMARY PREVENTION

Overall health benefit and reduced risk of sedentary lifestyle-related diseases were the focus of the original 1995 American College of Sports Medicine (ACSM)/CDC guidelines for physical activity: at least 30 minutes per day of moderate intensity physical activity most, preferably all, days of the week. The primary ACSM recommendation to the US public has since been revised, but it is still directed at general health benefits and risk prevention, not the specific treatment or prevention of obesity. How much physical activity does it take to reduce the risk of becoming overweight or obese? The 2009 ACSM position stand suggests that 150 to 250 minutes per week of physical activity (an EE of 1200–2000 kcal) should provide a stable weight profile, but this will, of course, depend upon an individual's caloric intake (10). Less than 150 minutes per week of physical activity is not adequate to prevent age-related increases in weight. Furthermore, it may also vary throughout life how much physical activity is needed to maintain a healthy body weight (10).

Minor weight fluctuations are normal based on hydration status, hormonal changes, clothing, time of day, and other factors. Therefore, prevention of weight gain or weight "stability" may actually be a range of absolute weights. Although still a debated topic, weight stability has been defined as a <3% change in body weight over time (11). Thus, although 150 minutes of physical activity per week may be sufficient to lower the risk of diseases such as diabetes, coronary artery disease (CAD), and hypertension, more than 150 minutes per week will be necessary in most people to maintain actual weight stability over a lifetime, which, in turn, affects the risk of these same diseases. The relationship among physical activity, body composition, weight, and risk of obesity and related diseases may result in a continuum of risk, or rather risk reduction, based on amount of physical activity participation.

PHYSICAL ACTIVITY AND WEIGHT LOSS

"Calories in = calories out" is an equation often discussed in weight loss interventions and obesity treatment. However, changes in energy intake versus EE are not equally effective at weight loss or prevention of weight gain. Exercise or physical activity as a sole intervention is less effective than diet alone or diet plus exercise in producing weight loss in short-term studies (10,12,13). Exercise alone has a widely variable affect and achieves only 3% to 23% of the weight loss that can be achieved by dieting alone and only 2% to 20% of the weight loss that can be achieved with dieting plus exercise (12,13). The length of an intervention or time spent on an attempt at weight loss and obesity treatment may play a role in the overall contribution of physical activity to the outcome of weight loss. Studies with a longer follow-up time of 12 to 18 months found that exercise was associated with better weight loss results (14,15).

The ACSM concluded that weight does indeed demonstrate a dose response to physical activity. Modest overall weight loss, defined as 2 to 3 kg (4.4–6.6 lb), would require 150 to 225 minutes of physical activity per week. In addition, 225 to 420 minutes of physical activity per week can yield greater weight loss at 5 to 7.5 kg (11–16.5 lb) (10). Put in the context of a patient's typical expectations, the amount of physical activity, required to achieve a 1 to 2 lb weight loss per week without dietary changes, is likely prohibitive in the daily schedules of most individuals (see also Novel approaches section for possible solutions). The estimated time commitment necessary to produce this affect is between 1.3 and 2.75 hours per day (16). The current body of research indicates that exercise or physical activity combined with decreased calorie intake, rather than physical activity alone or calorie restriction alone, will produce the greatest change in weight and more quickly meet an individual's weight loss and obesity treatment expectations. Therefore, physical activity should be paired with adjusted caloric intake to achieve optimal weight loss and body composition.

PHYSICAL ACTIVITY AND WEIGHT MAINTENANCE OR PREVENTION OF WEIGHT REGAIN

Once an individual has reached their maintenance or goal weight and body composition, the role of physical activity versus caloric intake shifts. Increased EE, or "calories out," contributes more significantly to weight maintenance or the prevention of weight regain.

Regular physical activity is associated with long-term weight loss maintenance (17–19). Predicting the amount or type of physical activity that will optimize this weight loss maintenance has yet to be accomplished. The National Weight Control Registry (NWCR), which is described in more detail below, reported that the majority of individuals who have successfully maintained a significant weight loss report high levels of physical activity (6,20). Weight regain in these individuals is associated with decreased physical activity (20). Unfortunately, most of the data on weight maintenance and physical activity are by self-report and often include retrospective categorization of participants in to high-, medium-, and low-activity groups. A minimum threshold of required physical activity to allow for weight maintenance or prevention of weight regain has yet to be truly determined. Theoretically, an individual could reduce caloric intake to the point that no physical activity is needed to maintain weight. However, this individual would not benefit from the many health improvements and reduced risk of chronic disease afforded by an active lifestyle. Furthermore, emerging data suggest that the fat-free mass loss associated with this approach may substantially lower the individuals resting metabolic rate, resulting in an increased risk of weight regain.

The NWCR is a self-reported database of individuals that have lost at least 13.6 kg ($\approx$30 lb) and maintained that loss for at least 1 year. Analysis of the NWCR data found that, on average, its participants were completing 60 to 75 minutes of moderate intensity physical activity or 35 to 45 minutes of vigorous activity per day (6). These data were, in part, used to help determine the new HHS guidelines on weight loss maintenance and physical activity. It is important to note that these are participation averages; the range of reported amount of activity from individual to individual was actually quite broad. Fifteen percent of entrants in the registry reported very low levels of physical activity, that is, levels even lower than those recommended simply for general health benefits (<30 minutes per day). And yet, they reported successful maintenance of weight loss. Alternatively, some participants reported very high levels of physical activity, greater than 90 minutes per day. However, overall the registry participants are still engaging in more daily physical activity than the average American. Approximately one-half of the entrants "meets or exceeds 60 min/day of moderate intensity physical activity" and "one-third meets or exceeds 90 min/day of physical activity" (6).

Several studies have demonstrated that like the NWCR participants, individuals who do more physical activity experience better weight maintenance. Jakicic et al. (15) found that individuals participating in more than 200 minutes of moderate-intensity physical activity per week tend to be more successful at weight maintenance. Another study found that individuals who lost more than 10% of their body weight after 2 years reported 275 minutes per week of physical activity (7). The 2009 ACSM position stand by Donnelly et al. (10) rates the evidence for physical activity prevention of weight regain as a category B based on National Heart, Lung, and Blood Institute categories of level of evidence.

To more accurately prescribe physical activity to an individual, randomized control trials that include randomization to physical activity levels for weight and body composition maintenance are needed. Few studies exist, and the range of actual EE in low, medium, and highly active groups in the available studies is so broad that a clinically significant conclusion regarding a threshold or minimum recommendation regarding amount of physical activity for maintaining a weight loss is difficult to make. After reviewing these and other studies, the ACSM position stand concluded that, on average, weight maintenance is likely to require approximately 60 minutes of moderate-intensity physical activity per day or about 420 minutes per week. This is almost 3 times the amount of physical activity recommended for "health benefits," regardless of weight status.

The importance of preventing weight regain is often underestimated. Unfortunately, many individuals cycle through major weight fluctuations from weight gain, to weight loss, to weight maintenance, to weight regain. Fluctuating weight has been associated with increased risk of cardiovascular disease and all-cause mortality (21,22). A successful weight loss attempt needs to be carefully monitored and supported to avoid these increased risks. Physical activity and nutritional, behavioral, and pharmacological tools all need to be optimized. Weight loss alone is not the ideal goal. The ultimate and optimal goal is weight loss and optimized body composition followed by successful maintenance.

A REVIEW OF THE CURRENT RECOMMENDATIONS

The US physical activity guidelines have multiple components and are geared at both health benefits in the general US population as well as weight loss and weight maintenance efforts to treat obesity. Confusion related to physical activity guidelines is predominately secondary to two issues: (1) multiple sets of guidelines exist from various different US and international public health and specialty organizations and (2) failure to differentiate between physical activity recommendations for overall health benefits versus recommendations specific to preventing or treating obesity by preventing weight gain, assisting in weight loss, and/or managing weight maintenance.

The 2008 HHS published their "Physical Activity Guidelines for Americans" for individuals aged 6 years and older. Previously, the HHS did not publish separate physical activity guidelines, but instead offered recommendations within the "Dietary Guidelines for Americans" that was published jointly by the HHS and the US Department of Agriculture. This was an opportunity to provide both nutritional and physical activity recommendations to the United States from a single source.

The HHS guidelines recommend 150 minutes per week of moderate-intensity physical activity, in at least 10-minute bouts, to gain the basic health benefits associated with physical activity. This is consistent with ACSM/American Heart Association (AHA) guidelines. These health benefits include decreased mortality and decreased risk of obesity-related comorbidities: heart disease, stroke, diabetes, and some cancers (21,22). Although the top-level basic HHS guidelines do not give specific recommendations for obesity treatment, the second-level recommendations indicate that "additional and more extensive health benefits" are provided by increasing moderate-intensity physical activity to 300 minutes per week (5).

The HHS Physical Activity Guidelines Advisory Committee recognizes that 150 to 300 minutes of physical activity per week may be necessary to avoid the 1% to 3% average yearly weight gain in most Americans. The committee also found that without dietary changes, approximately 45 minutes per day of moderate physical activity would be needed to obtain at least a 5% weight loss over the long term. This is greater than 300 minutes per week of physical activity as well. Finally, in patients who have already lost weight, even more physical activity may be necessary. To prevent weight regain after successful weight loss, HHS guidelines recommend that individuals need to participate in approximately 60 minutes of walking or 30 minutes of jogging daily (or an equivalent physical activity). This is 420 minutes per week of moderate-intensity physical activity or 210 minutes of more vigorous physical activity. However, the summary recommendations simply indicate that greater than 300 minutes may be necessary (5).

The above-mentioned recommendations may be surprising given that physical activity guidelines originally put forth by the ACSM and the CDC in 1995 were much lower. This outdated ACSM/CDC recommendation was that adults "should accumulate 30 minutes or more of moderate intensity exercise on most, preferably all, days of the week" (23). This is the sound bite or mantra that Americans can typically recall. Unfortunately, these guidelines are specific to the amount of physical activity necessary to improve health and reduce the risk of disease. They were not written with the intention of weight control or the treatment of obesity. These recommendations were revised in 2007. Although the baseline recommendation is still 150 minutes per week, the current guidelines are more specific. They recommend 30 minutes of moderate-intensity, specifically cardiovascular, exercise 5 days per week and strength training an additional 2 days per week. These remain the current ASCM basic guidelines published in conjunction with the AHA, not the CDC, and are again the recommendations to "maintain health and reduce the risk of chronic disease" without any specific intent of weight change or obesity treatment. Beyond basic health benefits, the ACSM/AHA recommendations go on to indicate that "to lose weight or maintain weight loss, 60–90 minutes of physical activity may be necessary" (24).

In 2009, the ACSM released an updated position stand that offered more specific recommendations regarding "appropriate physical activity intervention strategies for weight loss and prevention of weight regain for adults" (10). The new ACSM position stand found that there was A level evidence, as defined by the National Heart, Lung, and Blood Institute, to support that 150 to 250 minutes of exercise per week is needed to prevent initial weight gain in most adults. The level of evidence is not as strong for the amount of physical activity needed for weight loss and weight maintenance. The amount of activity required for substantial weight loss (5–7.5 kg [11–16.5 lb]) is 225 to 420 minutes per week. This is up to 60 minutes all days of the week to achieve 11 to 16.5 lb of weight loss (10). ACSM rates the level of evidence associated with this statement to be category B.

Finally, the amount of activity required for preventing weight regain after weight loss appears even less clear. The position stand indicates that it cannot definitively comment because correctly designed studies are lacking. However, the available information indicates that 200 to 300 minutes of exercise per week is likely necessary (10).

The updates and expansion of the guidelines to include more specific recommendations for the treatment of obesity by both ACSM and HHS were triggered by increasing research and observational data that suggested that weight management in general requires more physical activity than was originally prescribed for overall health. The increased physical activity requirement for weight management and obesity treatment was previously suggested by many other groups, including the International Association for the Study of Obesity Stock Conference report in 2002, the Institute of Medicine Committee on Dietary Reference Intakes report in 2002, and the researchers from the NWCR. Although some differences remain, these two sets of guidelines that are available in the United States now are consistent in that they recognize a much larger volume of physical activity is necessary when weight management and obesity treatment are the key treatment variables.

Finally, a set of guidelines specific to a subset of individuals struggling with obesity is also under development. This set of guidelines will refer specifically to physical activity recommendations for individuals before and after obesity surgery. The American Society of Metabolic and Bariatric Surgeons and the ACSM have established an expert panel to develop pre- and postoperative recommendations for physical activity. At the time of press, these guidelines are yet to be completed and published. The goal will be to identify special needs of the individual who has undergone obesity surgery and how physical activity can optimize his or her surgical outcome. For an excellent review on physical activity and obesity surgery, please see King and Bond (25). As a highlight, in a review of 17 studies, obesity surgery patients who participated in regular physical activity had a 3.6 kg (7.9-lb) greater weight loss. Patients who did not participate in regular physical activity had a 2.3 times greater odds of unsuccessful weight loss (26).

VOLUME VERSUS INTENSITY OF PHYSICAL ACTIVITY AND WEIGHT

Individuals trying to address weight control and the disease of obesity often ask whether it is more important to focus their efforts on a higher volume of physical activity at a lower intensity or a lower volume of physical activity at a higher intensity. In other words, are the calories burned equivalent, which would allow an individual to reduce their total time requirement by increasing their physical activity intensity?

Physical activity intensity can be described in terms of metabolic equivalents (METs). The amount of oxygen consumed or metabolic work done during quiet sitting is defined as "at rest" and is equal to 1 MET. Physical activity intensity has been classified as light, <3 METs; moderate, 3 to 6 METs; and vigorous, >6 METs (23). The reference to light, moderate, and vigorous are therefore specific, and the previously discussed guidelines specifically refer to these levels of intensity. Researchers have quantified 605 activities based on their MET requirement in the "Compendium of Physical Activities" (27). This compendium, although initially developed for researchers, is useful to clinicians as well. Clinically, it can assist a health care provider in prescribing appropriate physical activity choices for their patients. A similar compendium has been developed specifically for youth (28).

Importantly, the compendium offers absolute intensity levels and does not take into account variations in weight, body mass index (BMI), or body composition. Researchers have demonstrated that the compendium values underestimate the energy cost or MET level of weight-bearing physical activity in individuals with overweight or obesity and overestimate the MET level of non–weight-bearing physical activity (29) (see also Exercise Testing for Exercise Clearance section for further discussion). Still, the compendium is useful as a guide and can help health care providers begin the conversation about level and intensity of physical activity, which then must be translated into an individualized exercise prescription.

The Cochrane review on "Exercise for Overweight or Obesity" from 2006 looked at physical activity intensity, volume, and changes in weight. The review examined the pooled effect of many studies. The review reported that in four randomized controlled trials, exercising at greater than 60% of maximal oxygen consumption (VO_2 max) is more effective at promoting weight loss than exercising at less intense levels (1.5 kg), when there were no dietary changes (30). Interestingly, when dietary changes were added to the analysis, exercise still contributed a modest amount to weight loss, but the intensity of exercise was no longer a factor. In other words, the effects of moderate-intensity physical activity were similar to those of vigorous physical activity when calorie restriction was added to the intervention. Keep in mind that the exercise involved in these pooled studies was, on average, 3 to 5 days per week and ranged dramatically from 10 to 60 minutes (30). This wide range in volume and intensity of physical activity across individuals may have made it impossible to separate out significant differences. Given what is currently understood about physical activity and weight loss or maintenance, this volume of physical activity may have been sufficient in subjects at the high end of frequency and duration (i.e., high volume), but insufficient at the low end to demonstrate significant results when combined with the known larger effect of diet.

Similarly, Jakicic et al. (15) found no difference in weight loss when the total volume of EE was kept constant, but intensity ranged from moderate to vigorous over the course of 12 months. There is some evidence to suggest that physical activity intensity may have very specific benefits to individual comorbid conditions of obesity. For example, increased exercise intensity was found to reduce fasting serum glucose to a greater extent than lower intensity exercise (30). Overall, the literature suggests that sufficient volume of physical activity is more important in achieving weight loss or weight maintenance goals and that intensity of physical activity can be left to individual choice and ability level and optimized to decrease risk of injury.

PHYSICAL ACTIVITY AND COMORBID CONDITIONS OF OBESITY

Physical activity is not only helpful in the long-term treatment of obesity but also has a positive effect on many comorbid conditions of obesity. Physical activity is inversely related to all-cause mortality (31–33). In adults, exercise decreases overall risk of early death, heart disease, hypertension, stroke, diabetes, hyperlipidemia, metabolic syndrome, colon and breast cancer, anxiety, depression, and falls (5). Physical activity also improves bone density, sleep quality, and cardiorespiratory endurance. In children, it results in improved metabolic health biomarkers, bone health, body composition, cardiorespiratory fitness, and muscular fitness and decreased anxiety and depression (5).

EXERCISE TESTING FOR EXERCISE CLEARANCE

The risk of an acute cardiac event during exercise from underlying CAD is increased in individuals with obesity, because obesity itself a risk factor for CAD (34). In addition, individuals affected by overweight or obesity tend to carry multiple risk factors for CAD beyond their elevated BMI. These individuals have an increased incidence of metabolic syndrome, diabetes, impaired fasting glucose, dyslipidemia, and hypertension (34). However, the risk of an acute cardiac event is lower in individuals with CAD that participate in regular physical activity than in those who do not (35,36). The AHA states that maintaining regular physical activity may reduce the risk of exercise-related cardiac events during heavy exertional activities (35). Individuals who were active four or more times per week had a much lower relative risk of an adverse event than those who were physically active less than four times per week (36). Although no specific testing is identified, the AHA statement also recommends preparticipation screening and avoidance of certain exercises in high-risk patients.

The ACSM provides a set of "Guidelines for Exercise Testing and Prescription" (37). Under these guidelines, ACSM recommends diagnostic exercise testing in patients based on an initial assessment of their CAD risk factors. Risk factors include the following: (1) family history of myocardial infarction before 55 years old in first-degree male relative or before 65 years old in first-degree female relative, (2) smoking within the last 6 months, (3) hypertension, (4) abnormal lipids, (5) impaired fasting glucose—greater than 100 mg/dL, (6) obesity—BMI ≥30, and (7) sedentary lifestyle. Exercise testing is recommended in asymptomatic patients with "moderate risk of CAD" who plan to participate in physical activity that is >75% of their maximal heart rate. Moderate risk is defined as any man ≥45 years and woman ≥55 years *or* two or more risk factors listed above. Physical activity that is >75% of the patient's maximal heart rate is considered vigorous. However in individuals with overweight or obesity, this could correlate with activities that are defined as "moderate intensity" according to absolute MET level. As discussed previously, the compendium of MET levels will underestimate an individual's relative intensity during land-based activities when they have the disease of obesity.

For example, if the fitness level of an individual is low due to deconditioning, exercises that would normally be considered at the high end of "moderate" physical activity (5–6 METs) would actually be "vigorous" physical activity for this individual (>6 METs). For example, walking at a 4.0 mph pace on a level, firm surface is considered 5.0 METs. This would be classified as moderate physical activity in absolute terms. However, if an individual with obesity is deconditioned, this same intensity of walking may actually be a vigorous activity when their individual capacity is taken into account. This scenario can occur frequently in patients with obesity and directly affects exercise prescription for these individuals. An algorithm to determine whether screening is needed prior to the initiation of an exercise regimen is available in the ACSM guidelines (37).

Exercise testing in patients affected by obesity may also require modifications to the testing protocols and the testing equipment. For example, most patients with overweight or obesity require either a large or even more often a thigh-sized blood pressure cuff. A blood pressure cuff that is too small can elicit an inaccurately elevated reading. Orthopedic limitations may require accommodation by adjusting the type of exercise testing equipment used for the test. Some clients will require arm or leg ergometry instead of a standard treadmill due to lower extremity arthritis or other orthopedic pathology. Finally, the actual stress test protocol may need to be adjusted. Some patients with obesity have such a low fitness capacity that a lower initial workload (measured in METs) and smaller increases in workload increments per stage of the testing protocol are required. The ACSM guidelines for exercise testing recommend that the initial workload may need to be decreased to 2 to 3 METs and the workload increments reduced to 0.5 to 1.0 MET in individuals with obesity (37).

Because of severely decreased functional capacity and orthopedic issues, individuals affected by overweight or obesity often cannot complete an "adequate" stress test. In other words, functional limitations often result in an inadequate test because the patient fails to reach 85% of their maximal predicted heart rate. Although this suboptimal result cannot rule out cardiac ischemia at higher levels of physical activity, it does provide the individual and the medical provider a level of reassurance within the scope of the individual's current functional capacity. This type of result is typically interpreted as "negative and inadequate." Maximal heart rate measured during the test can be used to calculate a targeted heart rate training range during prescribed physical activity. It is unlikely that an individual will exert his or herself to a greater extent during a regular workout than during the exercise stress test.

In addition to standard treadmill exercise stress testing, sometimes testing with imaging modalities is required. In the population with overweight or obesity, a few additional details must be considered. Nuclear imaging may or may not be possible secondary to table weight limitations for the computed tomography scanner. Most standard tables have a 350 lb weight limit. Nuclear imaging may require two consecutive days of testing secondary to the increased body mass. A stress echocardiogram can also be used, but results may be affected by body habitus interference that can diminish the quality.

In general, individuals affected by overweight or obesity are more likely to require exercise testing than the general population because they are more likely to have related comorbidities that increase their risk for CAD. As functional capacity increases with decreased weight, improved cardiorespiratory fitness, and typically improved orthopedic limitations, repeat cardiac testing should be considered to obtain an "adequate" test at 85% of predicted maximal heart rate. Exercise testing not only provides reassurance for an individual's safety to participate in physical activity but also can help guide exercise prescription. During weight loss and weight maintenance, exercise testing data can provide a measure of maximal functional capacity in MET levels guide submaximal exercise prescription.

EXERCISE OR PHYSICAL ACTIVITY PRESCRIPTION

An exercise prescription should include the five fundamentals of physical fitness regardless of BMI classification: cardiovascular endurance, muscular strength, muscular endurance, flexibility, and body composition. Eventually, a comprehensive exercise program should address and improve all the five fundamentals. To build this program, individuals need instructions that are clear, simple, and based on measurable goals. These instructions come in the form of an exercise or physical activity prescription.

At a minimum, prescriptions should cover the five components of physical activity that are outlined within the abbreviation "FITTE": frequency, intensity, time, type, and enjoyment. Initially, individuals should be assessed for their current level of physical activity participation. This information will directly affect the volume and intensity of exercise prescribed. Then, to meet the requirements of FITTE, a prescription should indicate how often, how hard, how long, and what kind of exercise will be done. FITTE should be completed for the four activity-related fundamentals of physical fitness, that is, cardio, strength, muscular endurance, and flexibility.

Optimally, exercise or physical activity prescriptions should include a few additional key components. Motivational interviewing techniques and stages of change research have demonstrated the importance of assessing an individual's readiness for change. The physical activity prescription and related goals for someone in contemplation about exercise will be very different from an individual who is in the action or maintenance stages. It is important to discuss appropriate and realistic goals. The prescribing provider will need to strategize with the individual about the techniques to handle lapses and relapses into sedentary habits. Ideally, the written prescription will have a place for the health care provider and the individual patient to sign. This allows the prescription to become a contract that is no longer passive, but now actively engages the commitment of the individual. A copy of the prescription should be retained in the patient record for review and modification at follow-up visits.

Finally, consider exposing the individual to the concept of "optimal default." In the United States today, we have successfully engineered most physical activity out of our lives. Individuals affected by obesity need to find ways to reincorporate as much physical activity back into their activities of daily living (ADL) as possible in an effort to accumulate the large volumes of physical activity described previously as required for success. Examples can be simple and creative: take the stairs, change the mode of transportation from passive (driving) to active (walking or cycling), park farther away, fidget more, initiate active hobbies, meet friends for a walk instead of a coffee, consider a standing or walking workstation, or stand whenever you take a phone call. If an individual's original physical activity plan for the day, week, or year runs into a barrier, have a default (not just a backup plan) that creates increased physical activity.

SPECIAL CONSIDERATIONS IN EXERCISE PRESCRIPTION

Equipment modifications

Individuals affected by overweight or obesity can require specialized exercise equipment. Strength training equipment is now available to allow appropriate access for individuals with obesity to enter and exit the equipment with ease. Cardiovascular equipment such as treadmills, elliptical trainers, and recumbent bicycles are available that have increased maximal weight limits. Recumbent bicycles often have larger more comfortable and appropriate seating. Upright stationary bicycles often do not have standard seat modifications, but the seat is often easily removable and an alternative wider seat can be attached. Physiology balls come in a variety of maximum static and dynamic weight capacities. These should be evaluated carefully based on an individual's needs. Physiology balls also come in varying shapes. Different shapes can increase or decrease the balance challenge requirement to help develop core strength skills safely when obesity or a previously sedentary lifestyle is a concern. In general, equipment used by clients with obesity, especially those in class III obesity or higher, requires clarification of weight limits.

Personal equipment and attire should also be considered carefully. Aqua belts need to have adequate buoyancy support. Athletic footwear often needs to be increased in shoe width to accommodate increased fat deposition, and/or lower extremity swelling from lymphedema. Individuals with large anterior fat deposition in the form of a pannus often require careful attention to skin care during physical activity. Clothing that is developed to pull moisture away from the body can help minimize candidal infections and skin breakdown in dependent skin folds. Waistbands need to be comfortable and nonrestrictive. Tight clothing in the lower torso can lead to meralgia numbness of the anterior leg (paresthetica) that, although unlikely to cause harm, can be uncomfortable and become a barrier to physical activity participation.

Monitoring physical activity in patients with obesity

Using tools to monitor physical activity can help determine an individual's compliance with and response to obesity treatment, weight loss, or weight maintenance program. Tracking individual progress can also assist with patient motivation. Individuals can use physical activity recall surveys, physical activity logs, pedometers, or accelerometers to keep track of their physical activity participation.

Physical activity surveys can be completed at regular intervals and reviewed by the patient and the medical provider. Surveys ask the individual to look back and estimate their physical activity participation or compliance. They are typically quick, but can be affected by the patient's ability to recall information correctly, termed *recall bias*. A physical activity log, if done daily, can be more accurate, but it still depends on the subjective assessment of the individual. Because these logs are done with more frequency, they are more labor-intensive. On-line programs can ease some of the burden and provide ongoing feedback to the individual that is often useful and motivational.

Direct measurement of physical activity is preferred; however, there are obstacles when obesity is present. Some older physical activity measurement devices may be less accurate in the population with obesity. Previous studies have demonstrated conflicting results. Initially researchers reported that pedometers, used to measure step counts, were less accurate in individuals with obesity (38,39). Other studies have reported that pedometer accuracy was unaffected by BMI (40,41). A more recent investigation by Crouter et al. (42) suggests that the type of pedometer may play a role in whether BMI classification, waist circumference, and position of the pedometer (due to increased abdominal fat) affect the accuracy of the results. In general, when an inaccuracy was found, it was typically an underestimation of actual steps (42).

Accelerometers, electronic motion sensors that detect changes in acceleration, can also be used to track physical activity. Accelerometers provide more in-depth information regarding physical activity than pedometers, the latter of which only count number of steps. Accelerometers record frequency, intensity, and duration of physical activity. Few studies exist that have looked at accelerometer use specifically in the adult overweight or obese population (43–45). A recent study found that the amount of time an individual with obesity must wear an accelerometer to get a reliable estimation of physical activity is probably less than originally expected. The researchers reported that 6 hours of monitored time per day for 4 days was sufficient to reliably estimate moderate-to-vigorous physical activity participation (43). In a nonresearch setting, using pedometers or accelerometers can provide individuals with immediate objective daily feedback on whether their physical activity intentions are consistent with their daily actions, and more importantly their obesity treatment plan and weight management goals. Advances in technology now allow for many relatively inexpensive accelerometry options that interface with computer websites and smart phones. These advances have reduced the monitoring burden for the individual and increased the ability to get objective data for the health care provider. Many platforms provide individuals with feedback, motivational cues, corrective advice, and opportunities to create an active network of friends. Overall, monitoring is essential and may be most useful in individuals who find physical activity less enjoyable or struggle with compliance for any reason. Monitoring can serve as a trigger to improve regular participation in physical activity.

Mobility issues and physical activity in individuals with obesity

Physical activity in individuals with overweight and obesity can be directly affected by underlying mobility issues. Obesity leads to increased functional limitations and disabilities with age in both men and women. These deficits range from mild to severe and include ADL and instrumental ADL (46). Degenerative joint disease, previous total joint replacements or other orthopedic repairs, and previous or active injuries may affect participation in physical activity. Weight-bearing exercises with increased impact, such as a moderate-to-high impact group exercise classes, jogging, and treadmill walking or running often need to be avoided or restricted until a substantial amount of weight is lost. Mobility in the population affected by obesity is frequently affected by spinal pathology and pain, lower extremity problems, and balance deficits.

For example, obesity is associated with increased rates of osteoarthritis in the knee. The risk of osteoarthritis of the knee is 6.8 times greater in the obese population than in the lean population (47). In addition, individuals with obesity and osteoarthritis of the knees are 9.8 times more likely to experience deterioration in physical function than lean individuals with no arthritis (48). Body mass is a major determinant of decreased mobility, termed *mobility disability*, in 55- to 74-year-old adults. Angleman et al. (49) measured mobility disability using a timed 8-ft walk and self-reported difficulty with variables such as walking 100 yards, getting up from a chair after extended time spent sitting, and climbing several flights of stairs without rest. Increased body mass was related to decreased mobility. From a measurement standpoint, waist circumference was found to be the best predictor for obesity-related mobility disability (49).

Overweight or obesity also leads to an abnormal gait secondary to multiple biomechanical changes, including forefoot positioning, shortened stride, and rear-foot motion (50). Individuals with obesity are 5 times more likely to experience heel pain and plantar fasciitis than individuals with a normal BMI (51). These are just select examples of many orthopedic issues that affect physical activity participation and exercise prescription in individuals struggling with obesity.

In older adults with a BMI greater than 30 kg/m^2, obesity is also related to decreased balance regardless of overall strength (52). Individuals affected by obesity report an increased fear of falling (53). The odds of sustaining an injury, including those from falls, is increased 15% in the overweight population and 48% in patients with class III obesity (BMI ≥ 40) compared to normal-weight individuals (54).

Finally, adipose tissue itself can be a physical barrier to effective movement. It can actually obstruct getting into proper exercise positions or executing movement. Abdominal adipose tissue, including a large pannus, can prevent full hip flexion in either the seated or supine position. This makes stretching the iliotibial band, medial gluteus muscle, hamstrings, and low back difficult. These body areas are among those commonly injured in newly active individuals if not stretched adequately in a comprehensive exercise plan. A large dependent pannus can also severely limit land-based physical activity due to uncomfortable tissue movement, rubbing, and skin tension. This may occur with treadmill, elliptical, stationary bicycle, and recumbent exercise equipment in addition to free-motion land movement.

Evaluating individuals for mobility deficits or barriers is essential in the process of successful exercise prescription and long-term physical activity participation.

Resources for physical activity prescription

There are many resources available as examples for physical activity prescription. The American Academy of Family Physicians (AAFP) has developed a provider toolkit that includes an exercise prescription pad, BMI calculators, a physician primer, and tools for patients as they embark on increased physical activity as a medical management approach to their weight and weight-related comorbidities. The toolkit is part of the AAFP initiative called Americans in Motion (AIM)-Health Interventions (HI). The "AIM to Change Toolkit" can be found on the AAFP website at www.aafp.org. The National Heart, Lung, and Blood Institute also has helpful resources that are targeted and family- and community-based resources; these resources can be found under the "We Can" program on the www.nhlbi.nih.gov/health website. Finally, the CDC is always expanding and adding to their physical activity–enhancing resources. See their website at www.cdc.gov. When reviewing resources, it is important to recognize and understand the continuum of "Stages of Change" and how it can be useful when helping patients increase their level of physical activity by giving information and direction that is stage specific.

The goals for physical activity and exercise prescription in the individuals with overweight or obesity go beyond the contribution to EE and weight loss or weight maintenance. Physical activity prescription in this population needs to include goals regarding fat-free mass preservation, mobility associated with ADL, reduced pain, increased overall flexibility, improved strength, and decreased risk of fall. All of these considerations are in addition to typical calorie expenditure and improved cardiovascular health expectations.

Novel approaches to increasing physical activity and interrupting sedentary behavior

Increasing physical activity in the United States, as one of many methods to treat overweight and obesity, requires a matrix of solutions to support the differences between people and their varied living environments. Health care providers, public health specialists, researchers, exercise specialists, policy makers, and entrepreneurs are all introducing novel approaches to increasing EE through physical activity. Some approaches include environmental changes like innovative city planning and developmental models to increase pedestrian activities. Others are more behaviorally focused, including mass marketing approaches such as the CDC's campaign to increase physical activity in children. Policy changes are slow in coming, but they are beginning to emerge. Americans now have the ability to claim their health club or wellness center membership dues as a tax deduction. Similarly, many larger US companies offer partial payment for health club memberships and employee bonuses for voluntarily meeting or improving upon basic physical fitness criteria.

Perhaps one of the more creative recent solutions revolves around a concept called nonexercise activity thermogenesis (NEAT). Although the acronym is novel, the underlying premise reverts back to the idea that not all physical activities that contribute to EE are in the form of exercise. Recalling the earlier discussion about the total energy equation, EE = REE + TEM + EEPA, nonexercise activity thermogenesis is equal to total EE from physical activity minus exercise (or EEPA; EE from exercise = NEAT). EEPA accounts for approximately 30% of total daily EE. Unlike resting EE or the thermic effect of food, it is largely modifiable and appears to be highly variable from person to person. Researchers estimate that EE from physical activity that does not include intentional exercise may vary by up to 2000 kcal per day. Highly active individuals expend 3 times more energy per day than inactive individuals (55).

In considering a solution to the obesity epidemic, how could an inactive individual be converted to highly active individual if his or her day does not allow for dedicated time to exercise? Consider that the average American spends 1000 to 2000 hours at work per year. Researchers believe that this extensive time spent sitting may play a key role in the development of and solution to obesity. Could physical activity be constructed and introduced such that it occurs simultaneously and without interrupting an individual's workday? A major determinant in answering this question depends on how a given individual's workday is constructed. For a commercial airline pilot, it would be difficult to redesign a cockpit to allow for increased physical activity. However, for the majority of workers in America who spend a large component of their day sitting at a desk, there may be many relatively simple solutions. Researchers have been examining the possibility of increasing daily physical activity by transitioning workers from a sedentary chair-dependent work environment to an active work environment.

One proposed solution is to replace an individual's chair-dependent workstation (i.e., a desk) with an active workstation that uses a treadmill or bicycle. However, the goal is not to exercise. Recall that exercise has a purpose: to increase or maintain physical fitness. The goal of an active workstation is not to improve or maintain cardiovascular fitness, but to increase EE throughout the day by making sedentary work tasks slightly active. For example, in an exercise bout, an individual might walk at a speed of approximately 4 mph. When walking at a treadmill workstation, an individual would walk at less than 2 mph. The MET level for walking at less than 2 mph is 2.0. This would be classified as light physical activity. In comparison, walking at 4 mph corresponds to a MET level of 5.0, or moderate-intensity physical activity. The goal of an active workstation is not to exercise; the goal is to increase EE while completing normal work tasks. Levine et al. (56) suggest that increasing standing or ambulating time by 2.5 hours per day could result in an additional 350 kcal per day of energy output. Depending on an individual as a responder versus a nonresponder, this could amount to 9 to 11.3 kg (20–25 lb) over the course of a year (56).

Keep in mind, this type of increased EE has been shown to improve weight over time, but it will not provide the same mechanical cardiovascular benefits of more moderate or vigorous physical activity but may provide improvements in other cardiovascular risk markers. NEAT may be found to play a significant role in decreasing the suggested volume of 300 minutes of physical activity per week (discussed herein in the review of guidelines) to a more manageable volume of exercise during nonwork leisure-time hours. See Table 6.2 for suggestions.

Many other approaches to increasing EE throughout the day can be considered. Maximizing pedestrian activity whenever possible by, for example, parking farther away from a destination when driving, bicycling for transportation, using the stairs instead of elevators or escalators,

Table 6.2 Reincorporating physical activity into activities of daily living

Take the stairs

Change your mode of transportation from passive (driving) to active (walking or cycling)

Park farther away from stores

Fidget more

Start an active hobby (bring fun into activity)

Meet friends for a walk instead of coffee or food

Consider a standing or walking workstation (desk)

Increase active family time: backyard Olympics, front yard baseball, family room dancing

Plan active vacations: checkout walking, cycling, and hiking vacations in United States and Europe

Take on a new sport: great for your brain and your weight

or avoiding horizontal people movers such as those found in airports. Have patients consider a "wake-up" walk on their lunch hour (Table 6.3).

Even personal time can become more physically active without necessarily spending time at the gym. Recreational activities can incorporate more movement. Spending time as a family can be transitioned away from sedentary activities such as television and movies and refocused on active options such as backyard Olympics, family-oriented 3k and 5k fun walks or runs, or block party baseball with the neighbors. Consider active vacations that can be individually developed, but are also now available through travel agencies. Companies now specialize in walking, hiking, cycling, kayaking, climbing, and many other active adventure vacations. Encourage patients managing obesity to participate in creative problem solving. There are infinite ways to increase physical activity throughout the day.

The other novel approach to consider is the concept of interrupting sedentary behavior. Interrupting sedentary behavior is a separate and complimentary approach to using moderate and vigorous physical activity to meet the physical activity guidelines. Interrupting sedentary behavior occurs when an individual moves from sitting to standing or light activity. Although the United States does not, some countries have established sedentary behavior guidelines in addition to physical activity guidelines. The growing volume of peer-reviewed publications on interrupting sedentary behavior demonstrates the increased focus of scientists in the area. The number of articles per year had increased from less than 200 articles in 1995 to more than 1200 articles in 2012 (57). One important driver as to why sedentary interruption may become increasingly important is evident when occupational data from 1960 to 2008 are evaluated. The percentage of jobs in the United States that would be classified as moderate-intensity occupations has dropped by more than one-half in the past five decades. At the same time, light and sedentary occupations have increased by approximately 20% and 10%, respectively (58).

In patients with obesity, sitting less is associated with a lower mortality rate (59). The mortality rate of individuals with obesity who reported sitting most of their day was 4 times greater than those that reported sitting from almost none of their day to up to half of their day. Thus, even cutting sitting time in half may substantially lower mortality risk. In a study by Duvivier et al. (60), individuals were asked to replace sitting time with standing or light activity. Compared to individuals who sat the majority of the day, but participated in 1 hour of moderate to vigorous cycling, individuals who converted approximately one-half of their day to interrupted sedentary behavior had more improvement in plasma lipids and insulin action. Finally, for every 15-minute increase in sedentary behavior over time there

Table 6.3 Energy levels required to perform some common activities

<3 METs	3–5 METs	5–7 METs	7–9 METs	>9 METs
Washing	Cleaning windows	Easy digging in garden	Sawing wood	Carrying load up stairs
Shaving	Raking	Hand lawn mowing	Heavy shoveling	Climbing stairs quickly
Dressing	Power lawn mowing	Climbing stairs slowly	Climbing stairs	Shoveling heavy snow
Desk work	Carrying objects (15–30 lb)	Carrying objects (30–60 lb)	Carrying objects (60–90 lb)	
Washing dishes				
Driving auto				
Light housekeeping				
Golf (cart)	Golf (walking)	Tennis (singles)	Canoeing	Handball
Knitting	Dancing (social)	Basketball, football	Mountain climbing	Ski touring
Hand sewing	Tennis (doubles)	Snow skiing (downhill)		
Walking (2 mph)	Level walking (3–4 mph)	Level walking (4.5–5.0 mph)	Level jogging (5 mph)	Running >6 mph
Stationary bike	Level biking (6–8 mph)	Bicycling (9–10 mph)	Bicycling (12 mph)	Walking uphill (5 mph)
Very light calisthenics	Light calisthenics	Swimming, breast stroke	Swimming, crawl	Rope jumping
			Rowing machine	Bicycling (>12 mph)

is a 0.13-cm increase in waist circumference (61). Although there is much more to learn, it has become clear that a combined effort of obtaining adequate moderate-to-vigorous physical activity as well as shifting other sedentary segments of everyday life to light activity will likely provide the most ideal benefits.

SUMMARY

In summary, physical activity is a vital component to weight and health management and essential in the long-term treatment of obesity. Armed with scientific evidence behind the current guidelines, tools for patient assessment, and a thorough physical activity prescription, medical providers can facilitate a patient's transition to a more active life. Become familiar with local resources, including recreational and athletic facilities, physical activity trainers, exercise physiologists, community experts, and physical therapists. These resources will help guide a patient as he or she transitions. Finally, keep in mind that advances in technology have engineered almost all physical activities out of everyday life. To aid in weight loss and succeed at obesity treatment and weight maintenance, an individual needs to re-engineer physical activity back into his or her life, perhaps in new and creative ways, AND participate in traditional exercise.

REFERENCES

1. Ogden CL, Carroll MD, Kit BK, Flegal KM. *Prevalence of Obesity among Adults: United States, 2011–2012.* NCHS data brief, no. 131. Hyattsville, MD: National Center for Health Statistics; 2013.
2. The State of Obesity Report: Better Policies for a Healthier America 2014. Robert Wood Johnson Foundation and Trust for America's Health. www.healthyamericans. org, accessed March 24, 2015.
3. U.S. Centers for Disease Control and Prevention. *One in Five Adults Meet Overall Physical Activity Guidelines* [Press Release]. 2013. http://www.cdc.gov/media/ releases/2013/p0502-physicalactivity.html, accessed March, 2015.
4. Behavioral Risk Factor Surveillance System. http://www.cdc.gov/brfss/
5. US Department of Health and Human Services. *2008 Physical Activity Guidelines for Americans.* www.health.gov/paguidelines/summary.aspx
6. Catenacci VA, Odgen LG, Stuht J, et al. Physical activity patterns in the National Weight Control Registry. *Obesity* 2008; 16(1): 153–161.
7. Jakicic JM, Marcus BH, Lang W, Janney C. Effect of exercise on 24-month weight loss maintenance in overweight women. *Arch Intern Med* 2008; 168: 1550–1559, discussion 1559–1560.
8. Caspersen CJ, Powell KE, Christenson GM. Physical activity, exercise, and physical fitness: Definitions and distinctions for health-related research. *Public Health Rep* 1985; 100(2): 126–131.
9. Tataranni PA, Larson DE, Ravussin E. Body fat distribution and energy metabolism in obese men and women. *J Am Coll Nutr* 1994; 13(6): 569–574.
10. Donnelly JE, Blair SN, Jakicic JM, Manore MM, Rankin JW, Smith BK. American College of Sports Medicine Position Stand. Appropriate physical activity intervention strategies for weight loss and prevention of weight regain for adults. *Med Sci Sports Exerc* 2009; 41(2): 459–471.

11. Stevens J, Truesdale KP, McClain JE, Cai J. The definition of weight maintenance. *Int J Obes* 2006; 30: 391–399.
12. Hagan RD, Upton SJ, Wong L, Whittam J. The effects of aerobic conditioning and/or calorie restriction in overweight men and women. *Med Sci Sports Exerc* 1986; 18: 87–94.
13. Wing RR, Vendetti EM, Jakicic JM, Polley BA, Lang W. Lifestyle intervention in overweight individuals with a family history of diabetes. *Diabetes Care* 1998; 21: 350–353.
14. Jakicic JM, Winters C, Lang W, Wing RR. Effects of intermittent exercise and use of home exercise equipment on adherence, weight loss and prevention of weight regain for adults. *JAMA* 1999; 282: 1554–1560.
15. Jakicic JM, Marcus BH, Gallgher KL, Napolitano M, Lang W. Effect of exercise duration and intensity on weight loss in overweight sedentary women. *JAMA* 2003; 290: 1323.
16. Jakicic JM, Otto AD. Treatment and prevention of obesity: What is the role of exercise? *Nutr Rev* 2006; 64(2): S57–S61.
17. Hill JO, Hyatt HR. Role of physical activity in preventing and treating obesity. *J Appl Physiol* 2005; 99: 765–770.
18. Fogelholm M, Kukkonen-Harjula K. Does physical activity prevent weight gain: A systematic review. *Obes Rev* 2000; 1: 95–111.
19. Jakicic JM. The role of physical activity in the prevention and treatment of body weight gain in adults. *J Nutr* 2002; 132: 3826S–3829S.
20. Thomas JG, Bond DS, Phelan S, Hill JO, Wing RR. Weight-loss maintenance for 10 years in the National Weight Control Registry. *Am J Prev Med* 2014; 46(1): 17–23.
21. Diaz VA, Mainous AG 3rd, Everett CJ. The association between weight fluctuation and mortality: Results from a population based cohort study. *J Community Health* 2005; 30(3): 153–165.
22. Blair SN, Shaten J, Brownell K, Collins G, Lissner L. Body weight change, all-cause mortality, and cause-specific mortality in the multiple risk factor intervention trial. *Ann Intern Med* 1993; 119(7 pt 2): 749–757.
23. Pate RR, Pratt M, Blair SN, et al. Physical activity and public health: A recommendation from the Centers for Disease Control and Prevention and the American College of Sports Medicine. *JAMA* 1995; 273: 402–407.
24. Haskell WL, Lee I, Pate RR, Powell KE, Blair SN. Physical activity and public health: Updated recommendation for adults from the American College of Sports Medicine and the American Heart Association. *Med Sci Sports Exerc* 2007; 39(8): 1423–1434.
25. King WC, Bond DS. The importance of preoperative and postoperative physical activity counseling in bariatric surgery. *Exerc Sport Sci Rev* 2013; 41(1): 26–35.
26. Egberts K, Brown WA, Brennan L, O'Brien PE. Does exercise improve weight loss after bariatric surgery? A systematic review. *Obesity Surgery* 2012; 22: 335–341.
27. Ainsworth BE, Haskell WL, Whitt MC, et al. Compendium of physical activities: An update of activity codes and MET intensities. *Med Sci Sports Exerc* 2000; 32(9 Suppl): S498–S516.
28. Ridley K, Ainsworth BE, Olds TS. Development of a compendium of energy expenditures for youth. *Int J Behav Nutr Phys Act* 2008; 5: 45.
29. Howell W, Earthman C, Reid P, Delaney J, Houtkooper L. Doubly labeled water validation of the compendium of physical activities in lean and obese college women (Abstract). *Med Sci Sports Exerc* 1999; 31: S142.
30. Shaw K, Gennat H, O'Rourke P, Del Mar C. Exercise for overweight or obesity. *Cochrane Database Syst Rev* 2006; (4): CD003817.

31. Paffenbarger RS, Hyde RT, Wing AL, Hsieh CC. Physical activity, all-cause mortality, and longevity of college alumni. *N Engl J Med* 1986; 314: 605–613.
32. Paffenbarger RS, Hyde RT, Wing AL, Lee I-M, Jung DL, Kampert JB. The association of changes in physical activity level among other lifestyle characteristics with mortality among men. *N Engl J Med* 1993; 328: 538–545.
33. Lee I-M, Rexrode KM, Cook NR, Manson JE, Buring JE. Physical activity and coronary heart disease in women. *JAMA* 2001; 285: 1447–1454.
34. Cho E, Manson JE, Stampfer MJ, et al. A prospective study of obesity and risk of coronary heart disease among diabetic women. *Diabetes Care* 2002; 25(7): 1142–1148.
35. Thompson PD, Franklin BA, Balady GJ, et al. Exercise and acute cardiovascular events placing the risks into perspective: A scientific statement from the American Heart Association Council on Nutrition, Physical Activity, and Metabolism and the Council on Clinical Cardiology. *Circulation* 2007; 115(17): 2358–2368.
36. Giri S, Thompson PD, Liernan FJ, et al. Clinical and angiographic characteristics of exertion-related acute myocardial infarction. *JAMA* 1999; 282(18): 1731–1736.
37. Whaley M, ed. *ACSM Guidelines for Exercise Testing and Prescription*. 9th ed. (Philadelphia: Lippincot, Williams & Wilkins) 2014.
38. Melanson EL, Knoll JR, Bell ML, Donahoo WT, Hill JO, Nysse LJ. Commercially available pedometers: Considerations for accurate step counting. *Prev Med* 2004; 39: 361–368.
39. Shepherd EF, Toloza E, McClung CD, Schmalzried TP. Step activity monitor: Increased accuracy in quantifying ambulatory activity. *J Orthop Res* 1999; 17: 703–708.
40. Swartz AM, Bassett DR Jr., Moore JB, Thompson DL, Strath SJ. Effects of body mass index on accuracy of an electronic pedometer. *Int J Sports Med* 2003; 24: 588–592.
41. Elsenbaumer KM, Tudor-Locke C. Accuracy of pedometers in adults stratified by body mass index category. *Med Sci Sports Exerc* 2003; 35: S282.
42. Crouter SE, Schneider PL, Bassett DR Jr. Spring-levered versus Piezo-electric pedometer accuracy in overweight and obese adults. *Med Sci Sports Exerc* 2005; 37(10): 1673–1679.
43. Jerome GJ, Young DR, Laferriere D, Chen C, Vollmer WM. Reliability of RT3 accelerometers among overweight and obese adults. *Med Sci Sports Exerc* 2009; 41(1): 110–114.
44. Fogelholm M, Hiiloskorpi H, Laukkanen R, Oja P, VanMarken Lichtenbelt W, Westerterp K. Assessment of energy expenditure in overweight women. *Med Sci Sports Exerc* 1998; 30: 1191–1197.
45. Jacobi D, Perrin AE, Grosman N, et al. Physical activity-related energy expenditure with the RT3 and TriTrac accelerometers in overweight adults. *Obesity (Silver Spring)* 2007; 15(4): 950–956.
46. Houston DK, Stevens J, Cai J, Morey MC. Role of weight history on functional limitations and disability in late adulthood: The ARIC Study. *Obesity Res* 2005; 13: 1793–1802.
47. Coggon D, Reading I, Croft P, et al. Knee osteoarthritis and obesity. *Int J Obes Relat Metab Disord* 2001; 25(5): 622–627.
48. Ettinger WH, Davis MA, Neuhaus JM, et al. Long-term physical functioning in persons with knee osteoarthritis from NHANES I: Effects of comorbid medical conditions. *J Clin Epidemiol* 1994; 47(7): 809–815.
49. Angleman SB, Harris TB, Melzer D. The role of waist circumference in predicting disability in periretirement age adults. *Int J Obes* 2006; 30: 364–373.

50. Messier SP. Obesity and osteoarthritis: Disease genesis and nonpharmacologic weight management. *Med Clin North Am* 2009; 93(1): 145–159.

51. Riddle DL, Pulisic M, Pidcoe P, et al. Risk factors for plantar fasciitis: A matched case-control study. *J Bone Joint Surg Am* 2003; 85(5): 872–877.

52. Jadelis K, Milller ME, Ettinger WH, et al. Strength, balance, and the modifying effects of obesity and knee pain: Results from the Observational Arthritis Study in Seniors (OASIS). *J Am Geriatr Soc* 2001; 49(7): 884–891.

53. Austin N, Devine A, Dick I, et al. Fear of falling in older women: A longitudinal study of incidence, persistence, and predictors. *J Am Geriatr Soc* 2007; 55(10): 1598–1603.

54. Finkelstein EA, Chen H, Prabhu M, et al. The relationship between obesity and injuries among US adults. *Am J Health Promot* 2007; 21(5): 219–224.

55. Black AE, Coward WA, Cole TJ, Prentice AM. Human energy expenditure in affluent societies: An analysis of 574 doubly-labelled water measurements. *Eur J Clin Nutr* 1996; 50: 72–92.

56. Levine JA, Vander Weg MW, Hill JO, et al. Non-exercise activity thermogenesis: The crouching tiger hidden dragon of societal weight gain. *Arterioscler Thromb Vasc Biol* 2006; 26: 729–736.

57. Comparison of search of SCOPUS database during 1995 to search of SCOPUS database in 2012, accessed July 2013, from www.scopus.com

58. Church TS, Thomas DM, Tudor-Locke C, et al. Trends over 5 decades in U.S. occupation-related physical activity and their associations with obesity. *PLoS One* 2011; 6(5): e19657.

59. Katzmarzyk PT, Church TS, Craig CL, Bouchard C. Sitting time and mortality from all causes, cardiovascular disease, and cancer. *Med Sci Sports Exerc* 2009; 41: 998–1005.

60. Duvivier BMFM, Schaper NC, Bremers MA, et al. Minimal intensity physical activity of longer duration improves insulin action and plasma lipids more than shorter periods of moderate to vigorous exercise when energy expenditure is comparable. *PLoS One* 2013; 8(2): e55542.

61. Saunders TJ, Tremblay MS, Despres J-P, et al. Sedentary behavior, visceral fat accumulations, and cardiometabolic risk in adults: A 6-year longitudinal study from the Quebec Family Study. *PLoS One* 2013; 8(1): e54225.

7

Behavioral modification

ERIN CHAMBERLIN-SNYDER

INTRODUCTION

Behavior and lifestyle changes are necessary for weight loss and maintenance (1,2). This chapter discusses the importance of behavioral evaluation that includes interviewing and other methods of assessing a patient's desire to change. Goal setting and self-monitoring (food, activity, and behavior diaries) are integral to treatment, and specific practical hints and resources are included for the clinician's use (3). The rapid growth of personal use of technology and social media (e.g., apps on smart phones, websites, blogs) for health information has spurred clinical trials to study the effectiveness of these tools. Types of behavioral therapies are reviewed and examples are applied to the overweight or obese patient (4). Emotional factors, along with the hormonal and neurochemical processes, play a large role in disordered eating patterns. Current research studies are exploring the influence of the neurotransmitters on the limbic system of the human brain and the implications this influence has for behavior modification in the overweight or obese patient.

Self-defeating lifestyle choices (i.e., lack of self-restraint in food choices or self-discipline with exercising) used to be viewed as a lack of personal willpower. Even if clients lost weight initially, shaming or negative approaches rarely resulted in long-term success with weight maintenance. Now, in light of the findings of research on hunger hormones, neurotransmitters, and the effect of genetics and the environment, it is evident that treatment of obesity requires behavior modification, as well as nutrition education, increase in physical activity, medical evaluation, and sometimes pharmacotherapy (5).

Food programs should serve as a template to be adjusted on an individual basis, based on information from the patient's food and behavior diary and ongoing weight loss success. Individual tailoring of a food plan according to the patient's goals, family commitments, and work situations works best, but it takes homework on the part of the patient and bariatric team to review the diary, devise workable strategies and implement with the patient.

Exercise or increased physical activity normalizes neurotransmitters (such as serotonin and norepinephrine), optimizes cardiovascular health, increases muscle mass, and improves metabolism of nutrients, leading to a lower chance of weight regain. This important lifestyle change is the subject of Chapter 6 and should be noted as a critical change necessary for most obese people to lose weight.

Most behavioral programs in the past focused on participants changing diet and exercise. Personality and behavior tests were often used (6,7). Several assessment tools have since been developed to evaluate a wide range of specific behaviors, including disordered eating and thinking that may be present in a bariatric patient (8,9). As medical bariatricians, our expertise lies not only in the evaluation of genetic and physical causes of comorbid illnesses but also in the medical treatment of obesity, along with supplying huge doses of patient education and emotional support. Some clinicians provide the education piece in group sessions. The groups themselves can provide some emotional support to the patient and are a more efficient use of clinician time. Alternatively, individualized lifestyle suggestions are appreciated and may be more likely to be internalized by the patient (10).

INITIAL EVALUATION

During the initial evaluation, the patient history form should include questions related to current lifestyle and questions that illuminate whether a patient has insight into causes of his or her excess weight and self-defeating actions. To be an effective bariatrician, it is important to spend time learning the factors in the person's life that may have contributed to weight gain (4).

Many useful patient evaluation forms are presented in Appendix B. The American Society of Bariatric Physicians (ASBP) patient history form/template is an excellent resource, designed specifically for medical bariatric evaluations. The Weight Loss Questionnaire, Assessment of Patient Readiness form, and Food and Activity Diary (also available on the American Medical Association website at www.ama-asn.org) were developed by bariatric medicine specialists, including leaders of the ASBP and Diplomates of the American Board of Obesity Medicine (formerly the American Board of Bariatric Medicine) (11). The Quality of Life Assessment (from the Lifestyles, Exercise, Attitudes, Relationships, Nutrition [LEARN] program) can be completed by the patient at the initial consultation and used at various points during the follow-up office visits. The Diet Readiness Test Questionnaire (from the LEARN program) gleans information from the patient that may indicate their insight into behaviors needing to be changed (12).

Goal setting should take place at the initial visit. A "weight loss goals list" should be included for the patient to complete, and the patient should be encouraged to make goals specific (personal), measurable (precise), time framed (present), and realistic (possible) (13). The goals should be positive and include short-, intermediate-, and long-term goals. The patient's goal (wish) list is a useful tool to use during follow-up appointments when discussing success reached and behaviors yet to be modified. Information gathered on the history form is valuable in assessing the patient's baseline regarding the necessary behavioral changes to be addressed. Weight loss behavioral goals that are self-determined are more likely to result in long-term behavior changes (14). Self-monitoring is integral to the success of weight loss, as well as long-term maintenance of healthier weight.

A food diary kept by the patient will also give clues as to why food choices are made. Several examples of food, activity, and behavior diaries are included in Appendix B and can be adapted to fit the individual needs and preferences of the clinician and patient. Depending on the food program chosen by the patient and clinician to meet the patient's specific metabolic and weight loss needs, a column for amounts, calories, and grams of carbohydrates, proteins, or fats to be recorded should be included. We ask our patients to record physical activity so we can estimate their macronutrient needs. Also, if a suboptimal food choice is made, we ask the patient to write down why that food was chosen. This enables the patient to gain insight into their actions or behaviors. Some of the reasons listed include habit, environment, mood, addiction, and lack of interpreting hunger cues (physiological), convenience, lack of boundary setting, advertising, and lack of portion or dietary knowledge (8). The patient may not know the "why" and, in fact, an automatic response, or "mindless eating," may be discovered by the patient (15). Later, emotional antecedents may be identified and the patient can be encouraged to develop strategies to deal proactively with similar high-risk situations in the future.

STAGES OF CHANGE

The transtheoretical model of change (16) includes five stages of change: precontemplation, contemplation, preparation, action, and maintenance (Table 7.1). Relapse was added to later versions of this model; the concepts of "spiral of change" (17) and "contemplation ladder" (18) were added to suggest that a patient may relapse from any given stage to a previous stage. Although the majority of patients may come to your office stating a readiness for preparation and action, they may still be in precontemplation or contemplation about changing a certain behavior (e.g., dining out frequently) to lose weight. Each of the stages is applicable to each self-defeating behavior and takes varied amounts of time to extinguish, depending on the individual. The clinician can determine what stage the patient is in by asking open-ended questions *and then listening to the answer*. For example, precontemplation can be discovered by asking the patient whether he or she wants to change; for example, "My wife (or husband) made me come here. I don't see a problem." At this stage, the clinician should give the client information and advice about the positive health reasons to make a change. When a patient is in contemplation, for example, "I would like to lose weight, but I don't believe I can lose or keep it off," the clinician should accept ambivalence and avoid argument. Even patients who enter at the preparation stage need your help with short-, intermediate-, and long-term goal setting and to design a plan individualized to their goals, which may not necessarily be the same as your goals for the patient.

In the action stage, the clinician assists the patient to find his or her own solution by reviewing eating cues and discussing patient recognition of triggers and consequences of actions chosen and taken. A helpful technique is to use the "ask-tell-ask" method; for example, "Why do you think you chose fast food? You could choose to pack your lunch. Do you think you could pack a lunch four out of five work days?"

Table 7.1 Applying the stages of change model to assess readiness

Stage	Characteristic	Patient verbal cue	Appropriate intervention	Sample dialogue
Precontemplation	Unaware of problem, no interest in change	"I'm not really interested in weight loss. It's not a problem."	Provide information about health risks and benefits of weight loss	"Would you like to read some information about the health aspects of obesity?"
Contemplation	Aware of problem, beginning to think of changing	"I know I need to lose weight, but with all that's going on in my life right now, I'm not sure I can."	Help resolve ambivalence, discuss barriers	"Let's look at the benefits of weight loss, as well as what you may need to change."
Preparation	Realizes benefits of making changes and thinking about how to change	"I have to lose weight, and I'm planning to do that."	Teach behavior modification, provide education	"Let's take a closer look at how you can reduce some of the calories you eat and how to increase your activity during the day."
Action	Actively taking steps toward change	"I'm doing my best. This is harder than I thought."	Provide support and guidance, with a focus on the long term	"It's terrific that you're working so hard. What problems have you had so far? How have you solved them?"
Maintenance	Initial treatment goals reached	"I've learned a lot through this process."	Relapse control	"What situations continue to tempt you to overeat? What can be helpful for the next time you face such a situation?"

Source: Adapted from Prochaska JO, DiClemente CC. Toward a comprehensive model of change. In: Miller WR, ed. *Treating Addictive Behaviors.* New York, NY: Plenum; 1986, 3–27.

Maintenance of healthier weight improves with ongoing support that results from periodic visits with the clinician or a trained staff member of the bariatric office (19). Increasing the length of the treatment phase, not necessarily the time spent at each visit, improves weight loss and maintenance. A supportive environment should be provided so the patient can create their own strategies for combating threats (i.e., plan a, b, and c) (20). Long-term contact with providers, whether by phone, in person, in groups, via telemedicine, or through the Internet, improves maintenance of a healthy weight (21). Social support studies show weight loss and maintenance are better when a patient uses like-minded friends rather than a significant other as the support system (22). Self-help for patients can include written media, radio, television, visual and audio (CDs, MPs, iPod) media, and the Internet (23). More recent studies are exploring the use of the Internet as a tool to reach those who are homebound to increase availability of information, treatment, and maintenance support (24). Although some randomized control trials show personal contact is more effective at weight loss and maintenance, when human e-mail counseling was added to Internet programs, patients were more likely to stay engaged (25). The use of personal digital assistants with dietary software and smart phone applications can enhance weight loss if combined with telephone coaching or an automatic feedback message. However, without the follow-up interaction, these devices showed no significant advantage over a paper diary or record (26). Individualized texts also increase the success for weight loss (27). Interreality uses virtual simulations of experiences and virtual communities followed by the use of bio- and activity sensors and devices to track real-time behaviors of the patient and provide specific suggestions (28). Numerous blogs and personal sites (e.g., Facebook) have been created to share weight loss information, but increasingly privacy concerns limit some aspects of social media (29).

It is important to teach the patient to recognize danger signals that old behaviors are returning and suggest strategies for the mind games other people in their lives might play (e.g., "You have lost so much weight/worked so hard, you DESERVE to eat (poorly) when you are with us, your overweight family/friends/coworkers."). When a patient relapses into old self-defeating behaviors, a regain in weight is often the only sign. The clinician should reinforce the positive by praising previous success (e.g., "You did it before, you can do it again."). Rather than becoming frustrated about the relapse, the clinician should be welcoming the patient's return for help and assist them in learning what antecedent event lead up to the relapse. The clinician can then help the patient develop the skills necessary to maintain success and prevent a future relapse (30).

The stages of changes model serves as a guide; it has limitations (31) in that matching specific interventions to certain stages has not proven to facilitate change as well as motivational interviewing (32,33).

MODES OF TREATMENT

The standard modes of treatments include the following: motivational interviewing (MI), interpersonal therapy (IT), behavioral therapy (BT), cognitive therapy (CT), cognitive behavioral therapy (CBT), maintenance-tailored therapy (MTT), and acceptance-based therapy (ABT). The older technique of operant conditioning (Pavlov's dogs) is not as applicable to humans for producing desired behavior changes, but it might help explain to the patient how past emotions and stored memories may have an influence on undesired behaviors (34).

Motivational interviewing

MI is a directive, client-centered counseling style for eliciting behavior change by helping clients to explore and resolve ambivalence (35). Physicians who use MI in preventative health and chronic disease visits improve a patient's efforts at weight loss (36). Also, individual MI results in more weight loss and maintenance (37,38). The goal is to increase intrinsic motivation by encouraging the patient to think about change rather than impose an external demand by telling the patient what to do. Collaboration instead of confrontation is key. Through open-ended questions, the clinician can discover the patient's own perceptions, goals, and values. Rather than acting as an authority who assumes the patient lacks knowledge, the clinician provides resources to facilitate the patient's realization of the benefits of changing a self-defeating behavior, as opposed to the probable outcome of not changing (39). A similar approach has been described by the acronym GRACE (40): Generate a gap, Roll with resistance, Avoid arguments, Can do, and Express empathy.

MI can be used at each patient encounter when a clinician notes a positive behavior is lacking (e.g., no exercise) or damaging (e.g., eating out frequently) (37). Specific phrases have been suggested to use in the framework of MI (41). To generate a gap, you, as a clinician, can point out discrepancy between the patient's goals and their present behavior by refreshing an awareness of the stated reasons for change (refer back to the patient's own written goal list). Roll with resistance by listening attentively and acknowledging the patient's feelings, attempts to cope, and right to choose or reject change. It may be helpful to say, "I know how you feel, I have felt the same way, and this is what I found." You personally may not have had the same issue as the patient, but you can empathize by saying, "I had a hard time changing (insert self-defeating behavior)." A simple statement that "Nothing will ever change until YOU decide to change" may assist the patient in acknowledging the discrepancy between the continued self-defeating behavior and achievement of his or her goals.

Show empathic warmth by asking open-ended questions. Avoid arguments; remember that "He that complies against his will, is of the same opinion still" (Samuel Butler, 1612–1680). We are not called to this profession to argue with patients about their choices. A better strategy is to emphasize the patient's strengths and encourage hope for success. Express empathy, offer more information when the patient requests it, acknowledge that change is difficult, and provide a supportive atmosphere for your patient (42).

Interpersonal therapy

Many studies have shown that IT can lead to weight normalization (43). IT has a more individualized focused approach to emotional triggers and reframing of previous experiences. Due to the high prevalence of depression as a coexisting condition with obesity, it is recommended that a depression screen be performed on initial exam (44). You may prefer to refer the patient to a skilled psychiatrist or psychotherapist for more in-depth counseling, especially if the patient has a past personal history of emotional, physical, or sexual abuse. Several other approaches to behavioral modification are available and can be used within your practice, particularly if you or a staff member or colleague has some psychotherapy training. But some simple brief interventions, focused on one behavior change per visit, can be implemented by a well-trained clinician within the constructs of brief follow-up visits.

Behavioral therapy

BT is designed to reinforce or extinguish a behavior. It is based on principles of learning and is intended to alter lifestyle through action or behavior changes. Positive reinforcement is the most effective therapeutic tool (8). This reinforcement can be verbal praise ("I knew you could do it"), tangible or visual recognition of success (certificates, buttons, before-and-after pictures on a bulletin board) (1), recognition of the improvement of a comorbid condition as a result of the weight loss ("Your knee pain is down to a level 3 from your previously stated level of 9 on a scale of 1 to 10"), or showing the patient an indirect positive to their behavior changes ("You saved $200 this month by not dining outside your home"). You can refer the patient back to his or her goal list to point out the positive achievements ("You are able to play with your grandchildren longer now that your knees are less painful" or "You can buy new smaller [or better] better-fitting clothes").

Negative reinforcement is generally not as effective as positive reinforcement, but it may work as a form of mini-intervention if the patient continues to deny harm from the behavior and the consequences are high (e.g., "The usual course of uncontrolled diabetes mellitus is renal failure, probable dialysis treatments, and possible loss of eyesight or amputation of a limb. Do you want to boat/fish/travel [per patient's goals] in your retirement years?"). Some earlier approaches used increased exposure to the action, behavior, or food, sometimes along with aversive association (6). This is a strong approach and better implemented by a clinician with intervention and addiction training. Yet, as primary care providers and medical bariatricians, we often develop the repertoire, albeit after months and years of clinical experience, to take an aggressive interventional approach such as this to save the life of a patient.

Cognitive therapy

CT includes techniques to alter ineffective thinking. The patient is encouraged to change habits over time, since it takes an average of 21 days to establish a habit and 2 years to make the habit more permanent (1). Reframing the patient's thoughts regarding a behavior may include clinician's statements such as "Eating a relative's sugar-loaded treat is not necessarily a sign of love for them." You can assist the patient with phrases to use as tools in those situations ("I am full, but may I please have the recipe"). Presenting alternatives to the patient may widen their perspective. An example would be suggesting they might take two bites of a treat instead of a whole portion. Visualization, as practiced by successful athletes who create an image of themselves successfully attaining their goal (e.g., for a basketball player, making a free throw) just before they actually attempt it, is a helpful practice. You can encourage your patient to visualize behaving as a leaner person when they find themselves in challenging situations.

Cognitive behavioral therapy

CBT combines behavior changes with cognitive understanding to enable the patient to identify the environmental and emotional triggers for his or her self-defeating actions or behaviors. Suggestions and tools are given to the patient to modify the nature of antecedent events that trigger unwanted eating behavior or the response to them, so the patient is better equipped to *choose* the action they wish to take. *Avoidance* of trigger foods or situations that lead to unwanted eating provides an important strategy for the patient. Encourage your patient to substitute a noncaloric, pleasurable reward instead of food. Pleasure, like beauty, is in the eye of the beholder and is the key characteristic of a substitute behavior. Doing work, such as washing the laundry or running on the treadmill, is unlikely to activate the pleasure centers of the brain's limbic system like the patient's trigger food does. Again, this is where the patient goal (desire list) may help identify pleasurable, substitute behaviors. Success is more likely if the patient plans for a food-centered event by eating a healthy snack prior to the event or having a "good-choice" food available by bringing it with them. A diary that records food intake, associated emotions, and information, such as "Why did I eat that?," promotes self-recognition of mindless eating (15), identifies triggers for behaviors, and assists the patient in devising strategies to eliminate or modify reactions to antecedent events. Success is best accomplished by taking a tailored approach that addresses the patient's specific challenges (42,43). Whether a patient needs to implement more effective time management (e.g., using a day planner, taking a time management course, or reading a self-help book) to help them create time for fun physical activity and healthy meal planning, or needs help developing healthy boundaries in interactions with others, the most successful approach by the clinician is assisting the patient to explore his or her own values and thoughts preceding an emotion that produces the response or behavior.

Maintenance-tailored therapy

MTT varies the behavioral strategies intermittently over time to prevent habituation by using different treatments tailored to the patient's expectations. Although MTT and standard BT produce similar overall weight loss, participants in MTT have shown longer time of stable weight (45).

Acceptance-based therapy

ABT focuses on developing a tolerance to internal cues such as sadness, fatigue, or boredom that may lead to cravings. Greater weight loss can be achieved when ABT is incorporated into a behavior program, particularly among patients with a high rate of emotional eating (46,47).

BIOLOGICAL FACTORS

Current data suggest biological factors such as hunger and antihunger hormones may be more powerful than other natural reinforcing factors, such as having more energy. Recent theory has suggested that mechanisms involving the dysregulation or misinterpretation of cues to the limbic system, as well as the possibility of addiction to behavior-induced neurotransmitters, may explain the difficulty humans have in achieving and maintaining a healthy weight (48–51).

Physiological responses can lead to an increase in the fight-or-flight hormone epinephrine (due to a relative cell hypoglycemia) (13) or a modulation or activation of the dopamine receptors, causing changes in appetite, thirst, sexual desire, or other pleasure centers in the limbic system of the human brain. Treating certain foods (or behaviors) as an addiction may work for some patients, but the physiological hunger must also be addressed, whether this is done pharmacologically or by reinforcing the proper amounts of micro- and macronutrient intake and balancing those nutrients with an enjoyable form of physical activity. A food addiction questionnaire (Appendix B) may be an illuminating tool (52). Food addiction has been studied, and fasting potentiates the consumption of food and self-administration of drugs, and even sucrose solutions (53). Addiction treatment would start with avoidance of stimulus and adding cues in the environment to prompt a new behavior. Do not buy trigger foods, plan ahead for healthier choices to be readily available, and change your routine to avoid stimulus (e.g., drive a different way home to bypass your favorite fast-food restaurant). Some patients benefit from applying the concepts of 12 steps of Overeaters Anonymous, including avoiding getting too hungry, tired, angry, or scared. Psychological effects can cause a change in the patient's present mental state (e.g., elated, anxious, more relaxed) based on his or her past experiences and memory storage and retrieval by the limbic system.

The limbic system of the brain (particularly the hippocampus and amygdale) functions to determine the emotional state of mind. It is a principal player in memory storage, recall, and emotional interpretation of events (54). The limbic system also modulates motivation and libido, controls appetite and sleep, and processes sense of smell. Behavior reinforcement pathways include hindbrain centers for taste and forebrain centers for cognitive interpretation.

The nucleus accumbens is at the crossroads of the systems in that it interprets the signals of taste from the prefrontal cortex (olfaction) and communicates with the motor system for action and with the globus pallidus and hypothalamus for appetite and motivation. The neurotransmitters involved include norepinephrine (NE), serotonin (5-HT), and dopamine (DA). NE *stimulates* feeding by activating α_2-noradrenergic (NA) receptors and *inhibits* via α_1-receptors. 5-HT suppresses food intake by inhibiting α_2-NA in the midhypothalamus. DA positively reinforces a behavior or action by generating appetite, want, and motivation and then reward and pleasure. It also promotes escape from aversive stimulus (i.e., being hungry, lack of pleasure) (55). Genetic defects in the DA receptors have been implicated in the development of obesity (56–59), resulting in a reward deficiency syndrome whereby the patient is at risk for using more and more of the substance (e.g., sugar) to get the same satisfied feeling (59,60). Another hypothesis of some studies is that overstimulation of receptors and then withdrawal of the substance (e.g., sugar) creates a relative depletion of the dopamine signal (61) and processes or behaviors similar to addiction (62). Also, along with hormonal factors such as leptin and insulin resistance (63), this process has been postulated as an evolutionary advantage in that the obese patient becomes a thrifty storer of energy as a survival mechanism, but it now becomes a negative in the environment of abundant food (energy input) and less physical activity required to survive (energy output) (64,65).

BEHAVIORAL FACTORS

Everyone behaves in certain ways and may not always know why. The antecedent thought, or anticipation of a specific behavior or behavioral outcome, for example, may produce neurochemicals that reinforce the behavior. Behavior may be modified by tracing those thoughts and actions that lead to the behavior (back-chaining) and then substituting new, healthier (or at least not self-defeating) behaviors (e.g., reading, playing a game, or engaging in some other pleasurable activity as opposed to doing work [laundry]) that give a reward, feeling, or neurochemical response in the limbic system of the brain. Insert a new behavior closest to the desired outcome (or extinguish the old behavior closest to the undesired outcome). Then, work backwards by changing each action step and linking it to the new action changed before it. It takes many repetitions of practice to change an imprinted behavior pattern. For example, if you always overeat a certain trigger food at a holiday event, think why (e.g., your relative is a "food pusher," or you did not eat before being presented with the trigger). Then, learn to decline the food (e.g., "No, thank you," or "No, I'm good"). You could plan ahead to have a small portion and eat plenty of healthy satisfying food beforehand. You could bring a nontriggering, acceptable substitution. You could choose to show up at the event after dinner is over or you could decline to attend altogether. Even bad habits are sometimes more comfortable than new habits and attempting to change the action will cause anxiety (remember NE), or, especially in the beginning, not give you the same pleasure (DA). Anticipating and planning ahead for what action you will take, as well as training and repetition, ensure more likelihood of success. Some common stress reduction techniques include relaxation training through biofeedback, listening to pleasing music, and deep breathing exercises. Hypnosis also has some success in reframing and retraining thoughts or feelings surrounding food choices.

As in our previous example, if it makes you anxious or nervous to decline a relative's famous dish, you could opt to say, "It looks very tasty, but I am so full. Could I please have the recipe?" You can also take a relaxing breath and repeat your answer, "No, thank you." Or excuse yourself to go talk to another relative away from the food table (avoidance) (66).

CONCLUSIONS

Assisting the patient in discovering the *why* (the thoughts and emotions surrounding and preceding the action or behavior) and *how* to change or override the neurotransmitter feedback may be the future key to long-term success (12). Individualization is the key to behavioral change (67). Well-trained medical bariatricians are in the best position to know, listen to, and advise obese patients on how to apply the most recent research findings on behavioral change strategies. Thus, they are also the best resource to help the obese patient achieve long-term, healthy weight maintenance and an improved quality of life (68,69). New research is needed to help achieve the goal of matching treatments to a patient's needs to improve weight loss and its maintenance, as well as manage obesity as a chronic disease. The Obesity Treatment Foundation was created in concert with the ASBP and the American Board of Obesity Medicine with this goal in mind.

REFERENCES

1. Wadden TA, et al. Lifestyle modification for obesity; new developments in diet, physical activity, and behavior therapy. *Circulation.* 2012; 125(9): 1157–1170.
2. Koop CE. A quest for the healing roots of medicine. *The Chronicle of Higher Education*, 1992, July A5.
3. The American Board of Family Medicine Practice Guidelines. Accessed at http://www.aafp.org/patient-care/clinical-recommendations/clinical-practice-guidelines.html
4. American Society of Bariatric Physicians. *Adding Magic to Medicine: Using Techniques from the Behavioral Sciences to Treat Obesity.* Denver, CO: American Society of Bariatric Physicians; 2002.
5. Stuart R. Behavioral control of overeating. *Behav Res Ther.* 1967; 5: 357.
6. Jackson DN. *Personality Research Form*, 6th ed. Research Psychologists Press, London, Ontario, Canada; 1997.
7. Jackson DH, Hoffman H. Common dimensions of psychopathology from the MMPI and Basic Personality Inventory. *J Clin Psychol.* 1987; 43(6): 661–669.
8. Williamson DA, Perrin LA. Behavioral therapy for obesity. *Obesity.* 1996; 25: 943–955.
9. Bray GA, Bouchard C. *Handbook of Obesity.* New York: Marcel Dekker; 2004.
10. Black DR, Cameron R. Self-administered interventions: A health strategy for improving population health. *Health Educ Res.* 1997; 12(4): 531–545.
11. Brownell KD, Wadden TA. *The Learn Program for Weight Control.* Dallas, TX: American Health Publishing; 1998.
12. Van Dorsten B. Behavioral modification in the treatment of obesity. In: Barnett AH, Kumar S (eds.). *Obesity and Diabetes*; London: Wiley, 2004.
13. Ludwig DS, et al. High glycemic index foods, overeating, and obesity. *Pediatrics.* 1999; 103(3): E26.
14. Teixiera PJ, et al. Motivation, self-determination, and long term weight control. *Int J Behav Nutr Phys Act.* 2012; 9: 22.

15. Wansink B. *Mindless Eating: Why We Eat More Than We Think*. New York: Bantam Dell; 2007.

16. Prochaska JO. *Systems of Psychotherapy: A Transtheoretical Analysis*. Homewood, IL: Dorsey Press; 1979.

17. Prochaska JO, et al. In search of how people change. Application to addictive behaviors. *Am Psychol*. 1992; 47(9): 1102–1114.

18. Biener L, Abrams DA. The contemplation ladder: Validation of a measure of readiness to consider smoking cessation. *Health Psychol*. 1991; 10: 360–365.

19. Wing R, Hall J. *National Weight Control Registry*. www.nwcr.ws

20. Jeffrey RW, et al. Prevalence of overweight and weight loss behavior in a metropolitan adult population. *Am J Public Health*. 1984; 74: 349–352.

21. Van Dorsten B. *Obesity Course. Maintaining Patient Motivation in Long-Term Weight Management: Combining Creativity with Genius*. Atlanta, GA: ASBP; 2005.

22. Wing RR, Jeffrey RW. Benefits of recruiting participants with friends and increasing social support for weight loss and maintenance. *J Consult Clin Psychol*. 1999; 67(1): 132–138.

23. Tate DF, Wing RR, Winett RA. Using Internet technology to deliver a behavioral weight loss program. *JAMA*. 2001; 285: 1172–1177.

24. Harvey-Berino J, et al. Internet delivered behavioral obesity treatment. *Prev Med*. 2010; 51(2): 123–128.

25. Webber KH, et al. Motivational Interviewing in Internet groups: A pilot study for weight loss. *J Am Diet Assoc*. 2008; 108(6): 1029–1032.

26. Burke LE, et al. The effect of electronic self-monitoring on weight loss and dietary intake. *Obesity (Silver Spring)*. 2011; 19(2): 338–344.

27. Patrick K, et al. A text message based intervention for weight loss. *J Med Internet Res*. 2009; 11(1): el.

28. Riva G, et al. Interreality: The experiential use of technology in the treatment of obesity. *Clin Prac Epidemiol Ment Health*. 2011; 7: 51–61.

29. Newman MW, et al. It's not that I don't have problems; I am just not putting them on Facebook. *ACM 2011 Conference on Computer Supported Cooperative Work*, March 2011, China, 341–350.

30. Byrne SM. Psychological aspects of weight maintenance and relapse in obesity [review]. *J Psychosom Res*. 2002; 53(5): 1029–1036.

31. DiMarco ID, Klein DA, Clark VL, Wilson GT. The use of motivational interviewing techniques to enhance the efficacy of guided self-help behavioral weight loss treatment. *Eat Behav*. 2009; 10(2): 134–136.

32. Temple JL, et al. Differential effects of daily snack food intake on the reinforcing value of food in obese and non-obese. *Am J Clin Nutr*. 2009; 90(2): 304–313.

33. Rollnick S. Behavior change in practice; targeting individuals. *Int J Obes Relat Metab Disord*. 1996; 20: s22–s26.

34. Pollak KI, et al. Empathy goes a long way in weight loss discussions. *J Fam Pract*. 2007; 56(12): 1031–1036.

35. West DS, et al. Motivational interviewing improves weight loss in women with type 2 diabetes. *Diabetes Care*. 2007; 30(5): 1081–1087.

36. Carels RA, et al. Using motivational interviewing as a supplement to obesity treatment: A stepped-care approach. *Health Psychol*. 2007; 26(3): 369–374.

37. Miller WR, Rollnick S. *Motivational Interviewing: Preparing People for Change*. New York: Guilford Press; 2002.

38. Ruback S, et al. Motivational interviewing: A systematic review & meta-analysis. *Br J Gen Pract.* 2005; 55(513): 305–312.
39. Houng V. Putting prevention into practice: Counseling patients to prevent and decrease obesity. *J Okla State Med Assoc.* 2005; 98(6): 252–254.
40. Sim MB, et al. Influencing behavior change in general practice—Part 1-Brief intervention and motivational interviewing. *Aust Fam Physician.* 2009; 38(11): 885–888.
41. Burke BL, et al. The efficacy of motivational interviewing: A meta-analysis of controlled clinical trials. *J Consult Clin Psychol.* 2003; 71(5): 843–861.
42. Roberts RE, et al. Prospective association between obesity and depression. *Int J Obes Relat Metab Disord.* 2003; 27(4): 514–521.
43. Perri MG, Corsica JA. Improving the maintenance of weight lost in behavioral treatment of obesity. In: Wadden T, Stunkard A (eds.). *Handbook of Obesity Treatment.* New York: Guilford Press.
44. Goldberg JH, Klernan M. Innovative techniques to address retention in a behavioral weight-loss trial. *Health Educ Res.* 2005; 20(4): 439–447.
45. Jeffrey RW, et al. A comparison of maintenance-tailored therapy & standard behavioral therapy for treatment of obesity. *Prev Med* 2010; 51(6): 457–459.
46. Forman EM, et al. Mind Your Health Project. *Obesity.* 2013; 21(6): 1119–1126.
47. Tsujino N, Sakurai T. Orexin/hypocretin: A neuropeptide at the interface of sleep, energy homeostasis and reward system. *Pharmacol Rev.* 2009; 61(2): 162–176.
48. Zheng H, Lenard NR, Shin AC, Berthoud HR. Appetite control & energy balance regulation in the modern world: Reward-driven brain overrides repletion signals. *Int J Obes.* 2009; 33(2): 8–13.
49. Stoeckel LE, et al. Effective connectivity of a reward network in obese women. *Brain Res Bull.* 2009; 79(6): 388–395.
50. Adam TC, Epel ES. Stress, eating and the reward system. *Physiol Behav.* 2007; 91(4): 449–458.
51. Shin AC, Zheng H, Berthoud HR. An expanded view of energy homeostasis: Neural integration of metabolic, cognitive, and emotional drives to eat. *Physiol Behav.* 2009; 97(5): 572–580.
52. Jay K. Food addiction and the weight-loss surgery patient. *Obesity Action Coalitions News,* 2007 January, 15–17.
53. Wang GJ, Volkow ND, Fowler JS. The role of dopamine in motivation for food in humans: Implications for obesity. *Expert Opin Ther Targets.* 2002; 6(5): 601–609.
54. Suyama S, et al. [Roles and functional interplay of the gut, brain stem, hypothalamus and limbic system in regulation of feeding]. *Nippon Rinsho.* 2009; 67(2): 277–286.
55. Thanos PK, et al. The effects of two highly selective dopamine D3 receptor antagonists (SB-277011A and NGB-2904) on food self administration in a rodent model of obesity. *Pharmacol Biochem Behav.* 2008; 89(4): 499–507.
56. Hajnai A, et al. Altered dopamine D2 receptor function and binding to obese OTETF rat. *Brain Res Bull.* 2008; 75(1): 70–76.
57. Hajnai A, et al. Dopamine D2 receptors contribute to increased avidity for sucrose in obese rats lacking CCK-1 receptors. *Neuroscience.* 2007; 148(2): 584–592.
58. Hajnai A, et al. Obese OLETF rats exhibit increased operant performance for palatable sucrose solutions and differential sensitivity to D2 receptor antagonism. *Am J Physiol Regul Integr Comp Physiol.* 2007; 293(5): R1846–R1854.
59. Comings DE, Blum K. Reward deficiency syndrome: Genetic aspects of behavioral disorders. *Prog Brain Res.* 2000; 126: 325–341.

60. Geiger BM, et al. Deficits of mesolimbic dopamine neurotransmission in rat dietary obesity. *Neuroscience*. 2009; 159(4): 1193–1199.
61. Reinholz J, et al. Compensatory weight gain due to dopaminergic hypofunction: New evidence. *Nutr Metab (Lond)*. 2008; 5: 35.
62. Avena NM, et al. Evidence for sugar addiction: Behavioral and neurochemical effects of intermittent excessive sugar intake. *Neurosci Biobehav Rev*. 2008; 32(1): 20–39.
63. Bello NT, Hajnai A. Alterations in blood glucose levels under hyperinsulinema affect accumbens dopamine. *Physiol Behav*. 2006; 88(1–2): 138–145.
64. Berthoud HR. Interactions between the "cognitive" and "metabolic" brain in the control of food intake. *Physiol Behav*. 2007; 91(5): 486–498.
65. Lenard NR, Berthoud HR. Central and peripheral regulation of food intake and physical activity: Pathways and genes. *Obesity*. 2008; 16(3): 11–22.
66. Epstein LH, et al. Food reinforcement and eating: A multilevel analysis. *Psychol Bull*. 2007; 133(5): 88.
67. Hsu A, Blandford A. designing for a psychological change. *J Med Internet Res*. 2014; 16(6): e138.
68. American Society of Bariatric Physicians. www.asbp.org
69. The Obesity Foundation, American Board of Bariatric Medicine. www.abbmcertification.org

8

Pharmacotherapy

ED J. HENDRICKS

INTRODUCTION

In the past few years, several new antiobesity drugs have been approved; thus, physicians caring for overweight and obese patients have more pharmacotherapeutic agents from which to choose. These antiobesity drugs include the older drugs phentermine, diethylpropion, phendimetrazine, and orlistat and the more recently approved drugs phentermine/topiramate (Qsymia®), lorcaserin (Belviq®), and naltrexone/bupropion (Contrave®). Expectations are that liraglutide (Saxenda®) will soon be approved and added to this list.

The older drugs, phentermine, diethylpropion, and phendimetrazine, are substituted phenethylamines, a group of both naturally occurring and synthetic compounds that contain a wide variety of drug classes, including central nervous system stimulants (e.g., amphetamine), antilipemics, bronchodilators, cardiotonic agents, vasodilators, calcium channel blockers, antidepressants (e.g., bupropion), neuroprotective agents, antiparkinson agents, and psychotropic drugs (e.g., hallucinogens). Phentermine, diethylpropion, and phendimetrazine are often referred to as amphetamines, but those who do so are apparently uninformed of the biochemistry of substituted phenethylamines.

The newer drugs, which are approved for long-term use, are most often recommended elsewhere simply because the Food and Drug Administration (FDA)–sanctioned long-term trials of a year or more have been conducted and published. The older drugs, phentermine, diethylpropion, and phendimetrazine, are ignored because these drugs were only "approved for short-term use." Actually, these older drugs were approved on two separate occasions. Both approvals occurred long before obesity was acknowledged to be a chronic illness and therefore occurred long before the FDA required long-term clinical trials for obesity drug approvals. The FDA approved these drugs first in 1959 after trials focused on their safety as mandated in the 1938 Food Drug and Cosmetic Act. The initial approved label did not mention a time limit for therapy. In similarity to nearly all other approved drugs in the pharmacopeia, duration of therapy was left to the prescribing physician. In 1962, the US Congress amended the Food and Drug Act to require proof of efficacy as a condition of approval, and subsequently the FDA required drug companies to repeat the clinical trials for the older antiobesity drugs. Eventually, after 200 additional trials in 10,000 subjects, in 1977 the FDA reconsidered and reapproved phentermine, diethylpropion, and phendimetrazine. Despite the fact that no evidence of addiction or addiction potential had emerged, either in the trials or after 18 years of widespread clinical use, some interested parties, convinced that the drugs were addicting, were highly critical of the reapprovals. In a compromise to deflect the critics, the FDA reapproved the antiobesity drugs but for short-term use only and the labels were required to prominently warn of addiction potential. Later, the FDA defined short term to mean 12 weeks. This was in 1977, 18 years before the FDA decided antiobesity drugs should have trials of 1 year or longer.

Although long-term clinical trials tailored to current FDA specifications have not been conducted for the older drugs, they have been tested practically through long-term use in hundreds of thousands of patients. In the opinion of experienced practicing bariatric physicians, the older drugs are as effective, or more so, than the newer drugs; they share very few characteristics with amphetamine; they are considerably less expensive; and they are just as safe as the new drugs, if not safer. When patients who pay for their own medications are allowed to try any of the antiobesity drugs, they most frequently choose one of the older drugs, most often phentermine.

Pharmacotherapy is a mainstay in obesity treatment, but it should always be used within the context of a comprehensive approach to treating the illness. Pharmacotherapy should never be used alone, but rather in combination with caloric restriction for weight loss or dietary control for maintenance, and behavior modification. An increase in exercise frequency and intensity are important behavior modifications for nearly all patients. For optimum effectiveness, pharmacotherapy should be long term; the patient and the physician should mutually agree that medications selected should be used for as long as the drug is effective, provided undesirable side effects are absent or, if present, manageable.

CAUTIONS FOR PRESCRIBING PHYSICIANS

Although the evidence on both older and new antiobesity drugs is that these drugs are safe, many nonbariatric physicians believe them to be inherently dangerous, perhaps more dangerous than the obesity for which they are prescribed, at least unless the patient is egregiously overweight. One reason for this opinion is that weight management drugs in general and anorectics in particular have had a history of unexpected adverse effects (1). Although there is little evidence in the medical literature that the dangers enumerated in the product labeling for the older drugs have actually occurred, neither is there much documentation of long-term safety and efficacy for the older weight management drugs. As a result, unproven conjectures based on chemical structural similarities to amphetamine regarding the sympathomimetic amine drugs phentermine, diethylpropion, and phendimetrazine persist, and the potential benefits of effective obesity pharmacotherapy with these older drugs have been greatly restricted.

In 2008, the American Society of Bariatric Physicians (ASBP) conducted a national survey examining how bariatric physicians use pharmacotherapy in obesity treatment (2). The survey revealed a discrepancy between how bariatric medicine physicians actually prescribe pharmacologic agents in treating obesity and published treatment guidelines. The obesity treatment guidelines promulgated by many academic medical societies follow closely the clinical guidelines of the National Heart, Lung, and Blood Institute (NHLBI) for the diagnosis and treatment of obesity issued in September 1998 (3). The expert committee, in formulating the NHLBI guidelines, decided that diagnosis and therefore treatment decisions should be predicted entirely upon body mass index (BMI) or waist circumference (WC) thresholds. This decision was controversial because it was based on opinion and not evidence and because it restricted treatment, especially obesity pharmacotherapy. The decision was opposed by some clinicians at the time the NHLBI guidelines were adopted and published (4). A consortium of the American Heart Association, the Obesity Society, and the American College of Cardiology recently revised the NHLBI guidelines; the revision did not change reliance on BMI and WC for diagnosis. More recently, several other obesity treatment guidance documents have emerged that put the focus on making pharmacotherapy treatment decisions on complication-centric rather than BMI-centric decision points (5,6). The ASBP guideline has placed emphasis on diagnostic thresholds other than the BMI or WC since its inception (7). This national society of clinicians practicing obesity treatment developed practice standards and obesity treatment guidelines long before obesity was officially recognized as a disease and long before the use of the BMI came into vogue. BMI, originally an epidemiology tool that correlates best with obesity mortality, is known to be an insensitive indicator of abdominal adiposity (8–10) and of the typical morbidities associated with obesity (11). In particular, BMI is an insensitive indicator for cardiovascular risk (12,13). Recently, the ASBP introduced the ASBP Obesity Algorithm that also puts more emphasis on treating the disease process rather than relying on static BMI thresholds in making treatment decisions (14).

Selection of patients for whom controlled substance anorectic medications can be prescribed has become increasingly controversial since FDA approval of dexfenfluramine in 1996 and the subsequent phentermine/fenfluramine crisis (15). The ASBP first formalized and published their Anorectic Usage Guidelines in 1990 following the 1985 National Institutes of Health (NIH) Consensus Conference that first defined obesity by BMI thresholds: BMI ≥ 27.2 in women or BMI ≥ 27.8 in men. The ASBP guidance emphasized that pharmacotherapy for the chronic progressive illness called obesity, in any individual patient, should be based on the physician's judgment and not on arbitrary thresholds. Subsequently, in 1995, an expert committee of the World Health Organization opined that obesity should be defined as a BMI ≥ 30, whereupon the FDA mandated BMI restrictions in clinical trials for antiobesity drugs and added BMI threshold restrictions to dexfenfluramine as it was approved in 1996. The FDA added the same BMI restrictions to sibutramine upon its approval in 1999 and, at the same time, extended BMI restrictions to the older drugs, including phentermine. After 40 years of safe use, the older drugs were suddenly declared unsafe by government fiat; physicians who prescribed the drugs to patients who did not fit the government-decreed thresholds were precipitously prescribing "off label." In 1998, the NIH published "Clinical Guidelines on the Identification, Evaluation, and Treatment of Overweight and Obesity in Adults. The Evidence Report." These guidelines have also been adopted by a variety of medical associations, including the Obesity Society (formerly North American Association for the Study of Obesity) (16), the American Medical Association (17), the American College of Physicians (18), and numerous other organizations (19). These associations all define obesity by BMI threshold and offer guidance to restrict treatment with antiobesity drugs to patients with BMI ≥ 30 or with BMI ≥ 27 if the patient has diabetes, hypertension, or hyperlipidemia. Although these treatments were offered only as guides, not intended to override the clinician's judgment, it is the (unfounded) view of many government agencies and state medical boards that the official guidelines are *the standard of practice*. Of course, the official FDA label for every antiobesity drug, both old and new, stipulates that these drugs are only "indicated" for a given patient when that patient's BMI exceeds the official thresholds. It appears that only the ASBP obesity treatment guidelines recommend that physicians use their own judgment in deciding when to initiate pharmacotherapy treatment irrespective of a patient's BMI. For example, a diabetic overweight patient with a BMI < 27 may significantly benefit from weight loss induced by an antiobesity drug. ASBP guidelines acknowledge the use of antiobesity drugs in other clinical situations where patients' may enjoy clinical improvement.

Be forewarned that although I believe that the ASBP guidelines regarding pharmacotherapy in patients with a BMI < 30 or 27 are sound and are in the best interests of your patients, not all physicians, medical boards, and insurance companies agree. Each physician has to decide which of the guidelines to use in his or her own practice and how much to prudently use the anorectic agents in an off-label manner. Although the physician may believe it not in a patient's best interests, the safest course for the physician to follow in protecting his or her right to practice medicine may be to prescribe weight management medications strictly in accordance with product labeling.

Bariatric physicians who are treating their patients by prescribing the medications off label expose themselves to the risk that a zealous pharmacist or other individual will report the physician to the state medical board for "overprescribing" a controlled substance. Some medical boards will accuse the physician of "indiscriminately prescribing controlled substances," an act that then may be considered grounds for suspending or restricting the offending physician's license to practice.

Physicians who dispense controlled substances in their offices may avoid this risk, but should make themselves aware of Drug Enforcement Administration (DEA) regulations and follow them scrupulously. The DEA requires that every pill that comes into and goes out of a physician's office be accounted for. Dispensing logs, patient records, and patient accounts must be kept in exact correspondence. The DEA also expects a precise inventory that must be in exact agreement with invoices of drugs received and with the dispensing logs. The DEA can levy significant fines for each and every discrepancy their agents can find. If the DEA agents suspect that a physician is deliberately deviating from their rules or is not cooperative, they have the authority to shutter the physician's office, seize every asset, and take the physician away in handcuffs. In contrast, physicians who follow the rules, keep meticulous records, and are cooperative have nothing to fear if DEA agents arrive unexpectedly.

The state medical boards vary in their regulation of office dispensing practices; practitioners who wish to dispense medications should be aware of local requirements. Nearly every state board requires a good faith examination of a patient before any medication is prescribed or dispensed. Patients on maintenance on any of the controlled medications should be seen at least once every 3 months.

WHY USE PHARMACOTHERAPY?

One might ask why pharmacotherapy is a treatment mainstay; why use pharmacotherapy at all if it is so controversial? There have been numerous clinical trials in the past of all the weight management drugs, and these trials have been reviewed in several extensive meta-analyses, all of which agree that pharmacotherapy is an effective addition to obesity treatment (20–24).

Several studies have shown that patients in weight loss programs who are placed on a weight management drug lose more weight than those on the same program without the drug, in both short-term trials and long-term trials. In a study by Wadden et al. (25), patients given sibutramine lost 12% of their original weight at 52 weeks, whereas those on the same program with no drug lost 6%. In a study from my clinic, patients on phentermine and a low-carbohydrate ketogenic diet lost significantly more than did phentermine-untreated patients over a 2-year time period ($P = 0.0144$) (26). Haddock et al. (27) reported that, compared to published long-term studies, both 52-week weight loss and patient retention were better when phentermine was combined with caloric restriction in a private practice setting (27).

Bariatric physicians who use pharmacotherapy are generally in agreement with the assertion of Haddock et al. (27) that the rate of patient retention is higher in patients placed on weight management medications than in those on no medication. Obesity is a chronic illness; obviously, the longer patients stay in therapy, the higher the likelihood of both short-term weight loss and long-term successful weight maintenance.

Pharmacotherapy can also produce beneficial effects other than weight loss and metabolic improvements produced by weight loss. There is evidence that quality of life (QOL) improves with weight loss (28) and evidence that suggests that pharmacotherapy, by producing greater weight loss, enhances QOL improvement (29).

WHEN SHOULD PHARMACOTHERAPY BE INITIATED?

Current dogma stipulates that pharmacotherapy is only "indicated" after obesity is diagnosed and that the diagnosis of obesity requires a patient have a BMI ≥ 30, or in the case of a patient with obesity comorbidities, a BMI ≥ 27. These indications are explicitly stated in the label of each and every FDA-approved medicine for obesity. This is indeed dogma, for the reality is that the chronic illness currently categorized as obesity is a dynamic pathophysiological process that begins as the patient starts to store excess fat. The earliest pathological change is infiltration of the expanding adipose tissue with inflammatory cells. These are macrophages and T cells that initiate release of inflammatory and proinflammatory molecules that, in turn, initiate pathological changes in other organs and tissues throughout the body, including the central nervous system. The disease pathology begins early, but diagnosis is delayed until a late stage of the chronic progressive disease. Following this pattern has meant that the use of pharmacotherapy has been restricted during the early stages of the disease, allowing irreparable damage to progress. Once the drugs are "indicated," the disease is incurable.

MEDICATIONS

Agents for weight loss and maintenance

PHENTERMINE

Phentermine has been the most widely prescribed antiobesity drug since the FDA first approved it for marketing 55 years ago. The drug's enduring popularity with physicians and patients alike is testament to the drug's effectiveness and safety. Surveys in 2008 and 2012 revealed that 97% of the responding bariatric physicians used pharmacotherapy in treating obesity and that 98% of them used phentermine as their first choice for an antiobesity drug (2) (Table 8.1).

Phentermine is a substituted phenethylamine derived from β-phenylethylamine. Phenethylamine is a naturally occurring monoamine alkaloid found in mammals and many other organisms; in many foods, including chocolate, legumes, nuts, and seeds; and all varieties of animal protein. The β-phenylethylamine skeleton is also the framework for the neurotransmitters epinephrine, norepinephrine, dopamine, and lots of other natural and synthetic compounds. Medicinal substituted phenethylamines include phentermine; albuterol and other bronchodilators; decongestants; antidepressants such as bupropion; and drugs used in children and adults for attention deficit, such as methylphenidate, atomoxetine, lisdexamfetamine, and amphetamine.

A principal central nervous system anatomic site of action and whether and how molecular action influences eating behavior, food intake, and ultimately body weight in humans are unknown. A recent FDA review of a New Drug Application for an orally disintegrating form of phentermine (30) stated, "Weight loss seems to occur due to a combination of anorectic (decreased food consumption), thermogenic (increased metabolic activity), and drug-induced increased physical activity." The references cited for this statement are from studies on rodents (31–33). There are no reports of investigations into phentermine mechanism of action in human subjects.

Phentermine is available in two forms: phentermine hydrochloride (HCl) and phentermine base attached to an ion-exchange resin. Generic phentermine in the United States is phentermine HCl and is available as 37.5 mg tablets and as capsules containing 15, 30, or 37.5 mg. Phentermine resin is available in Australia, Costa Rica, the Dominican Republic, El Salvador, Guatemala, Honduras,

Table 8.1 Percentage of bariatric medicine physicians prescribing specific drugs for weight management in what percentage of their patients according to 2008 and 2012 American Society of Bariatric Physicians surveys of bariatric physicians prescribing practices

Drug prescribed	2008		2012	
	% MDs	% Pts	% MDs	% Pts
Phentermine	97	50	99	46
Diethylpropion	64	15	63	18
Phendimetrazine	60	18	60	20
Sibutramine	49	4	—	—
Topiramate	50	4	53	9
Orlistat	43	8	43	6
Zonisamide	8	2	11	1
Bupropion	28	7	61	9
Metformin	41	16	85	28
Naltrexone	25	1	16	3
Exenatide	—	—	38	2
Liraglutide	—	—	22	2

Source: Data from the American Society of Bariatric Physicians.
Note: % MDs, percentage of bariatric medicine physicians prescribing specific drugs for weight management; % Pts, percentage of patients prescribed drugs according to 2008 and 2012 American Society of Bariatric Physicians Surveys of Bariatric Physicians Prescribing Practices.

Hong Kong, Malaysia, New Zealand, Panama, Singapore, and South Africa. The molecular weights of the two formulations differ: phentermine HCl, 185.7 and phentermine base, 149.3. Because of this difference, a 30 mg dose of phentermine base is equivalent to 37.5 mg of phentermine HCl. Doses discussed below are for phentermine HCl.

In clinical use, phentermine has several distinctly different therapeutic effects. The first and most obvious is appetite suppression. The other effects are subtler at first, but they become increasing obvious with long-term continuation. These effects are improvements in a variety of harmful eating behaviors and detrimental eating cognitions. Improvements in eating behavior and cognition as determined with the Eating Behavior Questionnaire (EBQ), a 10-question psychometric scale of eating cognition and behaviors, persist in phentermine-treated patients even after the patient has been taking phentermine for years (34,35). Examples include measurable improvements in stress and emotional eating, improvement in eating control, less tendency for rapid, out of control eating, control over grazing, diminution of cravings, and better ability to adhere to an eating plan. Many patients, but not all, will notice that their perceived strength of these effects diminishes with time. This is truer of the effect on appetite than of the other effects. Typically, if the drug is discontinued, as the labeling advises, hunger and all prior harmful cognition and eating behaviors reappear, leading to weight gain, even though the patient struggles to continue to diet. When patients complain that the drug has become less effective in controlling their hunger and eating, consideration should be given to an increase in dose rather than to discontinuing the drug treatment. Increasing dose using a method known as dose-to-effect titration is discussed below in the Dose section.

The long-term effects of phentermine (and, in fact, of all other antiobesity drugs) have long been ignored, but they are clearly the basis for better success with long-term maintenance when phentermine is included in a maintenance regimen (26,27). One long-term effect observed by significant numbers of patients is a diminution of carbohydrate cravings. Such cravings typically disappear quickly in the early stages of a weight management program, especially if the caloric restriction component also restricts carbohydrate intake. Very-low–carbohydrate diets with daily carbohydrate restricted to 20 g or less work best in this regard. Carbohydrate cravings disappear promptly on such diets when no weight management medications are used, and it is impossible to tell whether phentermine helps much in allaying cravings after the first 3 days on such a diet. Patients having carbohydrate intakes greater than 20 g daily without phentermine will sometimes still complain of carbohydrate cravings, and it is in these patients that the addition of phentermine will sometimes produce diminution of cravings. If, later in the course of weight loss or during maintenance, carbohydrate cravings become a problem, the addition of phentermine or an upward adjustment of phentermine dose may alleviate cravings. The addition of 5-hydroxytryptophan combined with carbidopa added to the phentermine, discussed below, may be helpful in patients with carbohydrate cravings.

Duration of action—Phentermine HCl and phentermine base are both long acting, with a biological half-life of about 24 hours.

Clinical effectiveness—Phentermine is still the most effective antiobesity agent. A recent study of long-term phentermine use found that 83% of patients had weight loss equal to or greater than 10 of initial baseline weight at 1 year (26).

Contraindications—Contraindications to prescribing phentermine include pregnancy, nursing an infant, and previous severe allergic reaction to phentermine. Although pregnancy is a contraindication now, phentermine and other anorectics were widely used to prevent excessive weight gain during pregnancy from 1959 until 1979 without any adverse effects on either the gestation or the fetus. After the FDA introduced Pharmaceutical Pregnancy Categories in 1979, and gave phentermine a category X rating, obstetricians stopped prescribing phentermine during pregnancy. There are no known teratogenic effects ascribed to phentermine. Patients can be advised to continue taking it while trying to get pregnant and then discontinue it once pregnancy is diagnosed.

Nursing mothers should not have phentermine prescribed since the drug may find its way into the breast milk, producing an anorectic effect in the infant. (This is apparently conjecture; there are no supporting data.)

Phentermine given to someone who has had a prior severe allergic reaction may induce anaphylaxis.

Ages—Although phentermine labeling states that the drug should not be used in patients aged 16 years and under, the drug has been used in children as young as age 3 without ill effects (36,37). Typically, guidelines for treating obesity in children and adolescents either omit mentioning the sympathomimetic amine anorectics or condemn their use (38). The 2008 ASBP survey revealed that 56% of practicing bariatric physicians would prescribe anorectics for adolescents (the question did not specify an adolescent age range). Some caution is advisable here since pediatricians seem to be uniformly opposed to using the older anorectics. It is indeed incongruous that the very same pediatricians who will willingly use schedule II amphetamines to treat attention-deficit hyperactivity disorder (ADHD) in their patients refuse to consider far less dangerous schedule IV substances such as phentermine and diethylpropion for treating obesity. Informed consent should be obtained from the parents before prescribing phentermine for an adolescent, and the parents should be forewarned that the patient's pediatrician would likely be opposed to the use of phentermine. There is no upper age limit for phentermine.

Dose—The normal starting dose of phentermine HCl for adults is 15 to 18.75 mg (half of a 37.5 mg tablet) once or twice daily, with the second dose before 3 p.m. if a second dose is needed. Although the drug has a biological half-life of 18 to 24 hours and once-daily dosing should be efficacious, some patients benefit from twice-daily dosing. Phentermine has stimulant effects, which typically are mild and fade quickly. In patients who have a history of overreacting to stimulants, or have panic or anxiety, a lower starting dose of 15 mg may be advisable. An even lower starting dose could be achieved by breaking the 37.5 mg tablet into quarters to achieve a dose of approximately 9 mg. Eight-milligram tablets, available before the phen-fen crisis in 1997, are no longer manufactured. The starting dose for younger adolescents should be either approximately 9 or 15 mg per day. Later in treatment, doses may be adjusted as discussed in the following section. One early study reported that patients given phentermine on an alternating month schedule had the same overall weight loss as patients given phentermine continuously (39). This practice is not recommended since it interrupts weight loss, sometimes with significant weight gain during the off months. Patients taken off phentermine often begin to gain in the first month, become discouraged and disillusioned with their treatment, and are thus lost to follow-up.

Dose ranging—Although some early clinical trials used dose-to-effect titration of phentermine doses (40), there are only a few modern papers reporting phentermine doses exceeding 37.5 mg per day for treating obesity. There is no modern, double-blind, randomized, placebo-controlled prospective phentermine dose ranging clinical trials in the medical literature. There are, however, several reports suggesting that dose-to-effect titration has been in use for phentermine for many years. Haddock et al. (27) in their study state, "In cases of excessive hunger, the initial starting dosage was doubled for phentermine HCl." Their starting dose was either 30 or 37.5 mg per day; so, evidently some patients were started on either 60 or 75 mg per day. Another report from a private obesity treatment clinic reports starting compounded doses of 40 mg phentermine with 5-hydroxytyptophan (5-HTP)/carbidopa per day that are often then titrated to phentermine 55 mg per day within the first month (41). The 2008 ASBP

Prescribing Practices Survey asked the question "… what are the lowest and highest doses you prescribed [of phentermine] …" and although the *average* high dose was reported as 56 mg per day, significant numbers of physicians prescribed more than the average high dose. The raw data from the survey revealed that although 5% of respondent physicians prescribed 56 mg per day as their highest dose, 11% prescribed 60 mg per day, 19% prescribed 75 mg per day, 3% prescribed 90 mg per day, 4% prescribed 112 mg per day, 1% prescribed 150 mg per day, and 1% prescribed 180 mg per day as their highest dose (2). The responses indicate that 44% of the physicians surveyed have titrated phentermine doses beyond the Physician's Desk Reference (PDR)–recommended highest dose. This practice, dose-to-effect titration of phentermine, is therefore very commonly used in bariatric medicine.

In phentermine dose-to-effect titration, the dose, perhaps set low initially to avoid undesirable stimulant side effects, is adjusted upward if the patient complains of hunger, if weight loss is less than expected, or if harmful eating behavior worsens. Increases in scores of the EBQ mentioned above can be used to determine changes in eating behaviors. Early in the course of phentermine therapy, if tachyphylaxis occurs, dose adjustments are made, focusing on phentermine anorectic effect. Later dose adjustments are made focusing on the long-term eating behaviors. Doses may be adjusted up or down at any time during the course of the treatment, depending upon the patient's weight response, his or her perception of hunger, side effects, or changes in eating behaviors. Some patients may comfortably stay at their starting dose for years, whereas others may need higher doses soon after starting, and still others may benefit from an adjustment up or down after many months. Anytime a patient reaches a plateau in weight loss in spite of good compliance, dose adjustment upward should be considered. Anytime the clinician or patient detects changes in eating behaviors, dose adjustments should be considered. Conversely, if side effects occur at any dose, dose reduction should be considered if side effects cannot be managed otherwise. If at any time the patient believes he or she no longer needs the drug or that phentermine is no longer effective, it should be discontinued. Often in such cases, after phentermine is discontinued, the patient finds that it was more helpful than realized. In such cases, the drug can always be restarted. Testing with the EBQ is sometimes helpful in making the patient aware of phentermine or other antiobesity drug effectiveness.

Dose-to-effect titration is a common practice in medicine and is used with a wide variety of pharmacologic agents. Dose-to-effect titration of amphetamine drugs is the standard of practice in treating ADHD where physicians use the following three approaches:

1. Prescribe a low dose, then judge effectiveness
2. Gradually titrate to higher doses until behavior improves
3. Ramp up until side effects occur, then reduce dose to the level before they occurred (42)

Wide ranges of amphetamine doses are used in ADHD patients; clearly, some patients tolerate higher doses than the recommended starting doses. The ASBP prescribing surveys did not specifically ask about dose-to-effect titration, but the ranges of starting doses and highest doses reported suggest that the physicians who adjust phentermine doses higher use an analogous approach. Although there is not an extensive literature on dose-to-effect phentermine titration, this approach has clearly been long used in practice without reports of problems, suggesting this strategy is safe and effective. There are also anecdotal reports that adult obese patients with ADHD require (and tolerate) higher doses of phentermine, which might be expected in view of the range of effective amphetamine doses observed in ADHD patients. Doses higher than the limit suggested on the label for the phenethylamine antiobesity drugs have been discussed in presentations numerous times in scientific sessions at the meetings of the ASBP and at the Annual Review Course of the American Board of Bariatric Physicians (43–55). That some patients benefit from doses of phentermine higher than the FDA label recommends has been discussed numerous times in the peer-reviewed medical literature (2,26,27,40,56–58).

Dose-to-effect titration seems to be safe and effective for the patient, but this approach can jeopardize the physician's license or his or her malpractice insurance in states where medical boards insist on strict adherence to FDA drug labeling.

Other beneficial effects—Obviously, the most important beneficial effect of phentermine therapy is additional weight loss, but there are others. Low energy is a frequent complaint of obese patients at initial evaluation. Weight reduction therapy, in general, improves energy level in these patients, but the addition of phentermine to their therapy often provides an added improvement. In some cases, patients on phentermine report an aroused interest in their daily activities and improvements in mood. These effects may be seen both in patients with previously undiagnosed depression and in patients already on antidepressant medication. This effect should not be surprising; after all, amphetamine was first approved for depression. Generally, patients with attention deficit disorder (ADD) or ADHD experience some improvement in their ADD or ADHD on phentermine. This is true for patients on no medication, but may also be true for patients already on a stimulant medication for ADD or ADHD. Although the combination of amphetamine and phentermine may cause too much stimulation for some patients, others find the phentermine helps with hunger and eating behavior more than the amphetamine. Occasionally, some patients experience beneficial anticholinergic effects. Since phentermine can produce decreased gastrointestinal motility, some patients with chronic diarrhea or who suffer from rapid gastrointestinal transit time notice improvement on phentermine. Women with stress incontinence may note symptomatic improvement.

Adverse side effects—Since phentermine works by increasing norepinephrine release that then acts through β-adrenergic receptors pervasive throughout the entire nervous system, it should not be surprising that the drug can produce a diverse variety of side effects. Some side effects may be beneficial, as noted above, whereas others limit the effectiveness of the drug. The adverse side effects discussed in the following paragraphs are those that have actually been observed in practice. Potential adverse effects, of theoretical interest, that have not been, or have rarely been, observed are discussed in the following section. Where possible, estimates of the rate of occurrence of each reaction described are included. The incidence rates apply if the patient is taking the medication as directed. Incidences of adverse reactions may increase if the patient is taking more than advised.

Phentermine is a mild stimulant; patients' reactions to the stimulant effects of phentermine vary widely. Some patients notice "feeling speedy" with initial doses of phentermine, but most patients do not notice or complain of this effect. Other patients report being pleasantly energized. Rarely, a patient becomes so stimulated that he or she cannot be persuaded to ever take phentermine again. Generally, any adverse stimulant effects occur early, are mild, and disappear with continued exposure to the drug. Most patients experience a modest beneficial stimulant effect, but a very few have such severe stimulation the drug must be discontinued. If stimulation is a problem, a useful antidote is to give such a patient a beta blocker such as pindolol, 5 mg once or twice daily; this dosage will mitigate the stimulation without interfering with the anorectic effect.

In some patients, undesirable mood altering effects occur. There are patients who will stop phentermine because they experience mood changes and do not like the way they feel. In some cases, increased irritability occurs while on the drug. Irritability in some patients can be controlled with pindolol; if not, discontinuation of phentermine may be advisable.

Insomnia, another stimulant effect, is reasonably common in the population of patients presenting for obesity treatment. Insomnia is frequent in the general population and may have already been a problem before phentermine was started. The clinician should always question patients about their sleep patterns before the initiation of phentermine. Insomnia characterized by sleep onset delay occurs early on in phentermine therapy. This is a stimulant effect that, if it occurs at all, is most often mild and disappears if the patient continues the drug. Sleep deprivation symptoms are rare. The incidence of insomnia is perhaps 3% 1 month after initiation of phentermine therapy. There is a second form of insomnia that can occur after the patient has been on phentermine for months or years in which the patient goes to sleep easily, but awakens after a few hours and cannot go back to sleep. Sleep deprivation symptoms can become problematic with this form of insomnia. The incidence of late-appearing insomnia is generally less than 1 in 1000 patients. Early-onset insomnia typically responds to pindolol at bedtime. Late-onset insomnia will sometimes respond to melatonin; if not, then pindolol or trazodone should be tried rather than a benzodiazepine. If all remedies fail, discontinuation of the phentermine may be required for resolution of the insomnia.

Undesirable anticholinergic effects include dry mouth, constipation, lightheadedness, and difficulty with urination. Many patients complain of mild dry mouth, generally so mild it only serves to remind them to drink the 64 oz of water daily that we recommend. A rare patient will have such severe dry mouth that mucosal erosions may occur; the incidence of such severe dry mouth is <1 in 1000 patients. If constipation occurs, it is usually due to the change in fiber intake with caloric restriction, or it may be due in part to the phentermine. Constipation usually responds to strategies to increase fiber intake. If not, a probiotic may be helpful. Lightheadedness or dizziness occurs in about 2% of patients; but in bariatric patients, these conditions are more often due to transient hypoglycemia invoked by caloric restriction or postural hypotension due to inadequate sodium intake when on a ketogenic diet or due to continued antihypertension medication that is no longer needed after weight loss, rather than being due to phentermine. Other, more serious anticholinergic effects, such as increased intra-ocular pressure, confusion, disorientation, and symptoms associated with delirium, have not been observed in practice.

Phentermine-induced mild bladder outlet sphincter contraction can be counteracted with tamsulosin 0.4 mg daily or twice daily. Headache, occurring in about 1% of patients, is usually of the tension type and responds favorably to therapy. Patients with migraine in whom stimulant medications provoke attacks may experience a migraine headache upon initiation of phentermine, but most patients with migraine tolerate phentermine initiation without headache.

Palpitations occur in a few patients, and although these heartbeat changes may be distressing enough for the patient to discontinue the medicine, they are seldom associated with any electrocardiogram finding more than benign extrasystoles. Occasionally, patients taking phentermine experience one instance of an increased heart rate above their baseline pretreatment heart rate, but the same occurs in overweight and obese patients on dietary treatment alone. Other uncommon side effects include allergic reactions, impotence, bruxism, and intensification of preexisting tremors. Allergic reaction to phentermine, most often manifest as urticaria, is uncommon, but it does occur in <1 in 1000 patients. Phentermine may aggravate bruxism; this side effect is seldom seen with diethylpropion. Intensification of preexisting tremor does sometimes occur, as can happen with any stimulant in this condition.

Potential or theoretical adverse effects—Adverse effects of phentermine that are most likely to be seen in clinical practice are enumerated in the paragraph above. In addition to these effects, phentermine labeling includes a long list of potential side effects. With rare exceptions, none of the other potential adverse side effects listed in phentermine labeling have actually been observed in practice. Most of these are *theoretical conjectures* and are not based on fact, but rather upon the supposition that since the phentermine molecule is similar to amphetamine, phentermine should have adverse effects identical to or similar to those of amphetamine. Phentermine has been in use for 55 years. If these potential problems have not surfaced as of yet, the potential risk of these theoretical adverse effects must be either vanishingly low or not exist. Phentermine effects and adverse effects *are not identical* to those of amphetamine or methamphetamine.

Phentermine labeling lists nine contraindications, including advanced arteriosclerosis, cardiovascular disease, moderate-to-severe hypertension, hyperthyroidism, hypersensitivity or idiosyncrasy to sympathomimetic amines, glaucoma, agitated states, and history of drug abuse. Phentermine labeling also includes warnings concerning use in combination with other weight loss drugs, use in combination with selective serotonin reuptake inhibitors (SSRIs), primary pulmonary hypertension, valvular heart disease, tolerance, and impairment in ability to drive or operate machinery. Finally, phentermine labeling includes a paragraph on drug abuse and dependence that discusses six issues implying that all of these are hazards of phentermine therapy: abuse, intense psychological dependence, severe social dysfunction, addiction, chronic intoxication, and psychosis. Although some of these issues are well-known problems associated with amphetamine, or more often, with methamphetamine, none have ever been observed with phentermine. Every one of these issues is theoretical and is based solely on the conjecture that phentermine adverse effects *must* be identical to amphetamine and methamphetamine effects. A literature search on PubMed reveals there are a few rare exceptions to these last two statements, but closer investigation of the exceptions reveals that most of them do not withstand careful scrutiny (51).

Space constraints prohibit detailed examination of each and every one of these accusations against phentermine, but a few of them should be rebutted. The most fearsome of these accusations are related to valvular heart disease, hypertension, pulmonary hypertension, and abuse or addiction. It is clear now that phentermine does not and never has produced valvular heart disease (59–61). Amphetamine may elevate blood pressure, and there is a widespread assumption that the same is true of phentermine. Evidence in the medical literature of phentermine-related blood pressure effects is scant but, aside from a few anecdotal cases to the contrary (40), the evidence from clinical trials (62) and from retrospective reports (26,27,41) suggests that blood pressure decreases in phentermine-treated patients in weight loss programs. Phentermine, in the dose ranges discussed here, does not appear to induce sustained elevations of blood pressure. In a study of phentermine and blood pressure in a weight management program, transient increases in blood pressure were observed at 1 week after initiation of phentermine therapy in less than 1% of patients, and more rarely, transient increases in blood pressure at 1 week after phentermine dose increases (26). When a patient in a weight management program is found to have a blood pressure ≥140 systolic or ≥90 diastolic, a prudent course of action would be to withhold phentermine until blood pressure is in control. If the patient is not on antihypertensive medications, either daily hydrochlorothiazide at 50 mg, or a daily dose of the combination of 25 mg of hydrochlorothiazide and 25 mg of spironolactone, will often bring blood pressure in control quickly. Once blood pressure is in control, phentermine may be initiated or resumed.

The incidence of primary pulmonary hypertension in patients on phentermine is lower than the incidence in the general population (63); phentermine has not and does not induce primary pulmonary hypertension (64).

The hallmark of substance addiction is intense craving for the substance (65). This is present both during chronic substance use and upon substance cessation. Neither patients on long-term phentermine nor patients who abruptly cease phentermine exhibit phentermine cravings, nor do such patients manifest amphetamine-like withdrawal (57). There is not a single literature report of abuse, addiction, or withdrawal with phentermine. Clearly phentermine is not an addicting substance; neither abuse nor addiction, as defined in the Diagnostic and Statistical Manual of Mental Disorders (DSM)-IV (66), nor substance use disorder, as defined in the DSM-V (67), occurs in the context of phentermine pharmacotherapy.

Combinations and drug interactions—Although some on-line chemical databases (68) list a variety of drug interactions, the listings are for drug interactions for amphetamine and not for phentermine. Phentermine can be used in combination with any drug; there are neither known drug interactions or known contraindications to combining phentermine with any other drug. Although the FDA label warns of combining phentermine with monoamine oxidase inhibitors because of the possibility of hypertensive crisis, there is no published evidence such an event has ever occurred, even though obesity itself is a risk factor for hypertensive crisis (69). Phentermine has insignificant effects on 5-hydroxytrypophan and serotonin metabolism (70) and can be safely used in patients taking selective serotonin inhibitor antidepressants (71).

Several combinations of phentermine with other drugs with effects on weight have been found useful and are discussed in the Useful Combinations section.

DIETHYLPROPION

Diethylpropion is a safe and effective weight management drug and is widely used. The ASBP medication surveys of 2008 and 2012 revealed that 64% and 63% of bariatric physicians used it for an average of 15% and 18% of their patients, respectively (Table 8.1), making diethylpropion the second most frequently prescribed drug for weight management.

Diethylpropion is another sympathomimetic amine derived from β-phenylethylamine, and its molecular structure also resembles that of amphetamine. The FDA has long presumed that all the sympathomimetic amines, including diethylpropion, have effects and adverse effects similar to, if not identical with, those of amphetamine. Thus, the product labeling for diethylpropion includes all the same conjectures discussed herein for phentermine. The mechanism of action is thought to be similar to that of phentermine.

Diethylpropion has therapeutic effects similar to those of phentermine. Patients on diethylpropion initially notice suppression of appetite. Later, they notice improvements in eating behaviors. With a short half-life and less potent stimulation effects, diethylpropion has been used safely and with good effectiveness in adults (72); the elderly (73); and in the past, in children (74).

Duration of action—Diethylpropion has a biological half-life of 4 to 6 hours. The clinical duration of action is about 4 hours. Plasma levels obtained with the 75 mg time-released diethylpropion formulation administered once daily indicated a more gradual release than the immediate-release formulation (three 25 mg tablets given in a single dose). After administration of a single dose of one 75 mg controlled-release tablet or diethylpropion hydrochloride solution (75 mg dose) in a crossover study using normal human subjects, the amount of parent compound and its active metabolites recovered in the urine within 48 hours for the two dosage forms were not statistically different (http://www.rxlist.com/tenuate-drug/clinical-pharmacology.htm).

Clinical usefulness—Diethylpropion is a very useful weight management agent. Because of its short duration of action, it can be administered later in the day when patients have trouble with evening hunger, cravings, or loss of control of eating behavior. Patients in whom phentermine produces insomnia are candidates for diethylpropion. Some patients can tolerate a low dose of phentermine in the morning and may benefit from a morning dose of phentermine and an afternoon dose of diethylpropion.

Contraindications—Contraindications to diethylpropion are similar to those of phentermine: pregnancy, nursing an infant, and prior allergic reactions to diethylpropion. The drug was frequently prescribed for prevention of excessive weight gain during pregnancy, with no known problems for 20 years after diethylpropion was approved in 1959 until 1979 when the FDA Pharmaceutical Pregnancy Categories were introduced. Since there have been no human clinical trials of diethylpropion during pregnancy, the drug was assigned a B category and the majority of obstetricians stopped prescribing the drug.

Ages—Diethylpropion labeling admonishes that the drug not be used in children under the age of 16 years. The situation is analogous to the situation with phentermine; pediatricians once used diethylpropion for children, but then they stopped for reasons unrelated to the diethylpropion itself. There is no upper age limit.

Dose—The drug is available as 25 mg immediate-release tablets and 75 mg controlled-release tablets. The usual dose with either is 75 mg daily. Some patients do well with 25 or 50 mg daily. Thirty percent of the bariatric physicians responding to the 2008 ASBP survey indicated that they sometimes used higher doses of 100 to 150 mg daily.

Adverse side effects—Diethylpropion has adverse effects similar to those of phentermine. In general, adverse effects due to diethylpropion are less frequent and have lower intensity than are those due to phentermine.

Potential or theoretical adverse effects—Again, the FDA presumes, without evidence, that the adverse effects of diethylpropion are identical to those of amphetamine and methamphetamine. Diethylpropion labeling includes all of the same theoretical objections listed in phentermine labeling.

Combinations—Although various databases list drug interactions with diethylpropion, the interactions are amphetamine interactions. These have not been observed with diethylpropion. Diethylpropion is very safe and may be used in patients taking any other drug, including other weight management drugs.

PHENDIMETRAZINE

Although phendimetrazine has been available since its approval in 1959, there are only a few reports of its use in the peer-reviewed literature (75,76).

Clinical usefulness—Fifty-six percent of bariatric physicians have found phendimetrazine to be a useful drug; those who use it do so in 18% of their patients. Phendimetrazine is another sympathomimetic amine derived from β-phenylethylamine, and its molecular structure also resembles that of amphetamine. The FDA has long presumed that all the sympathomimetic amines, including phendimetrazine, have effects and adverse effects similar to, if not identical with, those of amphetamine. Thus, the product labeling for phendimetrazine includes all the same conjectures discussed for phentermine. The mechanism of action is thought to be similar to that of phentermine.

Phendimetrazine has therapeutic effects similar to those of phentermine. Patients on phendimetrazine first notice suppression of appetite and then later they notice improvements in eating behaviors.

Contraindications—These are the same as for phentermine.

Mechanism of action—In the body, phendimetrazine is converted to phenmetrazine, the active metabolite. Phenmetrazine is a sympathomimetic with anorectic properties.

Dose—The typical dose is 35 mg three times daily. The maximum dose listed in package labeling and PDR is 70 mg three times daily.

Dose ranging—Some patients tolerate more than the typical dose. The 2008 ASBP survey found that only 51% of bariatric physicians prescribed phendimetrazine at the recommended daily dose of 105 mg. Of the remainder, 16% prescribed 140 mg per day, 5% prescribed 175 mg per day, 26% prescribed 210 mg per day, and 1% each prescribed 280 and 315 mg as their highest dose.

Beneficial effects, adverse side effects, and potential or relative contraindications—These are all similar to those of phentermine. Phendimetrazine can be used in combination with the same drugs as is phentermine.

ORLISTAT

Clinical usefulness—Orlistat has not proven to be very useful in clinical practice because few patients tolerate the gastrointestinal side effects. Although 44% of medical bariatric specialists prescribe orlistat, these physicians only use it in 6% to 8% of their patients. Orlistat is a very safe, but only modestly effective, weight loss drug. It is an intestinal lipase inhibitor that prevents absorption of some of the fat a patient consumes for a few hours after taking the drug. Its effectiveness is limited by its unpopularity with the majority of patients. Some patients find it useful for maintenance. It is available as a prescription 120 mg capsule marketed as Xenical® and also as an over-the-counter 60 mg capsule (Alli®).

Dosages—Either 60 mg or 120 mg three times daily.

Adverse reactions and side effects—The most common side effects of orlistat are abdominal discomfort, oily stools, oily diarrhea, and increased flatus. Other side effects are listed in the PDR.

Management of adverse reactions and side effects—Severe adverse reactions are virtually unheard of, but the gastrointestinal side effects are very common. Most patients learn to skip the drug if they plan to eat a fatty meal. Adverse effects to orlistat can be lessened by lowering the amount of fat ingested during meals.

PHENTERMINE/TOPIRAMATE

The FDA first approved topiramate in 1996 as a treatment for refractory epilepsy. At that time, since most epilepsy drugs in use induced weight gain, many of the patients treated were either overweight or obese. Observations of weight loss among epilepsy patients treated with topiramate quickly led to weight loss trials in humans (77–80) that demonstrated both significant weight losses and successful weight loss maintenance. These reports, together with others indicating effective use of topiramate in the treatment on binge eating disorder (81–83), led to trials combining topiramate with phentermine (29).

Following a series of clinical trials demonstrating safety and efficacy (84–86), the FDA approved the combination of phentermine with topiramate (Qsymia) in 2012. Approval was controversial; the FDA had asked the sponsoring company, Vivus, Inc. (Mountain View, CA), to provide additional safety data. Despite the controversy, the 2012 ASBP prescribing practices survey, performed a few months before FDA approval, revealed that 61% of the bariatric physicians were already using phentermine combined with generic topiramate for some of their patients and that 43% indicated they would prescribe Qsymia were it to be approved.

Duration of action—Twenty-four hours.

Clinical usefulness—The various Qsymia trials proved the combination is an effective antiobesity medicine; 47% of patients on the high daily dose lost 10% or more of their baseline weight at 1 year. Weight loss at 1-year averaged 12.8% of baseline weight and 11.4% at 2 years.

Contraindications—Women taking topiramate during the first trimester of pregnancy have an increased risk of their baby having craniofacial defects, primarily cleft palate. Topiramate is found in the milk of nursing mothers and since the effects on newborns are unknown, topiramate is not recommended during breastfeeding. An acute closed-angle glaucoma syndrome is a very rare idiosyncratic reaction to topiramate. Although this usually responds to prompt treatment, it is probably best to avoid topiramate in patients with established angle closure glaucoma unless the patient's ophthalmologist agrees and will monitor eye pressure frequently.

Ages—The use of Qsymia in patients under the age of 18 years has not been evaluated and is therefore not recommended. Both phentermine and topiramate have been used individually in adolescents and children without problems peculiar to the ages; so, physicians and patients can draw their own conclusions. Since only 7% of the patients in the clinical trials were age 65 years and older, the FDA recommends being cautious in patients in this age group, even though no differences in efficacy or safety were observed. Again, both phentermine and topiramate have been used as individual drugs in this age group.

Dose—As a part of the FDA-mandated Risk Evaluation and Mitigation Strategy program, Qsymia is available only through pharmacies certified as trained in Qsymia dispensing by the FDA. The drug comes in capsules of four strengths (Table 8.2).

Phentermine strengths are expressed as phentermine base. The equivalent phentermine doses expressed as phentermine HCl are approximately 4.7, 9.3, 14, and 18.75 mg. The topiramate is an extended-release form of topiramate, with a peak plasma level at 9 hours. The resin form of phentermine has a half-life of 24 hours. Patients who have been on the usual dose (7.5 mg phentermine/46 mg topiramate) for 12 weeks and have lost 3% or less of initial body weight should have the dose escalated to 11.25 mg/69 mg for 14 days and then increased to the high dose (15 mg/92 mg).

Adverse side effects—Common side effects are multiple and are primarily due to the topiramate component. These side effects include paresthesia, headache, dizziness, dysgeusia, insomnia, constipation, and dry mouth. Less frequent side effects include short-term memory loss, dyslexia, nausea, and depression. Acute angle closure glaucoma can occur but is very rare and is thought to be an idiosyncratic reaction to the imbedded sulfur atom in the molecule. In practice, the combination phentermine/topiramate is not well tolerated long term by patients; more than one-half of patients discontinue the combination because of side effects mainly due to the topiramate (87).

Potential or theoretical adverse effects—The label indicates these include all of the potential or theoretical adverse effects listed herein for phentermine and topiramate. Metabolic acidosis is also a potential topiramate adverse effect.

Combinations—Dose levels of phentermine, but not of topiramate, in all Qsymia capsules are below typical adult doses used by physicians treating obesity. Vivus selected the phentermine dose levels based on weight loss effects in a 12-week trial. Their study showed that, although there was greater weight loss at phentermine doses greater than 15 mg phentermine base per day, there was an inflection in the dose-to-weight loss curve at 15 mg with a proportional decrease in the weight loss-to-dose ratio, leading them to conclude 15 mg per day was an optimal dose (Wesley Day, personal communication, Mountain View, California, April, 2013).

Table 8.2 Dosage forms of commercially available phentermine/topiramate combinations

Capsule	Phentermine (mg)	Topiramate (mg)
Starting	3.5	23
Usual	7.5	46
Escalation	11.25	69
High	15	92

This conclusion, therefore, did not take into consideration long-term effects of phentermine on eating, on eating behavior, or on eating cognition. Some patients find their eating control is improved when a supplementary dose of phentermine is added.

Generic phentermine HCl and generic topiramate can be combined, and in so doing, doses of either or both drugs can be adjusted. Generic topiramate is immediate release and is not the same as the slow-release topiramate in Qsymia. The result is that patients have to take two or more pills rather than one daily. An advantage to the generic combination is that some patients do better with higher phentermine and lower topiramate doses than Qsymia provides.

Table 8.3 compares the effectiveness of Qsymia (as well as lorcaserin and Contrave, discussed below) with both phentermine and topiramate monotherapy.

LORCASERIN

Lorcaserin (Belviq) is a selective serotonin 2C receptor agonist with minimal activity at other serotonin receptors, including the 2B heart valve receptors. After it was established that fenfluramine, acting as a serotonin 2B receptor agonist on heart valves, induced valvulopathy (88), Vivus initiated a search for specific serotonin 2C receptors. After establishing that lorcaserin was a potent 2C receptor agonist, but did not activate 2B receptors, a clinical development process was initiated. During the ensuing clinical trials, the FDA required that multiple echocardiograms be obtained on subjects. At 1 year, 2.2% of placebo-treated patients developed cardiac valvulopathy whereas 2.3% of lorcaserin-treated subjects did so. The difference was not statistically significant. The valve changes were predominantly mitral and aortic regurgitation of the sort seen in aging populations. No changes in pulmonary artery pressure were noted (89).

Forty-seven percent of lorcaserin-treated subjects in the clinical trials achieved a 5% weight loss at 1 year and 22.5% achieved a 10% or greater loss. Weight loss at 1 year averaged 6%, but placebo-adjusted weight loss was about 4%. The FDA is requiring Arena Pharmaceuticals (San Diego, California) to conduct a postmarketing 5-year long-term cardiovascular outcome trial (NCT02019264). Many physicians are already prescribing combinations of Belviq and phentermine in treating obesity and, as this text is written, Arena is conducting a safety trial of Belviq and phentermine (NCT01987427).

Duration of action—Twenty-four hours.

Clinical usefulness—It remains to be seen whether lorcaserin alone will be useful. Initial reports of the combination phentermine/lorcaserin suggest that it is quite effective, perhaps as effective as was the combination phentermine/fenfluramine.

Contraindications—The drug is rated as pregnancy category X.

Ages—The drug has not been tested in adolescents and children.

Dose—Ten milligrams twice daily.

Adverse side effects—The most common adverse side effects were headache, dizziness, nausea, and diarrhea. The number of patients who discontinued the drug in clinical trials because of side effects was low.

Potential or theoretical adverse effects—The DEA has decided the drug is potentially addicting and has deemed it a category IV controlled substance. This development came despite a DEA-requested study "… conducted according to standard abuse-potential guidelines …" evaluating the addiction potential of lorcaserin in polydrug users, which concluded that "… lorcaserin has a very low potential for abuse …", "… the subjective effects of supratherapeutic doses of lorcaserin were, on balance, negative, thereby confirming lorcaserin's low risk for abuse," and "The AEs reported in the current study also indicate that supratherapeutic doses of lorcaserin are associated with negative side effects that would mitigate the risk of abuse" (90) (ClinicalTrials.gov identifier NCT00828659).

Table 8.3 Effectiveness of new drugs compared to phentermine and topiramate monotherapy

Drug	Dose (mg/day)	Categorical weight loss 5%	Categorical weight loss 10%	Categorical weight loss 15%	Completers at 12 months (%)	Weight loss at 12 months (%)
Lorcaserin		63	35	NA	59	8
Qnexa	Phentermine 15, topiramate 96	84	60	43	59	15
Contrave		56	33	15	52	8
Phentermine compared, Haddock et al. (27)	30	84	61	NA	24	13–14
Topiramate, Astrup et al. (79)	96	96	78	49	31	17

Note: All data, with percentages rounded to whole numbers, are from company reports of clinical trials. The data selected are best case when several trials were conducted. Weight loss at 12 months is observed weight loss in completers without placebo subtraction. Haddock et al. (27) data are from a 12-month retrospective study in a fee-for-service private practice, not from a clinical trial. NA, not applicable.

SSRIs, serotonin and norepinephrine reuptake inhibitors, bupropion, tricyclic antidepressants, and monoamine oxidase inhibitors were excluded from the trials. One patient taking dextromethorphan developed serotonin syndrome. It seems prudent to watch for serotonin syndrome in patients on antidepressants. Since patients on long-term lorcaserin experience age-related aortic and mitral valve regurgitation at the same rate as do untreated patients, physicians should observe treated patients closely for the development of new murmurs. Physicians prescribing Belviq should familiarize themselves with the approved FDA label for the drug and with the clinical trial data (89,91–93).

Combinations—Early reports of using phentermine once daily combined with once daily Belviq have reported good success.

CONTRAVE

Contrave is a combination of bupropion, an antidepressant that is a weak inhibitor of neuronal reuptake of norepinephrine and dopamine, and naltrexone, a μ-opioid receptor antagonist originally approved for the treatment of alcohol and opiate addiction. Bupropion stimulates hypothalamic proopiomelanocortin (POMC) neurons to release α-melanocyte-stimulating hormone (α-MSH). α-MSH is an agonist of melanocortin 4 receptors that initiates a cascade leading to decreased energy intake and increased energy expenditure, resulting in weight loss. As POMC neurons release α-MSH, they also release a μ-opioid receptor agonist that induces diminution of α-MSH release. Naltrexone blocks this negative feedback, working synergistically with bupropion, thereby amplifying the weight loss effect. Bupropion is a substituted phenethylamine, but there have been no suggestions of addiction potential. The combination is not classified as a controlled substance.

Duration of action—Twelve hours.

Clinical usefulness—Forty-nine percent of Contrave-treated subjects in the clinical trials achieved a 5% weight loss at 1 year and 25% achieved a 10% or greater loss. Weight loss at 1 year averaged 6% to 8%, depending on the trial. The FDA required a preapproval, 5-year, long-term cardiovascular outcomes trial, but approved the drug in 2014 before the trial was completed, based on favorable preliminary data.

Contraindications—Uncontrolled hypertension, seizures, use of other bupropion-containing products, opioid or opioid antagonist use, monoamine oxidase inhibitor use, and pregnancy are contraindications. The drug is also contraindicated in nursing mothers.

Ages—Adults only; the drug combination has not been tested in children and adolescents.

Dose—Contrave tablets are available at 4 mg/90 mg naltrexone/bupropion and 8 mg/90 mg naltrexone/bupropion. The recommended daily dose is 32 mg naltrexone and 360 mg bupropion. Since nausea due to the naltrexone component is a common side effect, patients should be started with one morning 8 mg/90 mg tablet for the first week and then have gradual dose escalation increasing by one tablet per day each succeeding week until a dose of 32 mg/360 mg naltrexone/bupropion is reached at week 4. If nausea occurs, the dose can be reduced by switching to the 4 mg/90 mg tablets or by slowing the timing of dose escalation or by using both techniques.

Adverse side effects—Common side effects include nausea, constipation, headache, vomiting, dizziness, insomnia, dry mouth, and diarrhea. In the clinical trials, 24% of patients on Contrave discontinued it because of adverse effects.

Uncommon adverse effects—Suicidal behavior, activation of mania, seizures, increases in blood pressure and heart rate, allergic reactions, and angle closure glaucoma may occur, but are not common. Both drugs in the combination have been widely used; naltrexone first approved in 1984 has been prescribed for more than 1 million patients; bupropion first approved in 1985 has been prescribed for more than 50 million patients. Physicians prescribing Contrave should familiarize themselves with the FDA-approved label and with the clinical trial data (94–96).

Combinations—Presently there are no studies reported combining this drug with other agents for weight loss.

TOPIRAMATE

Shortly after this sulfamate-substituted monosaccharide was introduced as an antiepileptic, topiramate was noted to produce weight loss in treated subjects. Clinical trials demonstrated weight loss comparable to the other antiobesity drugs (77,79), and currently 45% bariatric medicine specialists prescribe topiramate for weight loss in their patients. Once a very expensive drug, the patent for topiramate has lapsed, and the drug is now available as a generic.

Clinical usefulness—Topiramate has been found to be very useful in treating binge eating disorder (82,97) and in treating drug-induced weight gain produced by antidepressants and some other psychiatric drugs (98). Topiramate can be used as a single agent, and since it is not a controlled substance, it can be used as an alternative to the older drugs. Obesity is not considered an indication for topiramate; the drug is not FDA approved for obesity, so its use in obesity is off label.

Absolute contraindications—Known sensitivity to sulfamates is an absolute contraindication.

Dose—Effective doses for weight management range from 25 to 200 mg per day. The typical starting dose for weight management is 25 mg at bedtime. If this dose does not produce the desired effect, the dose can be slowly increased in 25 mg increments using dose-to-effect titration. By increasing the dose once every 2 weeks or at monthly intervals, any annoying side effects can often be avoided. Most patients do not need more than 100 mg per day in the first year or two of treatment. Some patients eventually require 200 mg per day.

Beneficial effects—Patients with binge eating often experience diminution in frequency and intensity of binge eating. Patients with iatrogenic drug-induced weight gain either lose weight or stop gaining weight. Other patients note a decrease in hunger, eating, or both. Patients who have trouble with after dinner cravings, hunger, or eating behaviors sometimes respond well to topiramate.

Adverse side effects—A greater number of patients experience adverse side effects with topiramate monotherapy than do patients on phentermine monotherapy. As a result, after 6 months of treatment, a greater number of patients on topiramate alone have discontinued the drug. Topiramate is a weak carbonic anhydrase inhibitor and can produce symptoms suggestive of peripheral neuropathy. These symptoms usually disappear if the drug is continued. Memory loss for recent events, psychomotor slowing, difficulty with concentration, depression, speech or language problems, and dysesthesias are common at doses used for epilepsy and can occur at doses for weight management, but they are less common. Patients sometimes complain of dysgeusia, particularly for carbonated beverages; in some patients, this is actually a beneficial side effect.

Patients started on topiramate should be warned about the eye symptoms of a glaucoma attack. Always discontinue topiramate immediately if the patient complains of eye pain or any change in visual acuity. Patients who present with eye symptoms should be immediately referred to an ophthalmologist, since untreated secondary angle glaucoma is an ocular emergency that can result in blindness. Neurologic reactions can often be alleviated with dose reductions.

Combinations—Phentermine/topiramate is an effective combination. Clinicians may prescribe either the FDA-approved combination (Qsymia) or prescribe the two drugs as generics. Approved phentermine/topiramate was discussed above.

The two drugs can be initiated simultaneously or in sequence. My preference is to initiate the drugs in sequence to deal with any adverse side effects in sequence. If sequential initiation is selected, typically phentermine is started first and weeks or months later topiramate is added.

ZONISAMIDE

Zonisamide is another antiepileptic drug that can induce weight loss. A clinical trial with zonisamide as monotherapy indicated a respectable weight loss (99,100), and other clinical trials have shown it useful in binge eating (101,102). Another clinical trial has shown good results with a combination of bupropion and zonisamide (103), and yet another suggests zonisamide is useful in preventing olanzapine-associated weight gain (104). Probably as a result of these reports, a few bariatric physicians now use zonisamide in a few of their patients (2).

LIRAGLUTIDE

Liraglutide is a glucagon-like peptide 1 (GLP-1) receptor agonist that is 97% homologous to native GLP-1. The native hormone is a postprandially released gut hormone that lowers blood sugar, slows gastric emptying, decreases appetite, improves satiety, and lowers caloric intake. The drug was approved for diabetes in 2010 and has since been used in more than 3 million patients, many of whom lost weight (105). An FDA Advisory Committee recently recommended approval of the drug at a 3.0 mg per day dose for weight loss, and it is expected that the drug will receive FDA approval.

Other pharmacological agents

Certain drugs are useful as adjuncts in obesity pharmacotherapy. Generally, these drugs have not proven to be effective in producing weight loss when used alone.

Metformin is an agent useful in treating diabetics or patients with insulin resistance. The addition of metformin in treating diabetes or insulin resistance can prevent or diminish the weight gain attendant to other drugs used in treating these conditions and will occasionally produce a modest weight loss. More often, there is minimal or no weight loss. Metformin offers no benefit to a patient with a normal fasting glucose and insulin levels.

Bupropion is a dopamine and norepinephrine reuptake inhibitor. When used as monotherapy, it can produce a modest weight loss that plateaus within a few months (106). Bupropion should be considered when obese patients require an antidepressant. This drug should also be considered when a patient is gaining weight on another antidepressant. The 2008 ASBP Prescribing Practices Survey indicated that 25% of bariatric physicians were using bupropion in 7% of their patients. Weight loss is more impressive when naltrexone is combined with bupropion (107).

GLP-1 receptor agonists (other than liraglutide [see above]), including exenatide and albiglutide, enhance insulin secretion, suppress glucagon, and slow gastric emptying. Clinical trials in patients with type 2 diabetes have demonstrated weight loss in the range of 1 to 3 kg over 26 to 52 weeks (108,109). Exenatide (Byetta®) is currently available in the United States, as is albiglutide (Tanzeum™). These agents are intended as add-on drugs for use in diabetics with poor glucose control and are not intended for monotherapy either for diabetes control or for weight loss.

Spironolactone will, in some women, inhibit premenstrual chocolate, sugar, and other carbohydrate cravings. Spironolactone at 25 mg daily for a few days prior to menses often reduces or eliminates cravings. The combination of hydrochlorothiazide and spironolactone, at 25 mg of each, is equally effective and is less expensive.

5-HTP is the immediate precursor of serotonin (5-hydroxytryptamine) and has long been known to have anorectic properties and the effect of relieving carbohydrate cravings (110). 5-HTP is converted to serotonin in the brain and activates the leptin–melanocortin anorexigenic signaling pathway (111). 5-HTP works because it crosses the blood–brain barrier and is then converted to serotonin in the brain. However, because of its rapid decarboxylation and conversion to serotonin in the gut, liver, and bloodstream, high oral doses of 5-HTP are required to produce even small increases in brain serotonin. If 5-HTP is given alone, high doses of up to 900 mg per day produce the best results. Many patients have nausea and other gastrointestinal side effects at such high doses, limiting the effectiveness of 5-HTP alone. A few patients do well with 150 to 300 mg 5-HTP per day, but for most patients low doses are not effective.

Carbidopa is a peripheral inhibitor of L-aromatic amino acid decarboxylation and inhibits premature decarboxylation of 5-HTP to serotonin before it can cross the blood–brain barrier. Carbidopa, at a 5-mg dose, has no other pharmacological effect. L-dopa/carbidopa combinations are used in treating Parkinson's disease. The carbidopa inhibits decarboxylation of the L-dopa, increasing its effectiveness. Combining carbidopa with 5-HTP increases the effectiveness dramatically. 5-HTP/carbidopa in combination has been used extensively in Europe as a treatment for depression, generally at higher doses of 5-HTP than needed for anorectic use (112).

Patients can be started on a dose of 5 mg 5-HTP with 5 mg carbidopa, taken three times daily with food. If the patient has a good response and no side effects, then the dose may be gradually increased, first to 10 mg, then to 15 mg, and eventually up to 20 or 25 mg 5-HTP, always with 5 mg carbidopa (2,41). Occasional patients benefit from a fourth, nighttime dose. 5-HTP can cause gastrointestinal side effects in higher doses. Carbidopa is not used alone therapeutically and has no known side effects. Side effects for carbidopa reported in the medical literature are those of the L-dopa with which the carbidopa is compounded. The only significant adverse side effects are gastric irritation or nausea when the 5-HTP/carbidopa medication is taken on an empty stomach. Neither serotonin syndrome nor cardiac valvulopathy has been reported in patients on 5-HTP at any dose level (113).

Thus, 5-HTP/carbidopa can be thought of as safe replacement for fenfluramine, and like fenfluramine, it is best when used in combination with phentermine. Patients treated with 5-HTP/carbidopa alone generally neither experience a significant weight loss nor notice a diminution of sugar or other carbohydrate cravings.

Useful combinations

Phentermine and 5-HTP/carbidopa is a useful combination with a mechanism of action similar to phen-fen, but with no risk of cardiac pathology. The 5-HTP tends to modulate the stimulant effect of the phentermine so that patients tolerate the phentermine with fewer side effects. Weight loss with the combination when both phentermine and 5-HTP/carbidopa are started in a new patient is similar to that seen with phen-fen (41). Some physicians prefer to start the patient on phentermine and add the 5-HTP/carbidopa at a later time. One report suggests a 16% weight loss at 6 months with phentermine and an optimum protein, restricted carbohydrate diet at which point the 5-HTP/carbidopa is added resulting in a 17% weight loss at 1 year (2).

Phentermine/topiramate is the combination used in Vivus's new drug Qnexa discussed above. Both drugs are currently available as generics and can be prescribed or dispensed by bariatric physicians. By prescribing these drugs in combination, the disadvantages of a fixed dose combination can be avoided, with the possible benefit of producing greater weight loss.

The 2008 ASBP survey found that 18% of the physicians who used combinations of antiobesity drugs used phentermine/topiramate.

Phentermine/diethylpropion is a combination useful for patients who benefit from phentermine but can only tolerate low early-morning doses and experience return of hunger and appetite in the late afternoon or evening. The addition of one or two doses of diethylpropion after noon may be of benefit. Diethylpropion used in this way seldom provokes insomnia or overstimulation because of its short duration of action.

Phentermine/fluoxetine, thought to be an effective combination by some (114), has not been found useful by most bariatric specialists. The 2008 ASBP survey found that 3% of physicians using combinations used phentermine/fluoxetine.

Bupropion/naltrexone is the combination of drugs in the new drug Contrave discussed above. Both individual drugs are available as generics.

Bupropion/zonisamide as a combination has shown some promise. Patients in an initial 12-week trial with this combination reportedly achieved an 8.5% weight loss (103). Both drugs have been approved, so some bariatric physicians are using the combination.

Phentermine/pramlintide as a combination produced an 11.3% weight loss at 24 weeks in one study (115).

Medications known to cause weight gain

The list of drugs, both prescription and over the counter, that are known to induce weight gain in some patients is long and continues to grow. In some cases, the patient is conscious of the culprit drug, but more often the patient is unaware that a drug is inducing weight gain. The classes of drugs with central nervous system effects most often involved include antidepressants, antipsychotics, anticonvulsants, mood stabilizers, and migraine preventatives. Drugs without a central nervous system action that can induce weight include beta blockers, calcium channel blockers, antidiabetics, steroids, clonidine, clofibrate, antihistamines, antiretrovirals, and some chemotherapy agents. A recent excellent review provides more detail (116).

RECOMMENDED PRESCRIBING PRACTICES

Practical considerations

Pharmacotherapy is one mainstay of obesity treatment; dietary treatment, motivation, behavior modification, and exercise are the others. A combination of all these considerations can produce greater weight loss and promote lasting success for compliant patients than can any single component.

A danger to carefully avoid, not previously mentioned in this chapter, in including antiobesity drugs is that of reducing hunger or appetite so much that the patient eats insufficient protein. Patients who lose weight on protein-deficient diets lose muscle mass. In my opinion, a patient on any antiobesity drug should have a prescribed protein intake quota and be continuously questioned about his or her protein intake to ensure the consumption of enough protein to avoid net muscle protein loss. *A patient who cannot or will not eat the required protein should have his or her antiobesity drug dose reduced or discontinued.*

The amount of daily protein intake suggested in the Recommended Dietary Allowance is inadequate and fails to recognize that dietary protein need is inversely proportional to energy intake (117). As a result of this failure, any diet that stipulates caloric restriction combined with setting protein intake to a percentage of caloric intake may be a *protein-deficient diet* (118).

Such diets for weight loss should be avoided. Recent studies suggest that a minimum threshold protein dose of 30 g is required for the initiation of muscle protein synthesis (119), leading to the recommendation that adults should consume this threshold dose three times daily (118).

In recognition of these recent developments in protein research, some bariatric physicians now prescribe a startup restricted carbohydrate diet with a minimum of 120 g of protein (more for women taller than 70 in. or men taller than 72 in.), combined with 20 g of low glycemic carbohydrates, and 25 g of fat. The same protein intake is maintained when carbohydrate intake is liberalized to a low-calorie diet or to maintenance. The danger of inducing insufficient protein intake with an anorectic is considerably lessened if such a diet is prescribed. A physician must still continue to ascertain that the patient is eating enough protein despite the anorectic.

After 3 days on such a diet, hunger and carbohydrate cravings typically disappear (120), and the patient may discover that an anorectic medication is superfluous. Even so, many patients are more comfortable continuing their medication.

One reason successful maintenance is difficult is that most patients enter a "weight-reduced" metabolic state characterized by decreased metabolic rate; decreased sympathetic tone; and low circulating leptin, thyroxin, and triiodothyronine levels (121). Continued phentermine, or phentermine and 5-HTP/carbidopa, usually enables the patient to comfortably eat less. Free thyroxin and triiodothyronine levels should be assayed, and if either value is low, consideration should be given to treatment to return the levels to normal. Research has shown that low-dose leptin reverses the syndrome (122). One day, perhaps, we will have leptin for our maintenance patients, but even though it has been FDA approved, it is currently extremely expensive and approved only for lipodystrophy (123).

Weight maintenance

Most patients will have better long-term success with weight maintenance if antiobesity drugs are continued indefinitely after weight loss. Pharmacotherapy should always be offered to patients who lost weight without it any time they begin to gain weight after weight loss. This is true both for medical weight loss and weight loss induced by bariatric surgery. Bariatric surgery patients typically lose weight for perhaps a year after surgery and then reach a weight plateau. Subsequently, after a variable interval, many of these patients begin to gain weight, sometimes reaching or exceeding their preoperative weight. The addition of weight management drugs at the point when the patient has regained a few pounds may prevent further weight gain and is preferable to allowing the patient to regain. Little has been published on this strategy, and surgeons seldom think of prescribing antiobesity drugs.

FUTURE DRUGS

We can be optimistic regarding future prospects for new antiobesity drugs since there are numerous drugs in the development pipelines of several drug companies (124). Research into manipulation of gut microbiome suggests this method, too, holds promise for antiobesity therapy (125).

REFERENCES

1. Colman E. Anorectics on trial: A half century of federal regulation of prescription appetite suppressants. *Ann Intern Med* 2005; 143: 380–385.
2. Hendricks EJ, Rothman RB, Greenway FL. How physician obesity specialists use drugs to treat obesity. *Obesity (Silver Spring)* 2009; 17: 1730–1735.

3. NHLBI (National Heart, Blood, and Lung Institute). Clinical guidelines on the identification, evaluation, and treatment of overweight and obesity in adults—The evidence report. National Institutes of Health. *Obes Res* 1998; 6 Suppl 2: 51S–209S.

4. Atkinson RL, Hubbard VS. Report on the NIH workshop on pharmacologic treatment of obesity. *Am J Clin Nutr* 1994; 60: 153–156.

5. Kuk JL, Ardern CI, Church TS, Sharma AM, Padwal R, Sui X, et al. Edmonton obesity staging system: Association with weight history and mortality risk. *Appl Physiol Nutr Metab* 2011; 36: 570–576.

6. Daniel S, Soleymani T, Garvey WT. A complications-based clinical staging of obesity to guide treatment modality and intensity. *Curr Opin Endocrinol Diabetes Obes* 2013; 20: 377–388.

7. ASBP. *Overweight and Obesity Evaluation and Management*. Aurora, CO: American Society of Bariatric Physicians; 2009.

8. Zhang C, Rexrode KM, van Dam RM, Li TY, Hu FB. Abdominal obesity and the risk of all-cause, cardiovascular, and cancer mortality. Sixteen Years of Follow-Up in US Women. *Circulation* 2008; 117: 1624–1626.

9. Pischon T, Boeing H, Hoffmann K, Bergmann M, Schulze MB, Overvad K, et al. General and abdominal adiposity and risk of death in Europe. *N Engl J Med* 2008; 359: 2105–2120.

10. Fox CS, Massaro JM, Hoffmann U, Pou KM, Maurovich-Horvat P, Liu C-Y, et al. Abdominal visceral and subcutaneous adipose tissue compartments: Association with metabolic risk factors in the Framingham Heart Study. *Circulation* 2007; 116: 39–48.

11. Bays HE, Gonzalez-Campoy JM, Bray GA, Kitabchi AE, Bergman DA, Schorr AB, et al. Pathogenic potential of adipose tissue and metabolic consequences of adipocyte hypertrophy and increased visceral adiposity. *Expert Rev Cardiovasc Ther* 2008; 6: 343–368.

12. Romero-Corral A, Somers VK, Sierra-Johnson J, Jensen MD, Thomas RJ, Squires RW, et al. Diagnostic performance of body mass index to detect obesity in patients with coronary artery disease. *Eur Heart J* 2007; 28: 2087–2093.

13. Romero-Corral A, Somers VK, Sierra-Johnson J, Korenfeld Y, Boarin S, Korinek J, et al. Normal weight obesity: A risk factor for cardiometabolic dysregulation and cardiovascular mortality. *Eur Heart J* 2010; 31(6): 737–746. doi: 10.1093/eurheart/ehp1487.

14. ASBP. Obesity Algorithm 2013 [cited 2014 September 23]. Available from: http://asbp.org/obesityalgorithm.html

15. Connolly HM, Crary JL, McGoon MD, Hensrud DD, Edwards BS, Edwards WD, et al. Valvular heart disease associated with fenfluramine-phentermine. *N Engl J Med* 1997; 337: 581–588.

16. NIH. Clinical guidelines on the identification, evaluation, and treatment of overweight and obesity in adults—The evidence report. National Institutes of Health. *Obes Res* 1998; 6 Suppl 2: 51S–209S.

17. Kushner RF. *Roadmaps for Clinical Practice: Case Studies in Disease Prevention and Health Promotion—Assessment and Management of Adult Obesity: A Primer for Physicians*. Chicago, IL: American Medical Association; 2003.

18. Snow V, Barry P, Fitterman N, Qaseem A, Weiss K, Clinical Efficacy Assessment Subcommittee of the American College of Physicians. Pharmacologic and surgical management of obesity in primary care: A clinical practice guideline from the American College of Physicians. *Ann Intern Med* 2005; 142: 525–531.

19. NGC. National Guideline Clearinghouse 2009 [cited 2009 October 14]. Available from: http://www.guideline.gov/

20. Glazer G. Long-term pharmacotherapy of obesity 2000: A review of efficacy and safety. *Arch Intern Med* 2001; 161: 1814–1824.

21. Haddock CK, Poston WS, Dill PL, Foreyt JP, Ericsson M. Pharmacotherapy for obesity: A quantitative analysis of four decades of published randomized clinical trials. *Int J Obes Relat Metab Disord* 2002; 26: 262–273.

22. Li Z, Maglione M, Tu W, Mojica W, Arterburn D, Shugarman LR, et al. Meta-analysis: Pharmacologic treatment of obesity. *Ann Intern Med* 2005; 142: 532–546.

23. Padwal R, Li SK, Lau DC. Long-term pharmacotherapy for overweight and obesity: A systematic review and meta-analysis of randomized controlled trials. *Int J Obes Relat Metab Disord* 2003; 27: 1437–1446.

24. Shekelle PG, Morton SC, Maglione MA, Suttorp M, Tu W, Li Z, et al. *Pharmacological and Surgical Treatment of Obesity.* Evidence Report/Technology Assessment No. 103. 2004, pp. 1–172.

25. Wadden TA, Berkowitz RI, Womble LG, Sarwer DB, Phelan S, Cato RK, et al. Randomized trial of lifestyle modification and pharmacotherapy for obesity. *N Engl J Med* 2005; 353: 2111–2120.

26. Hendricks EJ, Greenway FL, Westman EC, Gupta AK. Blood pressure and heart rate effects, weight loss and maintenance during long-term phentermine pharmacotherapy for obesity. *Obesity (Silver Spring)* 2011; 19: 2351–2360.

27. Haddock CK, Poston WS, Foreyt JP, DiBartolomeo JJ, Warner PO. Effectiveness of Medifast supplements combined with obesity pharmacotherapy: A clinical program evaluation. *Eat Weight Disord* 2008; 13: 95–101.

28. Fullerton G, Tyler C, Johnston CA, Vincent JP, Harris GE, Foreyt JP. Quality of life in Mexican-American children following a weight management program. *Obesity* 2007; 15: 2553–2556.

29. Gadde KM, Kolotkin RL, Peterson CA, Day WW. Changes in weight and quality of life in obese patients treated with topiramate plus phentermine 272P. *Obesity* 2007; 15: A85.

30. Summan M. *Pharmacology/Toxicology NDA Review and Evaluation: NDA 20-2088 Phentermine ODT.* In: FDA/CDER (ed). Silver Spring, MD: Food and Drug Administration; 2010.

31. Roth JD, Rowland NE. Anorectic efficacy of the fenfluramine/phentermine combination in rats: Additivity or synergy? *Eur J Pharmacol* 1999; 373: 127–134.

32. Arch JR. The contribution of increased thermogenesis to the effect of anorectic drugs on body composition in mice. *Am J Clin Nutr* 1981; 34: 2763–2769.

33. Roth JD, Rowland NE. Efficacy of administration of dexfenfluramine and phentermine, alone and in combination, on ingestive behavior and body weight in rats. *Psychopharmacology (Berl)* 1998; 137: 99–106.

34. Hendricks EJ. *The Eating Behavior Questionnaire. Obesity Course: Diagnosis to Treatment.* Philadelphia, PA: American Society of Bariatric Physicians; 2014.

35. Hendricks EJ, Schmidt SL, Greenway FL, Istratiy Y, Hendricks MJ. *Eating Behavior Questionnaire: Treatment-Induced Changes in EBQ Scores. Overcoming Obesity Course.* Austin, TX: American Society of Bariatric Medicine; 2014.

36. Lorber J. Obesity in childhood. A controlled trial of anorectic drugs. *Arch Dis Child* 1966; 41: 309–312.

37. Rothman RB. Treatment of a 4-year-old boy with ADHD with the dopamine releaser phentermine. *J Clin Psychiatry* 1996; 57: 308–309.

38. Spear BA, Barlow SE, Ervin C, Ludwig DS, Saelens BE, Schetzina KE, et al. Recommendations for treatment of child and adolescent overweight and obesity. *Pediatrics* 2007; 120: S254–S288.

39. Munro JF, MacCuish AC, Wilson EM, Duncan LJ. Comparison of continuous and inter- mittent anorectic therapy in obesity. *Br Med J* 1968; 1: 352–354.

40. Douglas A, Douglas JG, Robertson CE, Munro JF. Plasma phentermine levels, weight loss and side-effects. *Int J Obes* 1983; 7: 591–595.

41. Rothman RB. Treatment of obesity with "combination" pharmacotherapy. *Am J Ther* 2010; 17(6): 596–603. doi: 10.1097/MJT.1090b1013e31818e31830da.

42. Manos MJ. Pharmacologic treatment of ADHD: Road conditions in driving patients to successful outcomes. *Medscape J Med* 2008; 10: 5.

43. Bruner DE, Richardson L, Steelman GM. *Use of Anorectic Medications. Eastern Regional Obesity Course*. Louisville, KY: American Society of Bariatric Physicians; 2006.

44. Hendricks EJ. *"Pharmacotherapy of Obesity." Annual Review Course*. Atlanta, GA: American Board Bariatric Medicine; 2001.

45. Hendricks EJ. *"Pharmacotherapy of Obesity." Annual Review Course*. Denver, CO: American Board Bariatric Medicine; 2002.

46. Hendricks EJ. *"Pharmacotherapy of Obesity." Annual Review Course*. Las Vegas, NV: American Board Bariatric Medicine; 2003.

47. Hendricks EJ. *"Pathophysiology of Obesity." Annual Review Course*. Scottsdale, AZ: American Board of Bariatric Medicine; 2004.

48. Hendricks EJ. *"Pharmacotherapy of Obesity." Annual Review Course*. Atlanta, GA: American Board of Bariatric Medicine; 2005.

49. Hendricks EJ. *"Pharmacotherapy of Obesity." Annual Review Course*. Lexington, KY: American Board of Bariatric Medicine; 2006.

50. Hendricks EJ. *"Pharmacotherapy of Obesity." Annual Review Course*. Nashville, TN: American Board of Bariatric Medicine; 2007.

51. Hendricks EJ. Adverse reactions to phentermine, evidence versus conjecture. *58th Annual Obesity & Associated Conditions Symposium*, American Society of Bariatric Physicians, Tampa, FL, 2008.

52. Hendricks EJ. Is phentermine addicting? *59th Annual Obesity & Associated Conditions Symposium*, American Society of Bariatric Physicians, Costa Mesa, 2009.

53. Steelman GM. *Controversies in the Use of Anti-Obesity (Anorectic) Medications. Western Regional Obesity Course*. Portland, OR: American Society of Bariatric Physicians; 2000.

54. Steelman GM. The art of tailoring drug therapy to your patients. *51st Annual Obesity and Associated Conditions Symposium*, American Society of Bariatric Physicians, San Diego, CA, 2001.

55. Steelman GM. *Difficult Decisions with Anorectic Use. Western Regional Obesity Course*. Denver, CO: American Society of Bariatric Physicians; 2002.

56. Hendricks EJ. Chapter 8: Pharmacotherapy. In: Steelman GM, Westman E (eds). *Obesity: Evaluation and Treatment Essentials*. New York: Informa Healthcare; 2010, pp. 81–99.

57. Hendricks EJ, Greenway FL. A study of abrupt phentermine cessation in patients in a weight management program. *Am J Ther* 2011; 18: 292–299.

58. Hendricks EJ, Srisurapanont M, Schmidt SL, Haggard M, Souter S, Mitchell CL, et al. Addiction potential of phentermine prescribed during long-term treatment of obesity. *Int J Obes* 2014; 38: 292–298.

59. Bonow RO, Carabello BA, Chatterjee K, de Leon AC Jr, Faxon DP, Freed MD, et al. 2008 Focused update incorporated into the ACC/AHA 2006 guidelines for the management of patients with valvular heart disease: A report of the American College of Cardiology/American Heart Association Task Force on Practice Guidelines (Writing Committee to Revise the 1998 Guidelines for the Management of Patients With Valvular Heart Disease): Endorsed by the Society of Cardiovascular Anesthesiologists, Society for Cardiovascular Angiography and Interventions, and Society of Thoracic Surgeons. *Circulation* 2008; 118: e523–661.

60. Roth BL. Drugs and valvular heart disease. *N Engl J Med* 2007; 356: 6–9.

61. Rothman RB, Baumann MH. Serotonergic drugs and valvular heart disease. *Expert Opin Drug Safety* 2009; 8: 317–329.

62. Kim KK, Cho HJ, Kang HC, Youn BB, Lee KR. Effects on weight reduction and safety of short-term phentermine administration in Korean obese people. *Yonsei Med J* 2006; 47: 614–625.

63. Hendricks EJ, Rothman RB. RE: Pulmonary hypertension associated with use of phentermine? *Yonsei Med J* 2011; 52: 869–870.

64. Rich S, Rubin L, Walker AM, Schneeweiss S, Abenhaim L. Anorexigens and pulmonary hypertension in the United States: Results from the surveillance of North American pulmonary hypertension. *Chest* 2000; 117: 870–874.

65. Heinz AJ, Epstein DH, Schroeder JR, Singleton EG, Heishman SJ, Preston KL. Heroin and cocaine craving and use during treatment: Measurement validation and potential relationships. *J Subst Abuse Treat* 2006; 31: 355–364.

66. American Psychiatric Association. *Task Force on DSM-IV. Diagnostic and Statistical Manual of Mental Disorders: DSM-IV-TR*, 4th edn. Washington, DC: American Psychiatric Association; 2000.

67. American Psychiatric Association. *DSM-5 Task Force. Diagnostic and Statistical Manual of Mental Disorders: DSM-5*, 5th edn. Arlington, VA: American Psychiatric Association; 2013.

68. INCHEM. *Phentermine: International Programme on Chemical Safety.* 2009 [cited 2009 October 14]. Available from: http://www.inchem.org/documents/pims/pharm/pim415.htm

69. Saguner AM, Dur S, Perrig M, Schiemann U, Stuck AE, Burgi U, et al. Risk factors promoting hypertensive crises: Evidence from a longitudinal study. *Am J Hypertens* 2010; 23: 775–780.

70. Zolkowska D, Rothman RB, Baumann MH. Amphetamine analogs increase plasma serotonin: Implications for cardiac and pulmonary disease. *J Pharmacol Exp Ther* 2006; 318: 604–610.

71. Rader WA, Steelman GM, Westman EC. Clinical experience using appetite suppressants and SSRIs. *J Okla State Med Assoc* 2008; 101: 180–181.

72. Cercato C, Roizenblatt VA, Leanca CC, Segal A, Lopes Filho AP, Mancini MC, et al. A randomized double-blind placebo-controlled study of the long-term efficacy and safety of diethylpropion in the treatment of obese subjects. *Int J Obes (Lond)* 2009; 33: 857–865.

73. Horie NC, Cercato C, Mancini MC, Halpern A. Long-term pharmacotherapy for obesity in elderly patients: A retrospective evaluation of medical records from a specialized obesity outpatient clinic. *Drugs Aging* 2010; 27: 497–506.

74. Stewart DA, Bailey JD, Patell H. Tenuate dospan as an appetite suppressant in the treatment of obese children. *Appl Ther* 1970; 12: 34–36.

75. Cass LJ. Evaluation of phendimetrazine bitartrate as an appetite suppressant. *Can Med Assoc J* 1961; 84: 1114–1116.
76. Le Riche WH, Van Belle G. Study of phendimetrazine bitartrate as an appetite suppressant in relation to dosage, weight loss and side effects. *Can Med Assoc J* 1962; 87: 29–31.
77. Bray GA, Hollander P, Klein S, Kushner R, Levy B, Fitchet M, et al. A 6-month randomized, placebo-controlled, dose-ranging trial of topiramate for weight loss in obesity. *Obes Res* 2003; 11: 722–733.
78. Astrup A, Toubro S. Topiramate: A new potential pharmacological treatment for obesity. *Obes Res* 2004; 12 Suppl: 167S–173S.
79. Astrup A, Caterson I, Zelissen P, Guy-Grand B, Carruba M, Levy B, et al. Topiramate: Long-term maintenance of weight loss induced by a low-calorie diet in obese subjects. *Obes Res* 2004; 12: 1658–1669.
80. Wilding J, Van Gaal L, Rissanen A, Vercruysse F, Fitchet M, Group O-S. A randomized double-blind placebo-controlled study of the long-term efficacy and safety of topiramate in the treatment of obese subjects. *Int J Obes Relat Metab Disord* 2004; 28: 1399–1410.
81. McElroy SL, Shapira NA, Arnold LM, Keck PE, Rosenthal NR, Wu SC, et al. Topiramate in the long-term treatment of binge-eating disorder associated with obesity. *J Clin Psychiatry* 2004; 65: 1463–1469.
82. Guerdjikova AI, Kotwal R, McElroy SL. Response of recurrent binge eating and weight gain to topiramate in patients with binge eating disorder after bariatric surgery. *Obes Surg* 2005; 15: 273–277.
83. Tata AL, Kockler DR. Topiramate for binge-eating disorder associated with obesity. *Ann Pharmacother* 2006; 40: 1993–1997.
84. Gadde KM, Allison DB, Ryan DH, Peterson CA, Troupin B, Schwiers ML, et al. Effects of low-dose, controlled-release, phentermine plus topiramate combination on weight and associated comorbidities in overweight and obese adults (CONQUER): A randomised, placebo-controlled, phase 3 trial. *Lancet* 2011; 377: 1341–1352.
85. Allison DB, Gadde KM, Garvey WT, Peterson CA, Schwiers ML, Najarian T, et al. Controlled-release phentermine/topiramate in severely obese adults: A randomized controlled trial (EQUIP). *Obesity (Silver Spring)* 2012; 20: 330–342.
86. Garvey WT, Ryan DH, Look M, Gadde KM, Allison DB, Peterson CA, et al. Two-year sustained weight loss and metabolic benefits with controlled-release phentermine/topiramate in obese and overweight adults (SEQUEL): A randomized, placebo-controlled, phase 3 extension study. *Am J Clin Nutr* 2012; 95: 297–308.
87. Neoh SL, Sumithran P, Haywood CJ, Houlihan CA, Lee FT, Proietto J. Combination phentermine and topiramate for weight maintenance: The first Australian experience. *Med J Aust* 2014; 201: 224–226.
88. Rothman RB, Baumann MH, Savage JE, Rauser L, McBride A, Hufeisen SJ, et al. Evidence for possible involvement of 5-HT(2B) receptors in the cardiac valvulopathy associated with fenfluramine and other serotonergic medications. *Circulation* 2000; 102: 2836–2841.
89. Arena. *Briefing document for FDA Advisory Committee Meeting: NDA 22-529 Lorcaserin.* In: FDA (ed). Silver Spring, MD: FDA; 2012, pp. 1–209.
90. Shram MJ, Schoedel KA, Bartlett C, Shazer RL, Anderson CM, Sellers EM. Evaluation of the abuse potential of lorcaserin, a serotonin 2C (5-HT2C) receptor agonist, in recreational polydrug users. *Clin Pharmacol Ther* 2011; 89: 683–692.

91. Smith SR, Prosser WA, Donahue DJ, Morgan ME, Anderson CM, Shanahan WR, et al. Lorcaserin (APD356), a selective 5-HT(2C) agonist, reduces body weight in obese men and women. *Obesity (Silver Spring)* 2009; 17: 494–503.

92. O'Neil PM, Smith SR, Weissman NJ, Fidler MC, Sanchez M, Zhang J, et al. Randomized placebo-controlled clinical trial of lorcaserin for weight loss in type 2 diabetes mellitus: The BLOOM-DM study. *Obesity (Silver Spring)* 2012; 20: 1426–1436.

93. Fidler MC, Sanchez M, Raether B, Weissman NJ, Smith SR, Shanahan WR, et al. A one-year randomized trial of lorcaserin for weight loss in obese and overweight adults: The BLOSSOM trial. *J Clin Endocrinol Metab* 2011; 96: 3067–3077.

94. Greenway FL, Dunayevich E, Tollefson G, Erickson J, Guttadauria M, Fujioka K, et al. Comparison of combined bupropion and naltrexone therapy for obesity with mono-therapy and placebo. *J Clin Endocrinol Metab* 2009; 94: 4898–4906.

95. Apovian CM, Aronne L, Rubino D, Still C, Wyatt H, Burns C, et al. A randomized, phase 3 trial of naltrexone SR/bupropion SR on weight and obesity-related risk factors (COR-II). *Obesity (Silver Spring)* 2013; 21: 935–943.

96. Verpeut JL, Bello NT. Drug safety evaluation of naltrexone/bupropion for the treatment of obesity. *Expert Opin Drug Saf* 2014; 13: 831–841.

97. Appolinario JC, McElroy SL. Pharmacological approaches in the treatment of binge eating disorder. *Curr Drug Targets* 2004; 5: 301–307.

98. Khazaal Y, Chatton A, Rusca M, Preisig M, Zullino D. Long-term topiramate treatment of psychotropic drug-induced weight gain: A retrospective chart review. *Gen Hosp Psychiatry* 2007; 29: 446–449.

99. Gadde KM, Franciscy DM, Wagner HR II, Krishnan KRR. Zonisamide for weight loss in obese adults: A randomized controlled trial. *JAMA* 2003; 289: 1820–1825.

100. Shin JH, Gadde KM, Ostbye T, Bray GA. Weight changes in obese adults 6-months after discontinuation of double-blind zonisamide or placebo treatment. *Diabetes Obes Metab* 2014; 16: 766–768.

101. McElroy SL, Kotwal R, Guerdjikova AI, Welge JA, Nelson EB, Lake KA, et al. Zonisamide in the treatment of binge eating disorder with obesity: A randomized controlled trial. *J Clin Psychiatry* 2006; 67: 1897–1906.

102. McElroy SL, Kotwal R, Hudson JI, Nelson EB, Keck PE. Zonisamide in the treatment of binge-eating disorder: An open-label, prospective trial. *J Clin Psychiatry* 2004; 65: 50–56.

103. Gadde KM, Yonish GM, Foust MS, Wagner HR. Combination therapy of zonisamide and bupropion for weight reduction in obese women: A preliminary, randomized, open-label study. *J Clin Psychiatry* 2007; 68: 1226–1229.

104. Wallingford NM, Sinnayah P, Bymaster FP, Gadde KM, Krishnan RK, McKinney AA, et al. Zonisamide prevents olanzapine-associated hyperphagia, weight gain, and elevated blood glucose in rats. *Neuropsychopharmacology* 2008; 33: 2922–2933.

105. Niswender K, Pi-Sunyer X, Buse J, Jensen KH, Toft AD, Russell-Jones D, et al. Weight change with liraglutide and comparator therapies: An analysis of seven phase 3 trials from the liraglutide diabetes development programme. *Diabetes Obes Metab* 2013; 15: 42–54.

106. Anderson JW, Greenway FL, Fujioka K, Gadde KM, McKenney J, O'Neil PM. Bupropion SR enhances weight loss: A 48-week double-blind, placebo-controlled trial. *Obesity Res* 2002; 10: 633–641.

107. Greenway FL, Whitehouse MJ, Guttadauria M, Anderson JW, Atkinson RL, Fujioka K, et al. Rational design of a combination medication for the treatment of obesity. *Obesity (Silver Spring)* 2009; 17: 30–39.

108. White J. Efficacy and safety of incretin based therapies: Clinical trial data. *J Am Pharm Assoc (2003)* 2009; 49 Suppl 1: S30–40.
109. Trujillo JM, Nuffer W. Albiglutide: A new GLP-1 receptor agonist for the treatment of type 2 diabetes. *Ann Pharmacother* 2014; 48(11): 1494–1501.
110. Garfield AS, Heisler LK. Pharmacological targeting of the serotonergic system for the treatment of obesity. *J Physiol* 2009; 587: 49–60.
111. Heisler LK, Jobst EE, Sutton GM, Zhou L, Borok E, Thornton-Jones Z, et al. Serotonin reciprocally regulates melanocortin neurons to modulate food intake. *Neuron* 2006; 51: 239–249.
112. Turner EH, Loftis JM, Blackwell AD. Serotonin a la carte: Supplementation with the serotonin precursor 5-hydroxytryptophan. *Pharmacol Ther* 2006; 109: 325–338.
113. Rothman RB, Baumann MH. Appetite suppressants, cardiac valve disease and combination pharmacotherapy. *Am J Ther* 2009; 16: 354–364.
114. Whigham LD, Dhurandhar NV, Rahko PS, Atkinson RL. Comparison of combinations of drugs for treatment of obesity: Body weight and echocardiographic status. *Int J Obes (Lond)* 2007; 31: 850–857.
115. Aronne LJ, Halseth AE, Burns CM, Miller S, Shen LZ. Enhanced weight loss following coadministration of pramlintide with sibutramine or phentermine in a multicenter trial. *Obesity (Silver Spring)* 2010; 18: 1739–1746.
116. Davtyan C, Ma M. Drug-induced weight gain. *Proc UCLA Healthcare* 2008; 12: 1.
117. Millward DJ. Macronutrient intakes as determinants of dietary protein and amino acid adequacy. *J Nutr* 2004; 134: 1588S–1596S.
118. Layman D. Dietary guidelines should reflect new understandings about adult protein needs. *Nutr Metab (Lond)* 2009; 6: 12.
119. Symons TB, Sheffield-Moore M, Wolfe RR, Paddon-Jones D. A moderate serving of high-quality protein maximally stimulates skeletal muscle protein synthesis in young and elderly subjects. *J Am Diet Assoc* 2009; 109: 1582–1586.
120. Martin CK, O'Neil PM, Pawlow L. Changes in food cravings during low-calorie and very-low-calorie diets. *Obes Res* 2006; 14: 115–121.
121. Rosenbaum M, Goldsmith R, Bloomfield D, Magnano A, Weimer L, Heymsfield S, et al. Low-dose leptin reverses skeletal muscle, autonomic, and neuroendocrine adaptations to maintenance of reduced weight. *J Clin Invest* 2005; 115: 3579–3586.
122. Rosenbaum M, Murphy EM, Heymsfield SB, Matthews DE, Leibel RL. Low dose leptin administration reverses effects of sustained weight-reduction on energy expenditure and circulating concentrations of thyroid hormones. *J Clin Endocrinol Metab* 2002; 87(5): 2391–2394.
123. Chan JL, Lutz K, Cochran E, Huang W, Peters Y, Weyer C, et al. Clinical effects of long-term metreleptin treatment in patients with lipodystrophy. *Endocr Pract* 2011; 17: 922–932.
124. George M, Rajaram M, Shanmugam E. New and emerging drug molecules against obesity. *J Cardiovasc Pharmacol Ther* 2014; 19: 65–76.
125. David LA, Maurice CF, Carmody RN, Gootenberg DB, Button JE, Wolfe BE, et al. Diet rapidly and reproducibly alters the human gut microbiome. *Nature* 2014; 505: 559–563.

9

Maintenance of weight loss

SCOTT RIGDEN

INTRODUCTION

Losing weight and keeping it off is a very difficult accomplishment in our society. Wadden's research team reported (1) that only 5% of patients maintained their full weight loss 5 years after treatment, whereas 62% had regained all of their approximately 15 kg loss. A review of the weight loss maintenance literature shows that weight regain is a problem regardless of the treatment used. Obese individuals in commercial weight loss programs do not seem to perform any better than those in research studies. A survey conducted by Consumer Reports (2) found that participants typically regained 30% to 40% of their weight loss 1 year after treatment; one-quarter regained all of it.

Weight maintenance studies are rare compared to the prolific number of weight loss studies. The commercialization of weight loss hardly ever includes a catchy announcement or advertisement regarding long-term maintenance. My experience has been that even bariatricians, who should be especially sensitive to maintenance of weight loss issues, prefer to discuss, almost exclusively, exceptional cases of weight loss. Perhaps the lack of excitement and emphasis on weight loss maintenance is a symptom of our society being oriented to fast, instant, and quick resolutions of problems. My experience as a veteran bariatrician is that very few new obese patients come in to the office with any thought of weight loss maintenance. All would agree that maintenance is not nearly as much fun and exciting as the initial weight loss with its associated positive feelings and physiological changes.

DEFINITION OF MAINTENANCE

One common definition of long-term weight loss that has been used in medical research is the intentional weight loss of at least 10% or more of the original weight and maintaining this weight loss for 1 year. The National Heart, Lung, and Blood Institute definition of success is at least 10% weight loss from baseline, <3 kg weight regain at 2 years, and sustained reduction in waist circumference of at least 1.6 in (3). Many bariatricians seem to agree with the criteria used by the National Weight Control Registry (NWCR), whose definition of "successful losers" is a minimum of 13.6 kg (30 lb) of weight loss maintained for a minimum of 1 year (4). No matter what criteria are favored by bariatricians, it is clear that overweight patients have very unrealistic goals for weight loss that may lead to disappointment and, ultimately, undermine their zeal to continue working intensely on their weight. A study by Foster et al. (5) on weight loss goals and expectations revealed most considered a hypothetical a 17% reduction disappointing; a 33% weight loss was a typical goal weight. Fortunately, maintaining a weight loss as little as 5% to 10% of the original weight can have very significant medical results (1).

Maintenance physiology

Many articles have identified compensatory physiological changes that the body makes after weight loss. These changes such as the stability of the number of fat cells, improved insulin sensitivity, decreased energy expenditure, and increased lipoprotein lipase activity are used to justify a pessimistic view that permanent weight loss is unlikely (6). However, Voelker (7) refutes the popular assumption that the overweight body is always destined to return to its set point weight. He discusses many studies that have not found an inappropriate decrease in resting metabolic rate for the reduced body size. My experience in bariatric practice certainly supports Volker's assertion. Table 9.1 shows four typical case studies of successful long-term maintenance from our practice; obviously, weight maintenance efforts were not overridden by some inevitable physiological set point in these cases.

Circulating angiotensin-converting enzyme (ACE) may become a valuable tool for predicting successful weight loss maintenance. Wang et al. (8) followed 125 overweight or obese healthy men who completed an 8-week weight loss program and then were followed for 6 months with serum ACE levels. They concluded that "a greater reduction of ACE during weight loss is favorable for weight maintenance in both men and women. This can offer useful information for personalized advice to improve weight-loss maintenance. It also confirms the role of ACE in metabolic pathways of weight regulation."

Maintenance and nutritional approaches

The inclusion of prepackaged food items in a planned menu as part of a 2-year weight loss and weight loss maintenance program was investigated by Rock et al. (9). The treatment program in the study involved in-person, center-based (structured group) or telephone-based, one-to-one (telephone group) weight loss counseling for the 2-year period. A control group was given prepackaged food items and had two individualized weight loss counseling sessions

Table 9.1 Four examples of successful long-term maintenance

Date (month/year)	Weight (lb)
Case study 1: 40-year-old female	
2/2001	159.4
8/2001	141
2/2002	137.6
5/2005	132.6
9/2005	126.8
7/2007	135.8
Case study 2: 42-year-old Native American male	
1/2007	474
7/2007	412.4
1/2008	398.6
6/2008	377.8
Case study 3: 48-year-old female	
6/2000	185
3/2001	184.2
4/2002	148.6
3/2003	151.8
3/2004	150.2
3/2006	155.4
3/2007	163.2
2/2008	149.6
Case study 4: 32-year-old female	
1/2002	266.8
6/2003	150.2
6/2004	177.8
6/2006	213.4
12/2007	155.8
6/2008	160

with a dietetics professional and monthly contacts. The structured group participants lost 7.4 kg or 7.9% of initial weight, the telephone group lost 6.2 kg or 6.8%, and the control group lost 2 kg after 24 months.

Toubro and Astrup (10) reviewed 1 year of maintenance among 43 subjects. One group of subjects was put on an ad libitum low-fat, high-carbohydrate diet; another group was put on a fixed calorie, exchange list diet. The mean weight loss of the participants was 12.6 kg prior to the maintenance period. During maintenance, the subjects attended sessions two to three times per month. At 1-year follow-up, 65% of the ad libitum low-fat group and 40% of the fixed calorie group had maintained a weight loss of 5 kg or more.

Reviewing multifaceted approaches to long-term weight maintenance, Perri et al. (11) concluded that one-on-one contact was superior to peer group support or "no-contact" conditions.

They recommended multifaceted maintenance programs, including ongoing professional contact, skills training, social support, and exercise.

After completing a very-low-calorie diet (VLCD), 210 subjects were followed for 15 months by Agras et al. (12). They found that use of prepackaged foods did not enhance successful maintenance. In fact, this strategy correlated with worse compliance and attendance in the maintenance condition.

Hartman et al. (13) conducted a long-term weight loss maintenance program after weight loss with supplemental fasting. More than 100 subjects were evaluated 2 to 3 years after treatment in a combined behavior therapy and VLCD program. Average weight loss was 27.2 kg; at follow-up the mean weight loss was 11.3 kg. Fifty-six subjects participated in the optional maintenance program, and 46 did not. Factors associated with long-term success were high levels of exercise and participation in the maintenance program for more than 8 months. The maintenance program consisted of regular group visits, occasional physician visits, review of nutrition and exercise topics, and visits to restaurants and grocery stores.

Walsh and Flynn (14) reported a 54-month evaluation of weight maintenance after a popular VLCD program. After initial weight loss for males of 27.2 kg and 19.3 kg for females, the average maintained loss 54 months after program entry was 5.1 kg. Twenty-six of 145 patients maintained a medically significant weight loss of 20% of their entry weight. As longer program attendance and continued exercise were the main correlates with successful maintenance, Walsh and Flynn (14) recommended at least 2 years of a maintenance program after reaching goal weight.

What happens in a prospective study of weight maintenance in obese subjects reduced to normal body weight without an associated weight loss training program? Hensrud et al. (15) directed 24 obese dieting women to diet until they lost 10 kg. They were not taught any weight management skills and then were followed until they attained their initial weight. At 1 year, they regained 42% of their weight loss, and at 4 years they had regained 87% of the weight previously lost. Ebbeling et al. (16) examined weight loss interventions and the effect of diet macronutrient composition on energy expenditure during weight loss maintenance. They reported results of a controlled feeding study that involved 21 overweight or obese adults who had achieved 10% to 15% weight loss and who consumed each of three isocaloric diets with differing macronutrient composition during a weight maintenance phase. They also found that declines in resting and total energy expenditure were greatest with a low-fat diet, intermediate with a low glycemic index diet, and least with a very-low–carbohydrate diet.

Maintenance and anorectic agents

Goldstein and Potvin (17) looked at long-term weight loss and the effect of pharmacological agents. They reviewed 20 weight-reduction studies on the effect of at least 6 months of pharmacological therapy on weight loss maintenance. The agents investigated included phentermine, mazindol, fenfluramine, dexfenfluramine, and fluoxetine. Ten of the clinical trials investigated the effect of therapy used intermittently or continuously for 6 months, and nine investigated the effects for more than 1 year. The conclusion of the article was that the long-range benefits of medication as an aid to weight loss maintenance exceeded the risks.

Weintraub's important publication (18) on long-term weight control was a meticulous 210-week study. The treatment plan was multimodal, with a combination of behavior therapy, nutrition counseling, exercise, and anorectic agents. His data clearly showed that whenever the drug treatment was discontinued, patients rapidly regained their lost weight despite adjunctive counseling.

A national task force on the prevention and treatment of obesity published its findings in 1996 (19). The two key points were as follows: (*1*) pharmacotherapy for obesity, when combined with appropriate behavioral approaches to change diet and physical activity, helps some obese patients lose and maintain weight loss for at least 1 year and (*2*) pharmacotherapy for weight loss maintenance is not recommended for routine use in obese individuals, although it may be helpful in carefully selected patients.

One issue that has been a concern about the use of anorectic agents in long-term maintenance is that their combination with serotonin selective reuptake inhibitors (SSRIs) would cause serotonin syndrome. In a survey of obesity medicine (20), physicians reported that there were no cases of serotonin syndrome reported in 1174 individual patients on this combination. More than 500 of these individuals were on phentermine plus an SSRI for more than 6 months. They concluded that "the monitored use of the combination of these medicines by trained practitioners is justifiable."

Another common objection regarding the long-term safe use of phentermine is the possibility of addiction potential and risk of amphetamine-like withdrawal symptoms. Hendricks et al. (21) reviewed the long-term use of phentermine in 117 patients who had been on this medication of an average of 8.35 years. The phentermine dose ranged from 18.75 to 112.5 mg daily. They reported that abrupt cessation of phentermine did not produce amphetamine-like withdrawal symptoms, even after a long duration of treatment with higher-than-recommended doses. They also found no phentermine cravings after stopping the drug, even on patients who had been taking the drug for 21 years.

It has been suggested that long-term use of phentermine could be detrimental to blood pressure and heart rate. Another study by Hendricks et al. (22) addresses the perception that phentermine pharmacotherapy for obesity increases blood pressure and heart rate, exposing treated patients to increased cardiovascular risk. Records of more than 300 obese patients were reviewed at 26 and 52 weeks. These data suggest phentermine treatment for obesity does not result in increased systolic or diastolic blood pressure or heart rate. Instead, weight loss assisted with phentermine treatment was associated with favorable shifts in blood pressure, and the researchers concluded that "phentermine treatment is associated with favorable shifts in categorical blood pressure and retardation of progression to hypertension in obese patients."

Obviously, clinicians who are using anorectic agents for long-term weight loss maintenance are urged to be judicious. Obtain informed consent, use medication only as an adjunct to a comprehensive program, regularly monitor the patient, individualize the dose to patient needs, and keep excellent records.

Based on years of clinical experience and the experience of many other bariatricians, I believe that pharmacotherapy can be a very effective tool during maintenance in carefully selected patients, when professionally monitored according to the American Society of Bariatric Physicians guidelines (23).

Maintenance and exercise

Wadden et al. (24) looked at successful maintainers and the average calories they burned per week in physical activities. Subjects in the Look AHEAD (Action for Health in Diabetes) study who had lost and maintained a 10% weight loss or greater over 4 years burned 1997.9 kcal per week with physical activity (24,25). This finding was significant at the $P < 0.005$ level. Subjects with a successful weight loss of 5% to 10% over 4 years burned 1406.2 kcal per week. The American College of Sports Medicine published guidelines (26) stating that between 200 and 300 minutes of moderate-intensity physical activity per week is likely to prevent weight regain. However, the US Health and Human Services 2008 guidelines state 300 to 420 minutes of moderate-intensity physical week is necessary to prevent weight regain (27).

Maintenance and the Internet

An example of the use of the Internet for weight maintenance can be found in Svetkey et al. (28), wherein they compared three strategies for sustaining weight loss. One thousand and thirty-two subjects were followed for 30 months after a 6-month weight loss phase. The average weight loss was 8.5 kg. Then, the subjects were divided into three maintenance groups: (1) a monthly personal contact group, (2) a group with unlimited access to an interactive technology-based intervention, and (3) a self-directed control group. The results showed that all three maintenance groups regained weight, but the personal contact group regained less weight (4 kg) than the self-directed and technology groups (5.5 kg). Interestingly, the interactive technology-based intervention provided early but transient benefit. Apparently the subjects were likely to "burn out" on using the Internet for their maintenance intervention.

In an attempt to examine social support in an Internet weight loss community and its effectiveness, Hwang et al. (29) conducted studies and interviews in a large Internet weight loss community. The members had major social support themes of encouragement and motivation, information and shared experiences; they valued convenience, anonymity, and the non-judgmental interactions as unique characteristics of their Internet-mediated support. These researchers conclude that the Internet weight loss community plays a prominent role in participants' weight loss efforts and merits further evaluation as a resource for clinicians to recommend to patients for long-term weight loss maintenance.

Maintainence and behavioral therapy

The National Institutes of Health–sponsored Diabetes Prevention Program (DPP) and Action for Health in Diabetes (Look AHEAD) studies were two recent landmark multiyear, multicenter research investigations (25,30). They compared the relative effectiveness of intensive behavioral and pharmacological approaches to treating body weight, diabetes status, and cardiovascular risk factors in adults with prediabetes and type 2 diabetes mellitus.

The DPP study interventions were intensive lifestyle, medication (metformin), and placebo. Each group had almost 1100 participants. The lifestyle intervention group featured an intensive course with the following specific goals: (1) >7% total body weight loss and maintenance of weight loss, (2) <25% of calories from fat, (3) a calorie goal of 1200 to 1800 kcal per day, and (4) >150 minutes of physical activity per week. The lifestyle intervention structure included a 16-session core curriculum over 24 weeks; a long-term maintenance program; supervision of each individual by a case manager; and access to a lifestyle support staff, including a dietitian, behavior counselor, and exercise specialist. Education and training in diet and exercise in addition to behavior modification skills were featured in the course. There was special emphasis on self-monitoring techniques, problem solving, individualizing programs, self-esteem, empowerment, and social support. There was frequent contact with the case manager and staff. After the core program, self-monitoring and other behavioral strategies were emphasized during monthly visits. Supervised exercise sessions were offered along with periodic group classes and motivational campaigns. The subjects were provided exercise videotapes and pedometers, and they were encouraged to enroll in a health club and/or cooking class. The retention and participation of the subjects in the intervention group was excellent, with an average follow-up of 2.8 years (range 1.8–4.5 years).

The study conclusively showed the results in the lifestyle intervention group to be superior to the metformin and placebo groups in increasing physical activity, losing weight, reducing the incidence of diabetes, and improving fasting glucose and hemoglobin A1c values. Seventy-four percent of the intensive lifestyle arm subjects achieved the study goal of >150 minutes of activity per week at 24 weeks. This group also had a more significant mean weight loss of 4.5 kg (9.9 lb) at 3 years. The researchers in the DPP study summarized that intensive lifestyle intervention reduced development of diabetes by 58%, compared to metformin reducing the development of diabetes by 31% ($P < 0.001$). They also confirmed that modest weight loss improves health, that modest increases in physical activity can be sustained, and that long-term adherence to lifestyle interventions is possible. The study clearly shows that people really will make lasting lifestyle changes with good maintenance strategies.

The Look AHEAD study is now in progress and also using lifestyle intervention to improve diabetes mellitus and to show health benefits such as decreased rates of cardiovascular death, nonfatal myocardial infarction, and nonfatal stroke. Using similar education and support sessions developed in the DPP protocol, the preliminary results after 1 year (19) were very exciting. At 1 year, the Look AHEAD intensive intervention resulted in a clinically significant weight loss of 8.6%, with the control group only losing 0.7%.

After 4 years, the Look AHEAD study (24,31) continued to show impressive results. Five thousand one hundred overweight participants with type 2 diabetes were randomly assigned to an intensive lifestyle intervention or a diabetes support and education group. At 1 year, in addition to superior weight loss as already noted, the intensive lifestyle intervention group produced significantly greater improvements in hemoglobin A1c, fitness, and numerous measures of cardiovascular disease risk. At year 4, participants in the intensive lifestyle intervention group maintained a loss of 4.9 kg in comparison with 1.3 kg in the support and education group, clearly demonstrating that long-term weight loss maintenance can be achieved with continued behavioral treatment. Participants in the study who maintained their weight loss, compared with those who did not, attended more treatment sessions and reported more favorable physical activity and food intake at year 4.

In 2012, Jakicic et al. (32) randomly assigned 363 overweight or obese adults to either a standard behavioral weight loss intervention or a stepped-care weight loss intervention that allowed modifications in the intensity and frequency of the behavior intervention components when weight loss goals were not met. They found that the stepped-care weight loss intervention resulted in a greater mean weight loss over 18 months.

Dr. John Foreyt, a faculty member in the Department of Psychology at Baylor Medical School, has contributed much to the understanding of the psychology of weight maintenance (33,34). He has found that consistent behaviors that correlate with successful maintenance include regular physical activity, self-monitoring, and continued contact with healthcare professionals. He reports that successful programs stress the importance of maintenance from the start of the weight loss program. Realistic goals need to be discussed with the patient from the initial appointment. The patients need to identify intrinsic health reasons why they want to have a healthier weight (e.g., improved energy, feel better about themselves). Extrinsic reasons such as losing weight for a class reunion seldom sustain motivation. Structured eating patterns with regular breakfast and several feedings a day are important. Health care professionals need to be a resource to help provide social support and help the patient solve problems. Weight regain is more likely to occur with inconsistent and restrictive dieting, elevated life stress, negative coping styles, and emotional or binge eating patterns.

Dr. Brian Wansink in the Department of Psychology at Cornell University has many helpful insights into long-term successful eating behaviors (35,36). Based on his behavioral research, Wansink reports that people make well more than 200 decisions about food every day. Unfortunately, these decisions are usually unconscious, robotic, and automatic. Therefore, much of our inappropriate eating is due to a variety of environmental stimuli and unconscious cues that could be improved with the development of new behaviors. For example, he has shown that overeaters will often consume smaller amounts of food, and feel just as full, if they use smaller plates and dishes.

The National Weight Control Registry

The NWCR is an observational cohort study of self-reported, long-term successful weight loss maintenance (4,37). Started in 1994, the NWCR is tracking more than 5000 individuals who have lost at least 13.6 kg (30 lb) and kept it off for at least 1 year. Registry members have lost an average of 30 kg (66 lb) and kept it off for 5.5 years. The weight losses have ranged from 13.6 to 136 kg (30–300 lb); the duration of successful weight loss has ranged from 1 year to 66 years. Some individuals lost the weight rapidly, whereas others lost weight very slowly, over as many as 14 years. The demographics show 80% of persons in the NWCR are female and 20% are male. The average woman is 45 years of age and currently weighs 66 kg (145 lb), whereas the average man is 49 years of age and currently weighs 86 kg (190 lb). About half of the participants lost the weight on their own, and the other half lost weight with the help of some type of program. Most of the registry participants had childhood onset obesity. Forty-six percent report being overweight by 11 years of age, 28.3% report being overweight by 12 to 18 years of age, and 28.3% report being overweight by 18 years of age. Forty-six percent report one parent was overweight, whereas 26.8% report both parents were overweight. Ninety-eight percent of these participants report they modified their food intake in some way to lose weight; 94% increased their physical activity, with the most frequently reported form of activity being walking.

By far, the highest single predictor of success in this group seems to be high levels of activity (38). Ninety percent exercise, on average, about 1 hour per day. The average energy expenditure per week is staggering, at almost 2700 kcal. In addition to aerobic activities, 24% of the males and 19.5% of the females included weight lifting in their regimen. Sixty-two percent watch less than 10 hours of television per week.

The current eating habits of registry participants show a low average caloric intake of 1380 calories; the macronutrient balance of their diet averages 24% fat, 19% protein, and 56% carbohydrate. The successful maintainers tend to eat five times daily; very few eat less than twice a day. Seventy-eight percent eat breakfast every day, and they eat out three times a week, on average. Interestingly, only 0.9% of subjects reported eating a diet less than 24% carbohydrate. Self-monitoring is used by a majority of the NWCR members. Seventy-five percent weigh more than once a week; 44% weigh once a day; 50% still count calories, and/or fat grams. Table 9.2 summarizes the successful weight maintenance strategies used by NWCR participants.

Table 9.2 Successful weight maintenance strategies by NWCR members

1. Low-fat diet
2. Low-carbohydrate diet
3. Low-calorie diet
4. High daily levels of physical activity, minimize watching television
5. Regularly eat breakfast, eat several times daily, avoid eating out
6. Frequent self-monitoring

Medication-related weight gain

An often overlooked problem in long-term weight loss maintenance is the frequent prescription of medications that cause weight gain as a common side effect (39). Since there are often alternative agents that do not cause such problems, it is hoped that prescribing professionals and patients will become more aware of this issue. As shown in Table 9.3, many different types of medications can lead to weight gain, including insulin, oral hypoglycemics, corticosteroids, antipsychotics, and antidepressants.

Obstructive sleep apnea

In multiple recent studies, body mass index has been shown to increase with sleep durations significantly less than 8 hours per night (40). Epidemiological studies have demonstrated a relationship between short sleep duration and increased risk of diabetes (40). Experimental studies have shown a strong relationship between acute sleep restriction and the development of abnormalities in glucose and insulin levels, serum cortisol, thyroid stimulation hormone, leptin, ghrelin, and sympathovagal balance (40). These physiological disturbances all contribute to weight gain. Bariatricians highly suspect obstructive sleep apnea when evaluating obese patients with central obesity, a neck circumference greater than 41 cm (16 in.), and an association with metabolic syndrome. Fortunately, these metabolic dysfunctions can be improved by treating obstructive sleep apnea with continuous positive airway pressure or similar technology. It is logical to include this important area for investigation and treatment to facilitate the probability of long-term successful weight loss maintenance. Table 9.4 contains some simple questions that can help the practitioner decide whether a sleep study evaluation is needed.

Table 9.3 Medications that can lead to weight gain

1. Anticonvulsants: valproic acid, carbamazepine
2. Antidepressants: tricyclic antidepressants, including amitriptyline (Elavil®); monoamine oxidase inhibitors, such as phenelzine (Nardil®); serotonin reuptake inhibitors, including paroxetine (Paxil®) and sertraline (Zoloft®); mirtazapine (Remeron®)
3. Anticancer agents: e.g., anastrozole (Arimidex®)
4. Corticosteroids: e.g., prednisone
5. Insulin: up to 17 lb weight gain can occur in an intensive 3-month treatment course
6. Lithium: gains can be 22 lb or more in 6 to 10 years
7. Oral contraceptives: e.g., ethinylestradiol (6, 100, 200 µg) leads to dose-dependent increases in body fat
8. Oral hypoglycemic agents (sulfonylureas): usual weight gain is more than 11 lb during 3 to 12 months of therapy
9. Antipsychotics: haloperidol, loxapine, olanzapine, and clozapine are the most likely culprits

Table 9.4 Sleep history questions

1. Do you snore?
2. Has anyone seen you stop breathing while you were asleep?
3. Has anyone observed long irregular pauses between breaths while you are sleeping?
4. Are you often too sleepy during the day?

FUTURE METABOLIC CONSIDERATIONS MAY INCLUDE GUT MICROBIOME

Future metabolic considerations for long-term successful maintenance might include manipulation of the gut microbiome. The human intestine is colonized by billions of microorganisms, the majority of which belong to the phyla Firmicutes and Bacteroidetes. Although highly stable over time, the composition and activities of the microbiota may be influenced by many factors, including age, diet, and antibiotics. Research shows that obesity is associated with the relative abundance of Firmicutes; conversely, Bacteroidetes are associated with leaner individuals. Researchers (41,42) have demonstrated through metagenomic and biochemical analyses that the metabolic potential of gut microbiota can be identified and manipulated, indicating that the obese microbiome (primarily Firmicutes) has an increased capacity to harvest energy from the diet. There have been numerous articles published in the past 5 years looking at the relationship between energy balance and gut microbiota. These animal and human studies suggest that the factors influencing the composition and the role of probiotics as a therapeutic modality may soon be available and useful.

PUTTING IT ALL TOGETHER

In my personal clinical experience, it is imperative to stress to the patient at his or her first appointment that a weight problem requires two strategies: phase A, a weight loss phase and phase B, a weight maintenance phase. Inform the patient that he or she will see the physician and staff at least once a month for 12 to 18 months after reaching goal weight, planting the seeds of a maintenance strategy from the start. Reiterate frequently that the program is "a marathon, not a sprint." Although that may sound trite and corny, our patients hear often and respond to "you are the little engine that could," "you are the tortoise that beats the hare," and "don't forget 'LSD'—long slow distance!" Throughout the weight loss phase, the key to long-term professional contact is personal bonding to the office and staff and physician; try to promote that bond by making visits enjoyable by frequently using laughter, humor, and awards to make the appointments a positive experience. All of our patients, while in the weight loss phase, receive a psychological and behavioral curriculum that goes beyond nutrition education and implementation of an exercise program. These curricula include modules on stress management, self-esteem, understanding eating triggers, self-nurturing, dealing with slumps, positive attitude, and mindful eating. It is important for patients to master the art of eating out and learn how to deal with holidays and special occasions. All patients are exposed to the ideas of relaxation breathing, stretching exercises, and pet therapy. To provide a manual for our patients, this information has been put together in a book (39).

In summary, the art and science of successful weight maintenance is still in its infancy. Most people underestimate the effort it takes to assist people in losing weight. Many breakthroughs are needed and expected in the next decade. At present, when all is said and done, persistence by the patient and physician seems to be the key. The importance of persistence was best stated by former president Calvin Coolidge: "Nothing in this world can take the place of persistence. Talent will not; nothing is more common than unsuccessful men with talent. Genius will not; unrewarded genius is almost a proverb. Education will not; the world is full of educated derelicts. Persistence and determination alone are omnipotent. The slogan 'press on' has solved and always will solve the problems of the human race."

REFERENCES

1. Wadden TA, Steen SN. Improving the maintenance of weight loss: The ten per cent solution. In: Angel A, Anderson H, Bouchard D, et al. (eds.). *Progress in Obesity Research*. London: John Libbey, 1996: 745–749.
2. Losing weight: What works. What doesn't. *Consumer Rep* 1993; 58: 347–353.
3. Wing RR, Hill JO. Successful weight loss maintenance. *Annu Rev Nutr* 2001; 21: 323–341.
4. Klem ML, Wing RR, McGuire MT, et al. A descriptive study of individuals successful at long-term maintenance of substantial weight loss. *Am J Clin Nutr* 1997; 66: 239–246.
5. Foster GD, Wadden TA, Kendall PC, et al. Psychological effects of weight loss and regain: A prospective evaluation. *J Consult Clin Psychol* 1996; 64(4): 752–757.
6. Leibel RL, Rosenbaum M, Hirsch J. Changes in energy expenditure resulting from altered body weight. *N Engl J Med* 1995; 332(10): 621–628.
7. Voelker R. Losers can win at weight maintenance. *JAMA* 2007; 298(3): 272–273.
8. Wang P, Holst C, Wodzig WK, et al. Circulating ACE is a predictor of weight loss maintenance not only in overweight and obese women, but also in men. *Int J Obes* 2012; 36: 1545–1551.
9. Rock CL, Flatt SW, Sherwood NE, et al. Effect of a free prepared meal and incentivized weight loss program on weight loss and weight loss maintenance in obese and overweight women. *JAMA* 2010; 304(16): 1803–1808.
10. Toubro S, Astrup A. Randomised comparison of diets for maintaining obese subjects' weight after major weight loss: Ad lib, low fat, high carbohydrate diet v fixed energy intake. *BMJ* 1997; 314(7073): 29–34.
11. Perri MG, Sears SF Jr., Clark JE. Strategies for improving maintenance of weight loss. Toward a continuous care model of obesity management. *Diabetes Care* 1993; 16: 200–209.
12. Agras WS, Berkowitz RI, Arnow BA, et al. Maintenance following a very-low-calorie diet. *J Consult Clin Psychol* 1996; 64(3): 610–613.
13. Hartman WM, Stroud M, Sweet DM, et al. Long-term maintenance of weight loss following supplemented fasting. *Int J Eat Disord* 1993; 14: 87–93.
14. Walsh MF, Flynn TJ. A 54-month evaluation of a popular very low calorie diet program. *J Fam Pract* 1995; 41: 231–236.
15. Hensrud DD, Weinsier RL, Darnell BE, et al. A prospective study of weight maintenance in obese subjects reduced to normal body weight without weight-loss training. *Am J Clin Nutr* 1994; 60: 688–694.
16. Ebbeling CB, Swain RD, Feldman HD, et al. Effects of dietary composition on energy expenditure during weight-loss maintenance. *JAMA* 2012; 307(24): 2626–2634.
17. Goldstein DJ, Potvin JH. Long-term weight loss: The effect of pharmacologic agents. *Am J Clin Nutr* 1994; 60: 6747–6657.
18. Weintraub M. Long-term weight control: The national heart, lung and blood institute funded multimodal intervention study. *Clin Pharmacol Ther* 1992; 51: 581–646.
19. National task force on the prevention and treatment of obesity. Long-term pharmacotherapy in the management of obesity. *JAMA* 1996; 276(23): 1907–1915.
20. Rader WA, Steelman GM, Westman EC. Clinical experience using appetite suppressants and SSRIs. *J Okla State Med Assoc* 2008; 101(8): 180–181.
21. Hendricks EJ, Srisurapanont M, Schmidt SL, et al. Addiction potential of phentermine prescribed during long-term treatment of obesity. *Int J Obes* 2014; 38(2): 292–298.

22. Hendricks EJ. Greenway FL, Westman EC, et al. Blood pressure and heart rate effects, weight loss and maintenance during long-term phentermine pharmacotherapy for obesity. *Obesity* 2011; 19(120): 2351–2360.
23. American Society of Bariatric Physicians. 2010. www.asbp.org
24. Wadden TA, Neiberg RH, Wing RR, et al. Four-year weight loss in the look AHEAD study: Factors associated with long-term success. *Obesity* 2011; 19(10): 1987–1998.
25. Look AHEAD Research Group. Reduction in weight and cardiovascular disease risk factors in individuals with type 2 diabetes: One-year results of the look AHEAD trial. *Diabetes Care* 2007; 30: 1374–1383.
26. Donnelly JE, Blair SN, Jakicic JM, et al. Appropriate physical activity intervention strategies for weight loss and prevention of weight regain for adults. *Med Sci Sports Exerc* 2009; 41(2): 459–471.
27. US Health and Human Services. *Physical Activity Guidelines.* 2008. www.health.gov/pagguidelines
28. Svetkey LP, Stevens VJ, Brantley PJ, et al. Comparison of strategies for sustaining weight loss: The weight loss maintenance randomized controlled trial. *JAMA* 2008; 299(10): 1139–1148.
29. Hwang KO, Ottenbacher AJ, Green AP, et al. Social support in an Internet weight loss community. *Int J Med Inform* 2010; 79(1): 5–13.
30. Diabetes Prevention Program Research Group. Reduction in the incidence of type 2 diabetes with lifestyle intervention or metformin. *N Engl J Med* 2002; 346: 393–403.
31. Wadden TA, Webb VL, Moran CH, Bailer BA. Lifestyle modification for obesity: New developments in diet, physical activity, and behavior therapy. *Circulation* 2012; 125: 1157–1170.
32. Jakicic JM, Tate DF, Lang W, et al. Effect of a stepped-care intervention approach on weight loss in adults. *JAMA* 2012; 307(24): 2617–2616.
33. Foreyt JP, Goodrick G. Attributes of successful approaches to weight loss and control. *Appl Prevent Psychol* 1994; 3: 209–215.
34. Foreyt JP, Goodrick GK. Evidence for success of behavior modification in weight loss and control. *Ann Intern Med* 1993; 119: 698–701.
35. Wansink B. Environmental factors that increase the food intake and consumption volume of unknowing consumers. *Annu Rev Nutr* 2004; 24: 455–479.
36. Wansink B, Sobal J. Mindless eating: The 200 daily food decisions we overlook. *Environ Behav* 2007; 39(1): 106–123.
37. Shick SM, Wing RR, Klem ML, et al. Persons successful at long-term weight loss and maintenance continue to consume a low-energy, low-fat diet. *J Am Diet Assoc* 1998; 98: 408–413.
38. Phelan S, Wyatt H, Nassery S, et al. Three-year weight change in successful weight losers who lost weight on a low-carbohydrate diet. *Obesity* 2007; 15: 2470–2477.
39. Rigden S. Weight gain with chronic illness and impaired liver detoxification. In: *The Ultimate Metabolism Diet. Eat Right for Your Metabolic Type.* Alameda, CA: Hunter House, 2008: 185–188.
40. Tatman J. *Impaired Sleep and Obesity. Obesity Course.* Phoenix, AZ: American Society of Bariatric Physicians, 2008: 176–190.
41. Havenaar R. Intestinal health functions of colonic microbial metabolites: A review. *Benef Microbes* 2011; 2(2): 103–114.
42. Brestoff JR, Artis D. Commensal bacteria at the interface of host metabolism and the immune system. *Nat Immunol* 2013; 14(7): 676–684.

10

Surgical treatment of the obese individual

JOHN B. CLEEK AND ERIC C. WESTMAN

INTRODUCTION

A discussion of the current treatment of obesity is not complete without a review of the surgical options. *Bariatric surgery* is the term used for the surgical treatment of obesity. The number of bariatric surgery operations has climbed steadily over the past 10 years to represent 193,000 cases in 2014. In recent reviews, Buchwald et al. (1,2) outline the research that demonstrates the reduction in obesity-related morbidity and mortality with the use of bariatric surgery. The bariatric surgery literature gives the best published view of how health can improve with weight loss. For example, hypertension is reduced or eliminated in 78.5% of patients, hyperlipidemia in 70% of patients, and obstructive sleep apnea is improved in 83.6% of patients. Analyses have now been published that show a reduction in mortality compared to usual care treatments. When compared with control groups that do not achieve substantial weight loss, there is a reduction in mortality in those who had bariatric surgery. In a retrospective study of 7900 patients with an average follow-up of 7.1 years, the mortality reduction at 7.1 years was 40%, including a 56% reduction in death from coronary artery disease, a 92% reduction in death from diabetes mellitus, and a 60% reduction in deaths from cancer. The overall reduction in mortality over a 10.9-year period was 29% (3,4).

WHO SHOULD HAVE BARIATRIC SURGERY?

With such dramatic outcomes, the question is which patients qualify for surgery? Current recommendations state that patients may be considered candidates for bariatric surgery if the body mass index (BMI) is greater than 40, and if the BMI is greater than 35 with other medical comorbidities such as hypertension, diabetes mellitus, and obstructive sleep apnea (5). The patient should have had a complete medical and psychological evaluation to rule out an endocrinological, psychiatric, or metabolic cause of obesity. Other reasons for candidacy include prior attempts at weight loss with no long-term success, commitment to regular healthcare follow-up, and long-term diet and exercise programs. Patients must be able to understand the surgical risks as well as their long-term commitment.

Contraindications to bariatric surgery are specific as well. Female patients who may wish to become pregnant in the 18 months postoperatively should not be considered for surgery. Patients with major psychiatric disorder, such as uncontrolled depression, suicidal ideation, and personality disorder, are not candidates for bariatric intervention. Active substance abuse is also an absolute contraindication to surgery.

Preoperative evaluation

The preoperative evaluations ensure that the patients meet the required criteria for surgery and help ensure patient safety (6). A thorough history and physical are necessary to optimize patient care, including identification of preoperative risk factors. Laboratory testing helps identify additional risk factors for surgical complications. The preoperative evaluations include psychological evaluation and often exercise evaluation as well.

A comprehensive history should include weight history and nutrition history. Prior weight-loss attempts should be recorded, including method used, results obtained, and length of success. Barriers to success need to be reviewed for correction preoperatively or postoperatively. Further history should address perioperative risks. For example, increased perioperative risk is associated with a history of thromboembolic events, smoking, sleep apnea, and unstable angina.

The physical examination should screen for causes of obesity as well as complications of obesity. Vital signs including blood pressure, heart rate, height, and weight should be documented. Skin should be inspected for striae suggestive of Cushing's syndrome. The oropharynx is evaluated for airway size and possible risk for sleep apnea. Pulmonary exam checks for pulmonary edema suggestive of uncompensated heart failure. Cardiac exam evaluates for murmurs and possible structural heart defects. Abdominal exam evaluates for hepatosplenomegaly associated with fatty liver disease. All other systems should also be checked for changes suggestive of unrecognized disease.

Laboratory testing should be comprehensive as well. Complete blood cell count, fasting blood sugar, comprehensive metabolic panel, and thyroid-stimulating hormone are drawn at a minimum. Many centers routinely screen for *Helicobacter pylori*, but this practice is not universal among bariatric surgery programs. Other laboratory testing should be based on the clinical situation of the individual patient.

No specific recommendations have been adopted for nutritional laboratory screening. In a series of patients reported by Flancbaum et al. (7), vitamin D deficiency was found in 68% preoperatively. In addition, iron deficiency was found in 43.9% and thiamine deficiency in 29% of the preoperative patients. Replacement of deficiencies needs to be undertaken prior to surgery, as replacement is problematic in the postoperative state.

Exercise evaluation is generally recommended preoperatively. Although the best exact testing modality is not known, the 4-minute walk test is commonly used. Patients with poor physical conditioning have twice the risk of serious postoperative complications compared to those with unlimited exercise tolerance. Patients with poor exercise tolerance may benefit from cardiology screening such as a dobutamine stress echocardiographic testing. Screening allows preoperative intervention to increase the operative safety.

Electrocardiograms are generally advised for men over age 45 years or women over age 55 years and for any patients with known or suspected heart disease. Patients with multiple risk factors, such as hypertension, diabetes mellitus, and dyslipidemia, should have a preoperative electrocardiogram, as should patients on diuretic therapy, due to the subsequent risk for electrolyte abnormalities.

Diagnostic chest radiographs should be obtained in patients with known pulmonary disease, history of congestive heart failure, or in patients more than 60 years of age. Many centers routinely screen every patient for sleep apnea as well.

A psychological evaluation is recommended for each patient; however, no standardized guidelines exist for this evaluation. Most bariatric surgery centers use a self-administered test such as the Beck Depression Inventory, Minnesota Multiphasic Personality Inventory, or Millon Behavioral Medicine Diagnostic, among other potential instruments. These instruments, in collaboration with the interview, are used to identify, in particular, eating disorders, major depressive disorders, suicidality, personality disorders, and substance abuse disorders. In a 2004 review by Herpertz et al. (8), 27% to 41% of preoperative patients have an Axis I diagnosis, whereas 22% to 24% have an Axis II disorder. In a review by Sarwer et al. (9), 62.2% of preoperative patients received a psychological diagnosis, and 31% of patients were referred for further evaluation and therapy prior to surgery. Mood disorders were the most common diagnosis, occurring in 19% to 60% of preoperative patients. Historically, 5% to 20% of patients are excluded from surgery based on their psychological evaluation.

A more controversial area of behavioral issues in the surgical candidate is the role of eating disorders, primarily binge eating disorder and nocturnal eating disorder, and subsequent outcome. Ten to 50% of patients presenting for bariatric surgery have binge eating disorder. Initially, this disorder was felt to be potential for poor weight loss results after surgery; therefore, patients were felt to be poor candidates. More recently, Fujioka et al. (10) showed at 12 and 24 months postoperatively, the excess weight loss is no different from controls. No change in perioperative complications is seen in this same period. Bocchieri-Ricciardi et al. (11) also demonstrate no difference between binge eaters and nonbinge eaters at 18 months in terms of weight loss. Eating disorders, especially binge eating, do not seem to be a contraindication for surgery at this time.

Up to 40% of patients presenting to a weight loss center have night eating syndrome. Night eating syndrome is characterized by anorexia in the morning, evening hyperphagia, nocturnal awakenings, and eating during the awakenings. Generally, more than one-half of consumed calories in the day are after 5 p.m. There is a lack of literature available relative to any role this disorder has in the approach to the surgical patient.

BARIATRIC SURGERY-RELATED TREATMENTS AND COMPLICATIONS

Preoperative treatment

A preoperative program may be required by the bariatric surgery center or by the patient's insurance provider, although there are no studies to support the use of these programs. Typically varying in duration from 3 to 12 months, these programs may include patient education regarding exercise, nutrition, and lifestyle changes. Compliance to the multiple visits of a preoperative program is thought to give a demonstration of the ability of the patient to comply with postoperative recommendations. Future research is needed to examine the importance of this type of program.

Preoperative weight loss is beneficial for improvement of operative complications as well for improved long-term weight loss. The more obese the patient is, the greater the risk of death or major perioperative complication when undergoing certain operative bariatric procedures. For medical comorbidities, as little as 10% total body weight loss improves multiple conditions, including obstructive sleep apnea, cardiovascular risk, thromboembolic risk, and elevated blood glucose. Because increased abdominal adiposity and enlarged liver are major factors in conversion to an open procedure from a laparoscopic procedure, reducing adipose tissue in the abdomen and liver fat before the surgery reduces the technical difficulty of the surgery. Preoperative weight loss is also associated with less intraoperative blood loss. Some data suggest that preoperative weight loss is predictive of postoperative weight loss.

Types of bariatric surgery

Although bariatric surgery started in the 1960s, a recent increase in surgeries has occurred due to the increased recognition of obesity as a serious medical problem, the use of minimally invasive surgery and laparoscopy, and increased reimbursement by insurance companies. Surgeries are generally classified based on the mechanism of action. According to the Society of American Gastrointestinal and Endoscopic Surgeons, the type of bariatric surgery can be categorized into (1) mostly restrictive, (2) mostly malabsorptive, and (3) purely restrictive.

Purely restrictive procedures include horizontal gastroplasty, silastic ring gastroplasty, vertical banded gastroplasty, and adjustable gastric band (12). Vertical banded gastroplasty consists of creating a fixed gastric pouch in the proximal stomach with a fixed band. The adjustable gastric band has been approved in the United States since June 2001 (Figure 10.1). The device has an inflatable cuff inside a silicone ring. A reservoir is attached to the inflatable cuff, allowing for the adjustment of the band circumference through saline injection into the reservoir. The reservoir is placed in a subcutaneous location, allowing for improved access. Anatomically, the reservoir or port is placed superior and left of the umbilicus. The band is placed around the gastric cardia, creating a 15 to 30 mL pouch. The wall of the stomach may be sutured over the top of the band to hold it in place. The band therefore creates a purely restrictive element to the gastrointestinal tract. The degree of restriction can be varied by the amount of saline placed in the reservoir and, hence, the cuff.

The currently most commonly performed bariatric surgery is a mostly restrictive procedure called the Roux-en-Y gastric bypass, or simply gastric bypass (Figure 10.2). In this procedure, the stomach is transected into two pieces: one piece is a pouch of 15 to 30 mL created from the cardia of the stomach, and the second part of the stomach is larger and sealed at the site of the transection and otherwise remains intact. The jejunum is divided approximately 91 cm (3 ft) from the gastric outlet. The end of the jejunum originating from the stomach, or Y limb, is reanastomosed to the jejunum 100 to 150 cm from the newly created end of the jejunum. This section is attached to the gastric pouch and is called the roux limb. A standard roux limb is 75 to 150 cm in length, while a long limb procedure creates a roux limb of 150 to 200 cm. The roux limb now carries incompletely digested food from the stomach pouch, while the Y limb carries digestive enzymes from the stomach and pancreas. The digestion proceeds in the common channel of the unchanged small intestine.

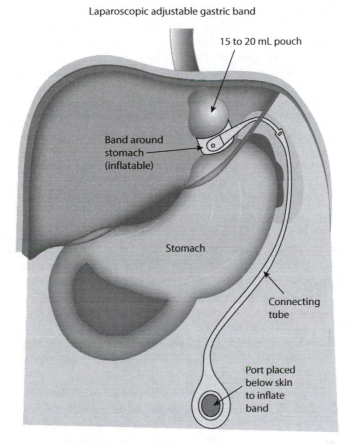

Laparoscopic adjustable gastric band

15 to 20 mL pouch

Band around stomach (inflatable)

Stomach

Connecting tube

Port placed below skin to inflate band

Figure 10.1 Example of gastric banding.

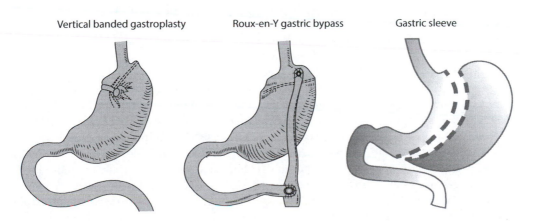

Vertical banded gastroplasty

Roux-en-Y gastric bypass

Gastric sleeve

Figure 10.2 Gastric bypass using Roux-en-Y.

Another restrictive procedure called the vertical sleeve gastrectomy, or gastric sleeve, has recently been introduced and seems to be as effective as gastric bypass over a 3-year period (13).

Mostly malabsorptive procedures include long limb gastric bypass and biliopancreatic diversion with or without duodenal switch. In a long limb gastric bypass, the roux limb is lengthened to 200 cm or longer. The increase in length of the roux creates a greater malabsorption. In the biliopancreatic diversion procedure, a partial gastrectomy is performed with a sleeve of lesser gastric fundus remaining intact, creating a 100 to 150 mL gastric pouch. The small intestine is transected in the first part of the duodenum. A new anastomosis is created with the new limb of the small intestine and the remaining intact duodenum. The common channel is created 50 cm from the ileocecal valve. In a biliopancreatic diversion with duodenal switch, the common channel is lengthened to 100 cm. These procedures are reserved for patients with a BMI greater than 50 due to the complications of the severe malabsorption.

Perioperative complications

Overall, the major risk factors for perioperative complications seem to include male sex, age more than 45 years, hypertension, diabetes, obstructive sleep apnea, unstable angina, congestive heart failure, and asthma. Risk factors for cirrhosis and pulmonary embolism increase perioperative complications. The super obese, with a BMI greater than 50, have a significantly higher risk for perioperative complications as well. Patients with limited exercise capacity, the inability to walk four blocks or two flights of stairs, have twice the risk of serious postoperative complications compared to those with unlimited exercise capacity.

Surgical mortality

The mortality rate is directly influenced by surgeon and hospital facility expertise. Published inpatient death rates range from 0.19% to 0.3%. High-volume bariatric centers performing more than 100 cases annually had 0.3% mortality rate compared to 1.2% mortality rate in those centers performing less than 50 cases annually. These same high-volume centers had lower complication rate at 10.2% compared to 14.5% in low-volume centers. The rationale for developing "centers of excellence" for bariatric surgery relate, in part, to the variability in these statistics.

Possible complications during hospitalization (Table 10.1)

Intraoperative complications include bleeding, injury to surrounding structures, and staple misfire. Bleeding complications occur from the staple line, anastomosis site, or mesenteric vessels, and they occur in about 4% of patients. Bleeding may be in the intestinal or gastric lumen, or intraperitoneal. Signs suggesting bleeding problems include hematemesis, bloody drain output, or a drop in hemoglobin. Treatment includes fluid resuscitation, transfusion as needed, and correction of any coagulopathy. Esophagogastroduodenoscopy (EGD) is indicated for intraluminal evaluation, but reoperation may be required for persistent intraperitoneal bleeding.

Anastomotic leak is an early postoperative complication of bariatric surgery. These leaks are reported in up to 3% of patients after gastric bypass. Anastomotic leaks are more common at the gastrojejunal anastomosis due to ischemia in the region felt to be due to tension in the sutures. Worsening abdominal pain, leukocytosis, fever, distress, oliguria, and tachycardia with a rate greater than 120 beats per minute suggest an intra-abdominal leak. Often, the presentation of the patient is tachycardia without other symptoms. Rapid surgical exploration of the abdomen is required.

Table 10.1 Possible postoperative complications for bariatric surgery patients

Possible complications during hospitalization

Intraluminal hemorrhage

Intraperitoneal hemorrhage

Anastomotic leak

Wound complications (ventral hernias, infection, and fascial dehiscence)

Deep venous thrombophlebitis

Pulmonary embolism

Pneumonia

Possible posthospital discharge complications

Protein malnutrition

Vitamin deficiencies: vitamin A, vitamin B1 (thiamine), vitamin B12, vitamin D, vitamin K, folate

Micronutrient deficiencies: iron, magnesium, zinc, calcium, copper, selenium

Steatorrhea

Dumping syndrome

Anastomotic stricture or ulceration

Internal and ventral hernias

Bowel obstruction

Fistulas

Cholelithiasis

Islet cell hypertrophy

Insufficient weight loss

Wound complications include ventral hernias, infection, and fascial dehiscence. Infection is more common in the obese, with a reported rate of 2.9% in laparoscopic gastric bypass. Ventral hernias or incisional hernias are reported in the same study as to occur in 0.45% of cases. Wound dehiscence happens in less than 1% of patients.

Obesity is linked to a higher risk of deep venous phlebitis and pulmonary embolism. The risk of venous thromboembolism increases with higher BMI, and the published rate is about 0.41%. Pulmonary embolism accounts for 50% of the early postoperative deaths. All patients should receive prophylaxis, including subcutaneous heparin. Strong consideration should be given to placement of a vena caval filter if the patient has multiple risk factors, including prior deep vein thrombosis, hypercoagulable syndrome, and venous stasis. A patient with tachycardia, shortness of breath, and oxygen desaturation should be evaluated for pulmonary embolus.

Pneumonia can occur after laparoscopic procedures, related to increased intra-abdominal pressure reducing diaphragmatic excursion. This condition also predisposes to pulmonary effusion. Dyspnea, fever, and leukocytosis suggest this possible problem. A chest x-ray can help confirm the diagnosis.

Possible posthospital discharge complications

Long-term complications of surgery include anastomotic strictures, cholelithiasis, intestinal obstruction, internal and ventral hernias, and gastrointestinal bleeding. Unique to the adjustable gastric band are band slippage, band erosion, and port problems. With respect to the duodenal switch with biliopancreatic diversion, steatorrhea is a common problem.

Anastomotic strictures develop in 2% to 27% of patients after gastric bypass. Strictures are more common when the stoma diameter is less than 1 cm. Presenting symptoms include dysphagia, nausea, and vomiting, or excessive weight loss. Most commonly, the stricture occurs at the gastrojejunal junction. Diagnosis of the stricture is made by upper gastrointestinal series or by EGD. The majority of cases are managed by simple balloon dilatation at the time of endoscopy. Rarely, surgical revision is required.

Anastomotic ulceration occurs is up to 20% of patients after gastric bypass. Ulceration usually occurs within the first 3 months. Symptoms include abdominal pain, nausea, vomiting, bleeding, and, rarely, perforation with an acute abdomen presentation. Ulcers are treated with proton pump inhibitors, sucralfate, and rarely surgical revision. These ulcers represent the most common cause of gastrointestinal bleeding.

Bowel obstruction is a later complication of surgery. Intraluminal causes of obstruction include blood clot; edema of the bowel wall or stoma; or in the case of adjustable gastric band, a band that is overly restrictive. Postoperative adhesions, incisional, or internal hernias can also cause late-onset bowel obstruction. Presenting symptoms include abdominal pain, nausea, and vomiting. A plain x-ray such as kidney, ureter, and bladder may aid in the diagnosis. Computerized tomography is more sensitive in diagnosis. Specifically, a swirl sign, in which the mesentery and perhaps intestine are visualized twisting through an internal mesenteric defect created during the surgery, is the most specific finding. Typically, surgery will be required to definitively treat the problem.

Cholelithiasis is common with any rapid weight loss and surgery is no exception. After bariatric surgery, from 38% to 52% of patients develop cholelithiasis within 1 year. Patients with gallstones at the time of surgery may have elective cholecystectomy at the time of their bariatric procedure. This technique is controversial and generally performed only with symptomatic gallstones at the time of bariatric intervention. Cholecystectomy is performed in 15% to 28% of patients within 3 years of a gastric bypass.

Steatorrhea is a problem in those patients having a malabsorptive procedure such as long-limb gastric bypass or biliopancreatic diversion with duodenal switch. The steatorrhea is generally due to the short common jejunal–ileal channel. If the common channel is less than 100 cm, then the risk for increased malabsorption and subsequent steatorrhea is increased. The only therapy for a common channel that is shorter than 100 cm with severe steatorrhea is surgical repair to create a longer common channel.

Complications unique to the adjustable gastric band procedure relate to the device itself. The band may erode into the stomach and even cause perforation. The band may slip, causing intolerance of the band with dysphagia or vomiting. The band may become infected, often with redness and drainage at the site of the port. The port may migrate or flip, making access difficult and causing a loss of the ability to adjust the band. The pouch may dilate, as well as the esophagus, if the patient continues to overfill the pouch. Generally, surgical removal is required to solve these issues.

Postoperative care is specialized to the bariatric patient, in particular for the gastric bypass patient. Adjustable laparoscopic band procedures are performed on an outpatient basis. The band needs to be adjusted at the first postoperative visit, usually 2 weeks after the surgical procedure.

The gastric bypass patient remains hospitalized for 2 to 3 days, and more stringent care is needed. To lessen the likelihood of pouch obstruction in the immediate postoperative period, no sustained release medications are given. Close blood sugar monitoring is required as medications need to be reduced rapidly. Most diabetics are discharged from the hospital no longer on diabetes medications.

Diet and, especially hydration, are monitored closely. Feeding may be started as soon as the nasogastric tube is removed. Continual sipping of clear liquids helps maintain hydration. The goal is to maintain 40 mL per hour of urine output after the first two postoperative hours. The diet for the first 2 days after surgery is clear liquids. On day 3, full liquids are initiated. During days 4 to 30, pureed foods with six small meals a day are included. A mechanical soft diet with five meals a day (½ cup of food at each meal) is recommended for days 31 to 60. Meals of ½ to ¾ cup, four times a day, are used from days 61 to 90. After day 90, regular food is consumed in three to five meals a day with each meal containing 1 to 1.5 cups. Patients are encouraged to drink at least 1.5 L of fluid daily. Recommendations include five to eight fruits and vegetables daily, no concentrated sweets, and 80 to 120 g of protein daily. Patients are asked not to drink fluids with meals as the fluid may empty the pouch more quickly and reduce satiety. Small bites, chewed thoroughly, are encouraged, with each meal lasting at least 30 minutes. Common food intolerances after surgery include bread, rice, pasta, chicken, milk, dairy foods, and carbonated beverages.

Patients require lifetime vitamin support (Table 10.2), especially after the malabsorptive or partial malabsorptive procedures (14). A general multivitamin is recommended daily, one or two tablets. Supplementation of calcium with calcium citrate at 1200 to 2000 mg daily is recommended. Citrate is better absorbed in the low-acid environment after any form of gastric resection. The dosage of vitamin D is not entirely agreed upon, although 400 to 800 IU has been the standard. Folate at a dose of one milligram daily should be taken. Elemental iron at 65 mg is recommended daily. Vitamin B12 at 500 μg is the minimum dose for daily supplementation.

Dumping syndrome generally occurs within 6 months of surgery. Seventy to 76% of patients will experience dumping syndrome on at least one occasion. When high-sugar foods are consumed, the patient may experience abdominal pain, nausea, vomiting, diarrhea, flushing, headache, weakness, dizziness, and syncope. Signs of dumping syndrome include tachycardia and hypotension. The etiology of dumping syndrome remains unclear, with some postulating an increase in glucagon-like peptide-1 (GLP-1), resulting in beta cell hyperplasia and a reactive hypoglycemia.

Nutritional deficiencies are common postoperatively, especially with the purely malabsorptive and partially malabsorptive surgeries. Purely restrictive surgery is less likely to cause nutritional deficits. The deficits arise due to reduction in the stomach size and the lower vitamin and mineral absorption due to malabsorption (15).

Fat-soluble vitamin deficiencies are more common after biliopancreatic diversion, but may also be a complication of gastric bypass. Vitamin A deficiency is reported in 52% to 69% of patients after biliopancreatic diversion and in 10% of patients after gastric bypass. A case report

Table 10.2 Suggested routine vitamin and mineral supplementation after bariatric surgery

Complete multivitamin, with iron daily (chewable, given early postoperative)
Calcium citrate 1200 to 1800 mg daily with vitamin D3 800 to 1000 IU daily
Ferrous sulfate 325 mg two to three times daily as needed
Oral vitamin B12 1000 μg daily
Folic acid 1 mg daily as needed
Zinc sulfate 100 mg as needed

of night blindness occurring 10 years after gastric bypass underscores the need for recognition. Oral replacement therapy is sufficient.

Vitamin K deficiency is reported in 51% to 68% of patients after biliopancreatic diversion with duodenal switch, and it is improved after vitamin K supplementation.

With respect to vitamin E, little evidence exists to support clinically significant changes in level. In study by Slater et al. (16), vitamin E levels did not change over a 4-year period after biliopancreatic diversion. Preoperative evaluation of micronutrients reveals an incidence of about 2% of vitamin E deficiency, but the importance of this is unknown.

Vitamin D has been extensively studied in the last several years. Vitamin D deficiency, as stated earlier, is evidenced in up to 68% of patients seen preoperatively. Malabsorption creates a risk for new onset or worsening of the vitamin D deficiency. In postoperative patients, the concern for inadequate vitamin D has surrounded bone loss. Vitamin D deficiency leads to secondary hyperparathyroidism, which may cause bone loss. Dexa scans for detection of bone loss are recommended at baseline and 1 year postoperatively.

Vitamin B deficiencies are a common postoperative nutritional complication. Folate is generally low because of reduced intake. Zero to 38% of patients after gastric bypass have folate deficiency. Folate deficiency may cause anemia and is of particular importance prenatally for reduction in neural tube birth defects.

Thiamine (vitamin B1) is lowered due to food intake restrictions, reduction in acidity from creation of the pouch, and duodenal exclusion (highest area of absorption). Thiamine deficiency is seen as early as 6 weeks postoperatively from malabsorptive procedures, especially in patients with recurrent vomiting. Beriberi may be seen at this early postoperative time. Thiamine deficiency may result in confusion, ophthalmoplegia, ataxia, and nystagmus, as in Wernicke's encephalopathy. Recognition of Wernicke's encephalopathy is critical for treatment to prevent long-term sequelae. Symptoms of beriberi may develop, not only early, but several years after surgery with symptoms of peripheral neuropathy, including pain and weakness of the lower extremities. Vitamin B12 deficiency is created by the achlorhydria, preventing nutrient release from food, by the low tolerance to milk and dairy, and by the reduced production of intrinsic factor. Deficiency of vitamin B12 may most commonly produce a megaloblastic anemia or peripheral neuropathy.

Micronutrient and mineral deficiencies are frequently observed postoperatively, especially after malabsorptive procedures. In particular, magnesium, zinc, iron, selenium, calcium, and copper may need to be evaluated postoperatively.

Iron deficiency is caused by the limitation in food intake, reduced acid production, and duodenal exclusion. The greatest proportion of iron absorption occurs in the duodenum. Iron deficiency is reported to occur from 13% to 52% of patients after gastric bypass 2 to 4 years after surgery, but up to 33% of patients may develop by the first year postoperatively. An anemia is recognized in up to 50% of patients after gastric bypass, with higher incidence in menstruating young women. Testing includes complete blood count, iron level, and ferritin. Ferritin is the most sensitive for detecting low iron.

Zinc absorption is impaired after malabsorptive procedures as zinc is absorbed primarily in the duodenum and proximal jejunum. Zinc deficiency results in dermatitis of the nasolabial folds and hands, reduced wound healing, and altered taste perception. Up to 50% of patients after biliopancreatic diversion will have zinc deficiency.

Magnesium deficiency is reported in just fewer than 5% of patients preoperatively. Patients may experience a loss of magnesium with excessive diarrhea or steatorrhea. A study by Johansson et al. (17) reports a slight increase in magnesium levels at 1 year after gastric bypass.

Magnesium should be checked in those patients with spasms or myalgias. No routine recommendation exists for checking levels in asymptomatic patients.

Calcium changes are common after malabsorptive surgeries. In a study by Newbury et al. (18), 25% of patients had hypocalcemia after biliopancreatic diversion. Attention should be given to calcium and ionized calcium levels in particular.

Copper deficiency can be seen after gastric bypass. Copper deficiency may cause a neuropathy that resembles vitamin B12 deficiency. Rarely copper can be an etiologic factor in anemia. Selenium deficiency is reported in up to 15% of patients after biliopancreatic diversion. Low selenium is reported in 3% of gastric bypass patients after 1 year. A case report by Boldery et al. (19) reveals a cardiomyopathy related to selenium deficiency in a patient after gastric bypass. Evaluation of selenium has not been a routine recommendation.

From a macronutrient standpoint, protein malnutrition is a postoperative risk. With greater amount of malabsorption, the risk of protein–calorie malnutrition increases. Reduced intake due to gastric restriction and food intolerance contributes to inadequate protein level. Signs of protein malnutrition include edema, anasarca, hair loss, and muscle wasting. Prealbumin and albumin levels are markers of protein stores. Severe inadequacy is marked by total protein of less than 5 g/dL and albumin less than 2.5 g/dL. Lowest levels of albumin occur 1 to 2 years after a gastric bypass. Treatment consists of increased intake of high-protein foods and protein supplements and may require enteral or parental nutrition.

Hypoglycemia is increasingly reported as a complication to surgery, specifically after gastric bypass. Neuroglycopenia appears to be related to islet cell hypertrophy. The hypertrophy origin is a point of controversy. The hypertrophy may be in response to weight gain, which necessitated the surgery, or be due to increase in incretin hormone GLP-1 response postoperatively. The common link is excessive insulin secretion in response to a meal with resultant delayed hypoglycemia. A portion of these symptomatic patients requires partial pancreatectomy, whereas most can be managed with diet and pharmacotherapy when needed.

The effects of surgery on gastrointestinal hormones are under intense scrutiny. The advantage of malabsorptive surgeries may rely on the changes in these hormones, such as peptide-YY (PYY), ghrelin, and GLP-1 in particular. The rapid resolution of diabetes mellitus in gastric bypass compared to adjustable gastric band suggests factors beyond weight loss account for the difference in effect. The gastrointestinal hormones are hypothesized to account for that difference in diabetic resolution as 80% to 100% of patients after gastric bypass have diabetes resolution compared to 30% to 70% of patients after gastric banding. In particular, patients after gastric bypass have an earlier rise in glucose after a meal compared to nonsurgical patients. This glucose rise precipitates a rise in postprandial insulin that is earlier and more pronounced than in nonsurgical patients. GLP-1 and PYY are enhanced postprandially in the surgical patient. The rise in PYY and GLP-1 may contribute to the satiety of the postoperative patient, as these hormones are known to be anorexigenic. PYY and GLP-1 are not increased with gastric band procedures and seem to account for the improved satiety after gastric bypass in comparison to gastric band. In addition, plasma ghrelin, orexigenic in nature, has a blunted response to weight loss in gastric bypass patients. This decrease in ghrelin contributes to the improved satiety after gastric bypass compared to gastric banding.

A long-term complication of surgery may be insufficient weight loss. Defined as a loss of less than 40% to 50% of excess weight, 15% to 17% of patients after gastric bypass and adjustable gastric band fail to lose expected amount of weight. The reasons for insufficient weight loss include lack of dietary adherence, lack of exercise, psychological causes, and surgical technique complications. From surgical standpoint, a large or dilated pouch, short roux limb, or gastrogastric fistula can create increased nutrient absorption. Surgical interventions may be the best treatment option in these cases.

Nonsurgical etiologies of insufficient weight loss are typically lifestyle related. In a study of 100 patients after gastric bypass, Elkins et al. (20) report 37% patients eat snacks, 2% drink sodas, 11% fail to take vitamin supplements, and 41% do not exercise. A program combining aerobic activity and strength training is recommended. The program should be a gradually progressive program, taking into account the patient's clinical status and physical ability. In a study by Evans et al. (21), participation in 150 minutes per week of moderate or higher intensity activity yields higher weight loss at 6 and 12 months postoperatively after gastric bypass.

With respect to pregnancy, women are encouraged to wait 1 to 2 years after surgery before planning pregnancy. With proper nutritional evaluation and support, minimal adverse effects have been noted. Specifically, iron, vitamin B12, vitamin A, folate, calcium, and vitamin D need to be followed closely as these nutrients have a direct impact on fetal development. A study by Weintraub et al. (22), in fact, shows that postsurgically treated women experience fewer diabetes and hypertension complications and have a reduced risk of neonatal macrosomia. A study by Sheiner et al. (23) of 298 patients reveals no increase in pregnancy or perinatal complications in women after weight loss surgery. A literature review by Grundy et al. (24) presents similar outcomes in terms of pregnancy morbidities.

Several other newer procedures are becoming increasingly used for weight reduction. Gastric sleeve surgery is the most common of these procedures. A gastric sleeve procedure is a restrictive procedure in which the stomach is resected along the greater curvature, leaving a tubular stomach of 60 to 80 cm. The antrum and pylorus of the stomach are preserved. The procedure has been performed in patients with Crohn's disease, ulcerative colitis, cardiomyopathy with low ejection fraction, and renal transplant patients. A review by Iannelli et al. (25) revealed a mean weight loss of 83% at 12 months, although Almogy et al. (26) revealed an excess weight loss of 45.1% at 12 months. Mortality rate in the reviewed studies by Iannelli et al. (25) is 0.9% and morbidity is 10.3%. This procedure is often used as part of a two-stage approach for the superobese patient with second-stage duodenal switch. Oberbach et al. (27) report using the gastric sleeve and gastric bypass in 10 adolescent cases.

Future surgical therapies may include gastric stimulator, intragastric balloon, endoluminal sleeve, and gastric pouch revision. The intragastric balloon, gastric pouch revision, and endoluminal sleeve are endoscopic procedures. Intragastric balloons are used for short-term weight loss, with 26% excess weight loss. The balloon promotes satiety. The potential complications include pressure ulcers, balloon rupture, and distal gastric obstruction.

Neuromodulation is a potential course of bariatric therapy. Variations include vagal pacemaker, sympathetic nerve stimulator, intragastric stimulator, implantable intestinal stimulator, and gastric implantable stimulator. By changing the nerve signals to the central nervous system, the hope is for significant reduction in intake and hence weight loss.

The endoluminal sleeve is endoscopically placed at the gastric outlet. The sleeve uncurls resulting in blockage of nutrient contact with the duodenum and proximal jejunum. Studies at this time do not extend beyond 6 months. The excess weight loss is 23.6%. Interestingly, four patients with diabetes had resolution of their diabetes.

In patients with gastric pouch dilatation, endoscopic revision has recently been undertaken. Revising from one type of surgery to another has been reported (such as from adjustable gastric band to gastric bypass). A variety of methods and procedures to improve the outcome from surgical intervention continue to evolve.

Compared to other weight loss approaches at this time, surgery has demonstrated the greatest excess weight loss, the greatest reductions in comorbidities, and the first demonstration of reduced mortality compared to those receiving usual care. The safety of the procedure has been significantly reduced, and the result is a large increase in bariatric surgical procedures over the past 5 to 10 years. The immediate future offers an increase in surgical interventions until prevention or other pharmacotherapy makes significant improvements. The care of the postoperative patient requires careful attention to nutritional status, but can be rewarding with the excellent results as described herein. Importantly, there has never been a randomized trial of bariatric surgery versus effective pharmacological or lifestyle modification treatment. This kind of study is needed to truly evaluate comparative effectiveness of these different therapies.

REFERENCES

1. Buchwald H, Avidor Y, Braunwald E, Jensen MD, Pories W, Fahrbach K, Schoelles K. Bariatric surgery: A systematic review and meta-analysis. *JAMA*. 2004;292(14):1724–37.
2. Buchwald H, Estok R, Fahrbach K, Banel D, Jensen MD, Pories WJ, Bantle JP, Sledge I. Weight and type 2 diabetes after bariatric surgery: Systematic review and meta-analysis. *Am J Med*. 2009;122(3):248–56.
3. Adams TD, Gress RE, Smith SC, Halverson RC, Simper SC, Rosamond WD, Lamonte MJ, Stroup AM, Hunt SC. Long-term mortality after gastric bypass surgery. *N Engl J Med*. 2007;357(8):753–61.
4. Sjöström L, Narbro K, Sjöström CD, Karason K, Larsson B, Wedel H, Lystig T, et al. Effects of bariatric surgery on mortality in Swedish obese subjects. Swedish Obese Subjects Study. *N Engl J Med*. 2007;357(8):741–52.
5. Jensen MD, Ryan DH, Apovian CM, Ard JD, Comuzzie AG, Donato KA, Hu FB, et al. 2013 AHA/ACC/TOS guideline for the management of overweight and obesity in adults. A report of the American College of Cardiology/American Heart Association Task Force on Practice Guidelines and The Obesity Society. *J Am Coll Cardiol*. 2014;63(25):2985–3023.
6. Mechanick JI, Youdim A, Jones DB, Garvey WT, Hurley DL, McMahon MM, Henberg LJ, et al. Clinical practice guidelines for the perioperative nutritional, metabolic and nonsurgical support of the bariatric surgery patient—2013 update: Cosponsored by American Association of Clinical Endocrinologists, The Obesity Society, and American Society for Metabolic & Bariatric Surgery. *Surg Obesity Relat Dis*. 2013;(9):159–91.
7. Flancbaum L, Belsley S, Drake V, Colarusso T, Tayler E. Preoperative nutritional status of patients undergoing Roux-en-Y gastric bypass for morbid obesity. *J Gastrointest Surg*. 2006;10(7):1033–7.
8. Herpertz S, Kielmann R, Wolf AM, Hebebrand J, Senf W. Do psychosocial variables predict weight loss or mental health after obesity surgery? A systematic review. *Obes Res*. 2004;12(10):1554–69.
9. Sarwer DB, Wadden TA, Fabricatore AN. Psychosocial and behavioral aspects of bariatric surgery. *Obes Res*. 2005;13(4):639–48.
10. Fujioka K, Yan E, Wang HJ, Li Z. Evaluating preoperative weight loss, binge eating disorder, and sexual abuse history on Roux-en-Y gastric bypass outcome. *Surg Obes Relat Dis*. 2008;4(2):137–43.
11. Bocchieri-Ricciardi LE, Chen EY, Munoz D, Fischer S, Dymek-Valentine M, Alverdy JC, le Grange D. Pre-surgery binge eating status: Effect on eating behavior and weight outcome after gastric bypass. *Obes Surg*. 2006;16(9):1198–204.

12. Folope V, Hellot MF, Kuhn JM, Ténière P, Scotté M, Déchelotte P. Weight loss and quality of life after bariatric surgery: A study of 200 patients after vertical gastroplasty or adjustable gastric banding. *Eur J Clin Nutr.* 2008;62(8):1022–30.

13. Schauer PR, Bhatt DL, Kirwan JP, Wolski K, Brethauer SA, Navaneethan SD, Aminian A, et al. Bariatric surgery versus intensive medical therapy for diabetes— 3-year outcomes. *N Engl J Med.* 2014;370(21):2002–13.

14. Malone M. Recommended nutritional supplements for bariatric surgery patients. *Ann Pharmacother.* 2008;42:1851–8.

15. Fujioka K, DiBaise JK, Martindale RG. Nutrition and metabolic complications after bariatric surgery and their treatment. *J Parenter Enteral Nutr.* 2011;35(5 Suppl):52S–9S.

16. Slater GH, Ren CJ, Siegel N, Williams T, Barr D, Wolfe B, Dolan K, Fielding GA. Serum fat-soluble vitamin deficiency and abnormal calcium metabolism after malabsorptive bariatric surgery. *J Gastrointest Surg.* 2004;8(1):48–55.

17. Johansson HE, Zethelius B, Ohrvall M, Sundbom M, Haenni A. Serum magnesium status after gastric bypass surgery in obesity. *Obes Surg.* 2009;19(9):1250–5.

18. Newbury L, Dolan K, Hatzifotis M, Low N, Fielding G. Calcium and vitamin D depletion and elevated parathyroid hormone following biliopancreatic diversion. *Obes Surg.* 2003;13(6):893–5.

19. Boldery R, Fielding G, Rafter T, Pascoe AL, Scalia GM. Nutritional deficiency of selenium secondary to weight loss (bariatric) surgery associated with life-threatening cardiomyopathy. *Heart Lung Circ.* 2007;16(2):123–6.

20. Elkins G, Whitfield P, Marcus J, Symmonds R, Rodriguez J, Cook T. Noncompliance with behavioral recommendations following bariatric surgery. *Obes Surg.* 2005;15(4):546–51.

21. Evans RK, Bond DS, Wolfe LG, Meador JG, Herrick JE, Kellum JM, Maher JW. Participation in 150 min/wk of moderate or higher intensity physical activity yields greater weight loss after gastric bypass surgery. *Surg Obes Relat Dis.* 2007;3(5):526–30.

22. Weintraub AY, Levy A, Levi I, Mazor M, Wiznitzer A, Sheiner E. Effect of bariatric surgery on pregnancy outcome. *Int J Gynaecol Obstet.* 2008;103(3):246–51.

23. Sheiner E, Balaban E, Dreiher J, Levi I, Levy A. Pregnancy outcome in patients following different types of bariatric surgeries. *Obes Surg.* 2009;19(9):1286–92.

24. Grundy MA, Woodcock S, Attwood SE. The surgical management of obesity in young women: Consideration of the mother's and baby's health before, during, and after pregnancy. *Surg Endosc.* 2008;22(10):2107–16.

25. Iannelli A, Schneck AS, Ragot E, Liagre A, Anduze Y, Msika S, Gugenheim J. Laparoscopic sleeve gastrectomy as revisional procedure for failed gastric banding and vertical banded gastroplasty. *Obes Surg.* 2009;19(9):1216–20.

26. Almogy G, Crookes PF, Anthone GJ. Longitudinal gastrectomy as a treatment for the high-risk super-obese patient. *Obes Surg.* 2004;14(4):492–7.

27. Oberbach A, Neuhaus J, Inge T, Kirsch K, Schlichting N, Blüher S, Kullnick Y, Kugler J, Baumann S, Till H. Bariatric surgery in severely obese adolescents improves major comorbidities including hyperuricemia. *Metabolism* 2014;63(2):242–9.

11

Medical treatment of pediatric overweight and obesity

ERIC C. WESTMAN

Treatment of overweight and obesity in children, and prevention of these conditions, is imperative. This is the first generation of children who may die before their parents due to the comorbidities of excess adiposity (1). The treatment of children is complicated because they are particularly susceptible to advertising and peer pressure, both at home and at school. Although the environment of a child may be difficult to control, the root cause of obesity is the same for children as it is for adults: hyperinsulinemia. The hormonal impact of insulin as a growth factor leads to macrosomia. Hyperinsulinemic children are not only obese but also large for their age. This can be seen in the infants of diabetic mothers who become hyperinsulinemic in the intrauterine environment due to maternal hyperglycemia.

Children have exposure both in school and via television and other electronic media, which define much of the social milieu today. It can be very difficult to control the source of food for children (Figure 11.1). This has led to the ingestion of large amounts of sugar, much of it as fructose. Advice on "healthy diets" has often been interpreted as license to eat primarily sugars

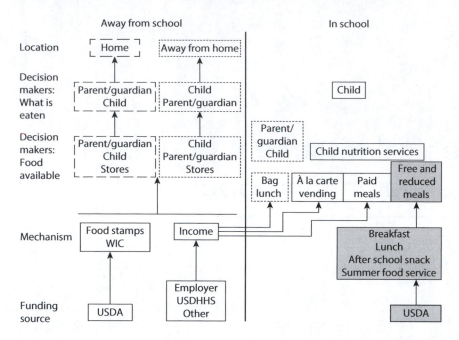

Figure 11.1 Factors influencing what a child eats. USDA = US Department of Agriculture; USDHHS = US Department of Health and Human Services; WIC = USDA Women, Infants, and Children Program.

and starches under the label of fruits and vegetables. (Until recently, ketchup was considered a "vegetable" in school lunch programs.) Especially troublesome is the reality that sugar-sweetened beverages are part of the social interaction of adolescents, and even infants are given juice and colas from the time they take a bottle. This sugar consumption leads to hyperinsu-linemia, the cause of the epidemic of type 2 diabetes and metabolic syndrome seen in children in the United States and other developed nations.

The role of parents in treatment of childhood obesity depends upon the stage of the child's development. In children younger than pubertal, parental support and engagement in lifestyle change are critical to the child's success. Pubertal and older teens often need to establish control over their bodies as evidence of individuation. In this case, helping the patient to strategize con-trol over his or her food may need to be done with parental support, but not parental responsi-bility. Only the clinician's judgment and relationship with the family can inform this approach.

DEFINITION OF OBESITY

Obesity in children is more difficult to define than in adults due to the changing height and normal growth of children. So, pediatric obesity is defined as excess adiposity relative to opti-mal growth parameters. Because of the relationship of weight gain to growth in children, body mass index (BMI), although the standard for defining obesity in adults, is not accepted uni-versally for use among children. The Centers for Disease Control and Prevention suggests two levels of concern for children based on the BMI-for-age charts (2):

1. At the 85th percentile and above, children are "at risk for overweight."
2. At the 95th percentile or above, they are "overweight."

Table 11.1 BMI categorization for children

BMI category	Traditional terminology	Newer terminology
<5th percentile	Underweight	Underweight
5th–84th percentile	Healthy weight	Healthy weight
85th–94th percentile	At risk of overweight	Overweight
≥95th percentile	Overweight or obesity	Obesity

Some experts consider those children above the 95th percentile as "obese," corresponding to a BMI of 30 (considered obese in adults) (3) (Table 11.1). The use of percentage of body weight that is fat mass is also a good marker of obesity. Using the body fat percentage, boys over 25% fat and girls over 32% fat are considered obese. Body fat percentage can be measured in the office, and obesity medicine specialists often have access to equipment that provides a measurement of percentage of body fat.

GOAL OF TREATMENT

The goal of treatment of pediatric obesity depends, in part, on the physiological age of the child. Although the reduction of excess adiposity in a safe, tolerable, and sustainable way is still the treatment goal, the clinician must assess the child's growth to develop the treatment plan. Because children reach a point in their growth and development where linear growth ceases due to epiphyseal closure, the urgency and intensity of treatment may be impacted by how close the child is to cessation of linear growth. If the child is within a year or so of epiphyseal closure as noted by bone age, and above the 90% BMI, then aggressive treatment options including carbohydrate and caloric restriction and even adjunctive anorectic medications may be appropriate. Certainly, in any child in whom a surgical option is being discussed, a trial of vigorous medical therapy is indicated.

WHAT IS HEALTHY NUTRITION DURING WEIGHT LOSS?

Dietary protein is critical for appropriate growth, including bone and muscle development. The protein requirement for children is age dependent, and the values are based on extrapolations rather than large population measurements (4). It appears that the protein concentration of breast milk (≈150 mg of protein/kg/day) is adequate for the first 6 months of life. After that, approximately 120 mg/kg/day appears sufficient by most standards. This is assuming that the protein is of high biological value (animal protein). If daily protein needs are fulfilled by lower biological value proteins, then the daily requirement may be larger. The need for water and minerals parallels adult humans. Carbohydrates and fats are used to supply the energy needed for growth and development.

DIETARY TREATMENT (CARBOHYDRATE OR CALORIE RESTRICTION)

The use of diets that induce nutritional ketosis in children is historically supported, both by populations eating primarily meat and fat (Inuit) and by the use of ketogenic diets to treat seizures. Children tolerate these diets well, and they are able to maintain appropriate growth and development. Therefore, in cases where ketogenic diets are needed to generate lipolysis of adipose stores, they have a history of safe use in children, with appropriate monitoring, of course. Children with less urgent or intense need for lipolysis may be able to "grow out of" their excess adiposity if sugary beverages and other forms of empty calories, primarily refined carbohydrates, are removed from the diet and replaced by adequate protein, leafy green vegetables and limited consumption of complex carbohydrates (i.e., those with lower glycemic indices). If ketogenic- or carbohydrate-restricted dietary approaches are used, then neither the amount nor the type of dietary fat is restricted. Calories are also unrestricted in this approach. If a balanced deficit diet approach is used, without carbohydrate restriction, then fat calories may be restricted as part of the calculated caloric deficit. If a balanced deficit diet approach is used, careful attention to ensure adequate protein intake is needed. Although dietary vitamins and minerals are required in small amounts and are found in food naturally, during any dietary approach to weight loss, a multivitamin is recommended as a safety net.

CLINICAL ASSESSMENT

The obesity medicine specialist caring for a child typically obtains an initial measurement of lipids, a chemistry profile, and fasting glucose and insulin levels. A 2-hour postprandial glucose and insulin level is appropriate if any concern exists about the possibility of type 2 diabetes mellitus and to assess the postglucose challenge insulin response. Teenagers can easily tolerate a 3-hour glucose tolerance test with insulin levels. Of course, topical anesthetic agents such as EMLA (lidocaine and prilocaine) cream should be used if possible, to decrease pain and anxiety. Abnormal laboratory values would be repeated at intervals—about 3 months is often adequate time for these abnormalities to correct. In addition, in all prepubertal patients, a bone age x-ray should be considered. If the bone age is more than 1 year ahead of the chronological age, then the urgency of treatment increases, especially as the child approaches puberty. Therefore, the Tanner rating scale is used to assess the developmental progress toward puberty (5,6). A Tanner 3 with advanced bone age may need intense treatment and close follow-up to slow the onset of puberty and to avoid premature epiphyseal closure.

Children are measured for height and weight at every visit, and percentiles are plotted. It is not uncommon for a linear growth spurt to occur as weight loss occurs, presumably because of improvement in chronic hyperinsulinemia. Measurement of percentage of body fat is also helpful, if available. Clothing sizes and belt and waist measurements can also help document progress.

MEDICATION TREATMENT

Anorectic agents or insulin sensitizers are not labeled for use in children, but some research has been done in this area (7–9). In contrast, children routinely receive medications for treatment of attention deficit disorder/attention deficit hyperactivity disorder that has chemical similarity to drugs used for appetite suppression. As mentioned, it seems reasonable that any child or adolescent considering a surgical procedure for treatment of obesity should be given a trial period of intense medical management that may include anorectic medication(s), if this is considered appropriate by the treating physician. The monitoring interval may be more frequent than the usual monthly visit, as determined by the clinician. All appropriate risk–benefit discussions are documented and consent forms are signed. Of course, anorectic medications must be prescribed within the regulatory confines of the state agencies supervising these medications.

DIETARY TREATMENT

Carbohydrate restriction

Dietary carbohydrate is the primary insulin secretagogue. Because pancreatic insulin secretion is stimulated by the glucose/amino acid ratio in the portal vein and in response to the rate of increase in blood glucose, a powerful way to lower insulin levels is to reduce dietary carbohydrate. When the dietary intake of carbohydrate is reduced to less than 50 g per day, most individuals excrete ketones in the urine, leading to the descriptive name of ketogenic diet. Several popular diets have used the recommendation of very low levels of carbohydrate (<20 g per day) in the early stages of the diet to enhance lipolysis (10–14). The presence of urinary ketones is an indicator of an increase in fat oxidation. Several research groups have referred to this approach as a very-low–carbohydrate ketogenic diet or low-carbohydrate ketogenic diet. When dietary carbohydrate is low (20 g per day), insulin secretion remains low—close to basal levels—and fat burning (lipolysis) and protein burning (gluconeogenesis) occur as glucagon levels rise. A low-carbohydrate diet is one that contains 50 to 150 g per day and is not typically associated with nutritional ketosis. When dietary carbohydrate is present in sufficient amounts for stimulating insulin secretion, fat storage will occur. This may even be true in situations where total energy intake is limited, resulting in fat storage and lean tissue breakdown. The dietary carbohydrate signals fat deposition, whereas the need for gluconeo-genesis in energy-limited diets results in lean tissue use. In general, the low-carbohydrate diet will raise high-density lipoprotein (HDL) cholesterol, lower triglycerides, and have little effect on low-density lipoprotein (LDL) cholesterol. The average weight loss over 6 to 12 months in clinical trials ranged from 5.1 to 12.2 kg, although in private clinical settings larger amounts of weight loss have been reported. Examples of popular carbohydrate-restricted programs include the Atkins Diet, the South Beach Diet, and the Protein Power Plan.

Several studies have been published that support the safety and effectiveness of carbohydrate-restricted diets in children. A randomized trial of 30 adolescents compared a low-carbohydrate diet to a low-fat diet over a 12-week period (15). The low-carbohydrate group was instructed to consume <20 g of carbohydrate per day for 2 weeks, then <40 g per day for 10 weeks. The low-carbohydrate group lost more weight (mean 9.9 kg vs. 4.1 kg, $P < 0.05$) and had improvements in non-HDL cholesterol levels ($P < 0.05$). Sondike et al. (15) concluded that the low-carbohydrate diet was effective for short-term weight loss and that the diet did not harm the lipid profile.

In another study, 37 obese elementary school–aged children from a Pediatric Endocrinology Clinic (Marshall University School of Medicine, Huntington, West Virginia) were recruited to follow either a carbohydrate-restricted diet or a calorie-restricted diet (16). The carbohydrate-restricted diet allowed <30 g of carbohydrate per day, with unlimited calo-ries, protein, and fat. After 2 months, the 27 children (mean age of 12 years) following the carbohydrate-restricted diet lost an average of 5.2 ± 3.4 kg ($P < 0.001$) and decreased their BMI by 2.4 ± 1.3 points ($P < 0.001$). After 2 months, the 10 children following the calorie-restricted diet gained an average of 2.4 ± 2.5 kg and 1.0 point on the BMI value ($P < 0.001$). In this study, the carbohydrate-restricted diet was superior to the calorie-restricted diet for weight loss in obese school-age children. Another study from the same clinic examined the effect of a carbohydrate-restricted diet on serum lipid profiles after 10 weeks in children aged 6 to 12 years (17). After 10 weeks, both the serum cholesterol and serum triglycerides showed significant improvements: −24.2 mg/dL in cholesterol and −56.9 mg/dL in triglycer-ides ($P < 0.02$ for both).

Another study tested the effectiveness of a carbohydrate-restricted diet in obese children aged 12 to 18 years in 11 community pediatric practices (18). A carbohydrate-restricted diet of <50 g of carbohydrate per day was used. In total, 38 teens completed the 6-month study and 84% lost weight, ranging from −23.9 to +5.5 kg. There was also a significant decrease in mean BMI (from 34.9 to 32.5 kg/m^2).

A different study examined the effect of a carbohydrate-restricted diet on cardiac function by using echocardiography (19). Thirty obese children (mean age 12.2 years) were followed for 6 months on a low-carbohydrate, nonrestricted calorie diet providing less than 30% of the total calories from simple carbohydrates, with an exercise recommendation. The mean weight change was 5 kg ($P < 0.0001$) and 5 BMI units ($P < 0.0001$). The echocardiographic results showed that the low-carbohydrate diet led to improvements in subclinical right and left ventricular diastolic dysfunction (20).

The ketogenic diet is a low-carbohydrate diet developed in the 1920s for the treatment of children with seizures refractory to medical treatment (21). A modified ketogenic diet, modeled after the carbohydrate-restricted diet used for weight loss, has also been studied for seizure control (22). Twenty children, aged 3 to 18 years, with at least three seizures per week, who had been treated with at least two anticonvulsants, were enrolled and received the carbohydrate-restricted diet (10 g/day plus vitamin and calcium supplements) over a 6-month period. After 6 months, 13 (65%) had >50% improvement in their frequency of seizures and 7 (35%) had >90% improvement (4 were seizure free). The diet was well tolerated without adverse effects. The study concluded that the modified ketogenic diet was an effective and well-tolerated therapy for intractable pediatric epilepsy.

Calorie restriction

In calorie-restricted diets, calories are explicitly limited, and instruction is given to either count calories or to follow a diet protocol that is low in calories. Calorie- and fat-reduced diets and balanced deficit diets generally do not achieve nutritional ketosis because they contain sufficient carbohydrate to prevent ketogenesis. Although calorie-restricted diets will lead to weight loss, they do not lead to the same pattern of cardiometabolic risk reduction or lean tissue sparing as low-carbohydrate diets. In general, the 30% fat calorie–restricted diet will lower LDL-cholesterol, modestly impact triglycerides, and modestly raise HDL-cholesterol. Examples of popular calorie-restricted diet programs include Weight Watchers, Jenny Craig, and Nutrisystem. There has been a general trend in calorie-restricted diets to also restrict carbohydrates in some way (low glycemic or low carbohydrate) (23).

Combination of calorie restriction and carbohydrate restriction

Very-low-calorie diets (VLCD), also referred to as supplemented fasting, are diets that provide between 300 and 800 kcal per day. VLCDs provide enough protein to meaningfully reduce lean tissue wasting and supply essential minerals and vitamins along with varying amounts of carbohydrates and fats (24). There are two general classes of VLCD: one class consists of common foods with dietary supplements of minerals and vitamins, and the other class consists of a defined formula providing all nutrients as beverages, soups, bars, or a combination taken three to five times per day. The food-based VLCD consists mostly of lean meat, fish, and poultry, whereas the formula VLCD usually requires the addition of carbohydrate as sugar or modified starch to enhance palatability. The food-based VLCD provides a modest dose of fat inherent in the food choices, whereas fat is not always provided in the defined formula diets.

Examples of formula-based VLCDs are Optifast, Medifast, Pro-Cal (R-Kane), and Robard New Direction.

A VLCD was included in a multidisciplinary weight reduction program for children that extended over 1 year and included a hypocaloric diet, exercise, and behavior modification (25). Fifty-six overweight children (aged 7–17 years) were enrolled into the weight management program and 62.5% successfully completed the 1-year program. There was a significant decrease in body weight and body fat, as assessed by weight determinations and skinfold measurements ($P < 0.0001$). The BMI decreased significantly from 32.7 to 28.7 kg/m^2 ($P < 0.0001$). The study concluded that a multidisciplinary weight reduction program that combines a VLCD, followed by a balanced hypocaloric diet, with a moderate-intensity progressive exercise program and behavior modification is an effective means for weight reduction in obese children and adolescents.

SIDE EFFECTS

There are two groupings of side effects based upon whether they occur early or late in the treatment process. VLCDs (400–800 kcal per day) probably have a higher incidence of side effects than carbohydrate restriction using food (1200–1500 kcal per day) due to the lower caloric intake. During adaptation to carbohydrate restriction and nutritional ketosis, the most common side effects are weakness, fatigue, and lightheadedness. Although there is a modest reduction in peak aerobic performance in the first week or two of a VLCD, orthostatic symptoms occurring during normal daily activities are the result of the combination of diet-induced natriuresis and an inadequate sodium intake. These symptoms can be prevented by the addition of 2 to 3 g per day of sodium (taken as bouillon or broth, for example) in all patients not requiring continued diuretic medication, along with attention to adequate dietary potassium, with supplementation as needed. Of course, diuretic medications may require downward adjustment during this period of natriuresis.

After the first few weeks of adaptation to carbohydrate restriction, the most common side effects are constipation and muscle cramps. The constipation may result in part from the lower fiber content of dietary intake, but it is also exacerbated by dehydration. If increasing fluid intake to a minimum of 2 L per day does not resolve the constipation, then 1 teaspoon of milk of magnesia at bedtime, bouillon supplementation, or a carbohydrate-free fiber supplement can be used. Muscle cramps can occur either early or late in treatment, and they are more common in people with a history of diuretic medication use or prior heavy ethanol consumption. In almost all cases, the muscle cramps respond promptly to supplementation with 1 teaspoon of milk of magnesia at bedtime or 200 mEq per day of slow-release magnesium chloride, suggesting prior depletion of this essential mineral as the root cause. Excessively brisk deep tendon reflexes suggest hypomagnesemia in neurologically intact individuals.

SURGICAL TREATMENT

Weight loss surgery for children is available in a few centers, but it is not generally recommended unless serious consequences of obesity are present (e.g., nonalcoholic fatty liver disease/nonalcoholic steatohepatitis) (26).

CONCLUSIONS

Childhood obesity is at crisis levels; the current generation of children may die before their parents due to the comorbidities of excess adiposity. Many effective treatments are available,

Table 11.2 Medical approaches to treat pediatric obesity

- Carbohydrate-restricted diet
- Calorie-restricted diet
- Very-low-calorie diet
- Combined medication and dietary therapy

including dietary and medical approaches with a unifying theme of restricting sugar, carbohydrate, and caloric intake (Table 11.2). Trained physicians developing comprehensive individualized treatment plans can be extremely effective in assisting children in improving their health by treating this serious health problem.

ACKNOWLEDGMENT

The author thanks Wendy Scinta for reading and providing suggestions for the first edition of this chapter.

REFERENCES

1. Olshansky SJ, Passsdssaro DJ, Hershow RC, Layden J, Carnes BA, Brody J, Hayflick L, Butler RN, Allison DB, Ludwig DS. A potential decline in life expectancy in the United States in the 21st century. *N Engl J Med* 2005;352:1138–1145.
2. Centers for Disease Control and Prevention, National Center for Health Statistics. Growth Charts. Updated August 4, 2009. Available at http://www.cdc.gov/growth-charts/clinical_charts.htm
3. Barlow SE, Expert Committee. Expert Committee recommendations regarding the prevention, assessment and treatment of child and adolescent overweight and obesity: Summary report. *Pediatrics* 2007;120:S164–S192.
4. Joint FAO/WHO/UNU Expert Consultation. *Protein and Amino Acid Requirements in Human Nutrition.* Geneva, Switzerland; 2002. http://whqlibdoc.who.int/trs/WHO_TRS_935
5. Marshall WA, Tanner JM. Variations in the pattern of pubertal changes in boys. *Arch Dis Child* 1970;45:13–23.
6. Marshall WA, Tanner JM. Variations in the pattern of pubertal changes in girls. *Arch Dis Child* 1969;44:291–303.
7. Berkowitz RI, Fujioka K, Daniels SR, Hoppin AG, Owen S, Perry AC, Sothern MS, et al. Effects of sibutramine treatment in obese adolescents: A randomized trial. *Ann Intern Med* 2006;145(2):81–90.
8. Glaser Pediatric Research Network Obesity Study Group. Metformin extended release treatment of adolescent obesity: A 48-week randomized, double-blind, placebo-controlled trial with 48-week follow-up. *Arch Pediatr Adolesc Med* 2010;164:116–123.
9. Boland CL, Harris JB, Harris KB. Pharmacological management of obesity in pediatric patients. *Ann Pharmacother* 2015;49(2):220–232.
10. Vernon MC, Mavropoulos J, Transue M, Yancy WS Jr, Westman EC. Clinical experience of a carbohydrate-restricted diet: Effect on diabetes mellitus. *Metab Syndr Relat Dis* 2003;1:233–237.

11. Vernon MC, Kueser B, Transue M, Yates HE, Yancy WS, Westman EC. Clinical experience of a carbohydrate-restricted diet for the metabolic syndrome. *Metab Syndr Relat Dis* 2004;2:180–186.
12. Westman EC, Feinman RD, Mavropoulos JC, Vernon MC, Volek JS, Wortman JA, Yancy WS Jr., Phinney SD. Low-carbohydrate nutrition and metabolism. *Am J Clin Nutr* 2007;86:276–284.
13. Nordmann AJ, Nordmann A, Briel M, Keller U, Yancy WS Jr., Brehm BJ, Bucher HC. Effects of low-carbohydrate vs low-fat diets on weight loss and cardiovascular risk factors: A meta-analysis of randomized controlled trials. *Arch Intern Med* 2006;166(3):285–293.
14. Shai I, Schwarzfuchs D, Henkin Y, Shahar DR, Witkow S, Greenberg I, Golan R, et al. Weight loss with a low-carbohydrate, Mediterranean, or low-fat diet. *N Engl J Med* 2008;359(3):229–241.
15. Sondike SB, Copperman N, Jacobson MS. Effects of a low-carbohydrate diet on weight loss and cardiovascular risk factors in overweight adolescents. *J Pediatr* 2003;142:253–258.
16. Bailes JR Jr., Strow MT, Werthammer J, McGinnis RA, Elitsur Y. Effect of low-carbohydrate, unlimited calorie diet on the treatment of childhood obesity: A prospective controlled study. *Metab Syndr Relat Dis* 2003;1:221–225.
17. Dunlap BS, Bailes JR Jr. Unlimited energy, restricted carbohydrate diet improves lipid parameters in obese children. *Metab Syndr Relat Dis* 2008;6(1):32–36.
18. Siegel RM, Rich W, Joseph EC, Linhardt J, Knight J, Khoury J, Daniels SR. A 6-month, office-based, low-carbohydrate diet intervention in obese teens. *Clin Pediatr (Phila)* 2009;48(7):745–749.
19. Zeybek C, Aktuglu-Zeybek C, Onal H, Altay S, Erdem A, Celebi A. Right ventricular subclinical diastolic dysfunction in obese children: The effect of weight reduction with a low-carbohydrate diet. *Pediatr Cardiol* 2009;30(7):946–953.
20. Zeybek C, Celebi A, Aktuglu-Zeybek C, Onal H, Yalcin Y, Erdem A, Akdeniz C, Imanov E, Altay S, Aydın A. The effect of low-carbohydrate diet on left ventricular diastolic function in obese children. *Pediatr Int* 2010;52(2):218–223.
21. Freeman JM, Vining EP, Pillas DJ, Pyzik PL, Casey JC, Kelly LM. The efficacy of the ketogenic diet-1998: A prospective evaluation of intervention in 150 children. *Pediatrics* 1998;102(6):1358–1363.
22. Kossoff EH, McGrogan JR, Bluml RM, Pillas DJ, Rubenstein JE, Vining EP. A modified Atkins diet is effective for the treatment of intractable pediatric epilepsy. *Epilepsia* 2006;47(2):421–424.
23. Armeno ML, Krochik AG, Mazza CS. Evaluation of two dietary treatments in obese hyperinsulinemic adolescents. *J Pediatr Endocrinol Metab* 2011;24(9–10):715–722.
24. Tsai AG, Wadden TA. The evolution of very-low-calorie diets: An update and meta-analysis. *Obesity* 2006;14:1283–1293.
25. Sothern, Udall JN Jr, Suskind RM, Vargas A, Blecker U. Weight loss and growth velocity in obese children after very low calorie diet, exercise, and behavior modification. *Acta Paediatr* 2000;89(9):1036–1043.
26. Nobili V, Vajro P, Dezsofi A, Fischler B, Hadzic N, Jahnel J, Lamireau T, et al. Indications and limitations of bariatric intervention in severely obese children and adolescents with and without nonalcoholic steatohepatitis: ESPGHAN Hepatology Committee Position Statement. *J Pediatr Gastroenterol Nutr* 2015;60(4):550–561.

12

Binge eating disorder: Etiology, assessment, diagnosis, and treatment

RALPH CARSON

The term *binge eating* first entered the clinical vocabulary in 1957 when it was cited as a condition with the behavioral characteristic of unrestrained eating (1). However, at that time, it required the intake of "large" quantities of food, but it did not have to occur at regular intervals. Then, binge eating received little clinical attention for nearly 40 years, remaining largely associated with gluttony and dismissed as a problem of overindulgence. In 1995, Fairburn's work, calling binge eating "a true problem," focused on the serious repercussions of the disorder in both health and other areas of life (2).

In 2013, binge eating disorder (BED) was given a stand-alone category in the Diagnostic and Statistical Manual of Mental Disorders (DSM)-V (3) under the designation of psychiatric disturbance. With new criteria regarding the frequency of the behavior required to make a diagnosis of BED, the DSM-V made the diagnosis applicable to a larger group of individuals. Instead of requiring the behavior to occur twice a week over 6 months, BED could be diagnosed when the behavior occurred at an incidence of once a week over 3 months.

INCIDENCE OF BED

About 5.5% of the population lives with BED. Although this may sound like a small number, it is the most common of all eating disorders and includes millions of individuals, men (2%) and women (3.5%) alike (4). Not only does binge eating occur in both men and women but also the numbers are increasing. In 1990, those suffering from BED accounted for just 1% to 3% of the population (5). Although obesity is more prevalent among those with BED than it is among the regular population (4,6,7), and many adults with BED have been overweight as children (8), obesity is not a predictor of BED. However, studies show that 18% to 46% of weight control programs' obese members suffer from BED (9).

There are cultural and emotional patterns associated with BED, including the characteristic emotional distress of postbinge shame, guilt, and disgust and a higher incidence of depression and anxiety common in binge eaters (10). Although we note typical weight fluctuations among binge eaters and recognize their body-image dissatisfaction, especially around the issue of weight, behavioral research is scant regarding complex analyses of the disorder and determination of causalities (11).

RISK FACTORS

Differences between the obese with and without BED may be fertile ground for further study. For example, although there is a similar personality profile between obese patients with and without BED, patients with BED showed lower scores in self-directedness (12). In addition, binge eaters intake more energy (positively correlated with body mass index [BMI]) (13) during a binge meal than do individuals of similar body weight without BED. When looking at risk factors stemming from childhood experiences, the retrospective study of Grilo and Masheb (14) of a series of 145 consecutive outpatients with BED showed that some kind of childhood mistreatment was present in a full 83% of subjects. This finding is supported in work by Striegel-Moore et al. (15). The type of mistreatment was less about sexual (30%) and physical abuse (36%) than about issues such as emotional abuse (59%), emotional neglect (69%), and to a lesser degree physical neglect (49%). Findings such as these could have ramifications in the treatment of BED.

In addition to childhood traumas, there are a host of other risk factors for BED reported in earlier findings by Striegle-Moore et al. (16) and corroborated later (17). Such factors include social pressures, such as low social support; pressures to be thin; low self-esteem (18); and criticism of weight and shape stigma. In addition, the work identified internal psychological pressures, such as difficulty expressing emotions; depression; impulsivity; social isolation or withdrawal to lifestyle patterns such as emotional eating, skipping meals, limiting food categories, dieting, and weight problems (19); and substance abuse. Other circumstantial risk factors included younger age of menarche, childhood obesity, parental obesity, parental depression, and genetic makeup.

COMPLICATIONS OF BED

In 2000, the National Task Force on the Prevention and Treatment of Obesity established that binge eating represents a clinically significant public health problem, impacting both medical and psychiatric care industries (20). That finding is borne out by observing the high rate of comorbidity among obesity (6,7,21), psychiatric disorders, and medical conditions (16,22,23). In the psychiatric realm, BED can commonly co-occur with major depressive disorder, personality disorder, bipolar disorder, substance abuse, body dysmorphic disorder, kleptomania, irritable bowel syndrome, fibromyalgia, or anxiety disorder (24,25).

In addition, some of our most prevalent national medical health issues are diseases associated with obesity. The same litany of issues comprises the major complications of BED; several of these issues are shown in Table 12.1. Further impact of BED can be seen in the degree of distress (marked distress per DSM-V) that binge eating brings to those with it. Furthermore, binge eating has even wider-reaching societal impacts. For example, people miss work, school, or social activities to binge eat. In the overwhelming majority of cases where the binge eater is struggling with obesity, the negative feelings they have toward themselves, the preoccupation

Table 12.1 Medical conditions associated with both obesity and binge eating

• Type 2 diabetes	• Poor female reproductive health
• High blood pressure	• complications of pregnancy
• High cholesterol levels	• menstrual irregularities
• Coronary heart disease	• infertility
• Congestive heart failure	• irregular ovulation
• Angina pectoris	• Cancers of the
• Stroke	• uterus
• Asthma	• breast
• Osteoarthritis	• prostate
• Musculoskeletal disorders	• kidney
• Gallbladder disease	• liver
• Sleep apnea and respiratory problems	• pancreas
• Gout	• esophagus
• Bladder control problems	• colon and rectum

with appearance, and the shame and desire to hide the problem cause binge eaters to avoid social gatherings. They are often so successful at hiding binge eating that close family members and friends do not know they binge eat.

DIAGNOSTIC CONSIDERATIONS

A copy of the DSM-V criteria for the diagnosis of BED, a list of assessment tools, and some other information about BED that might be interesting to the clinician are present in the Table 12.2.

Inherent problems with the definition and assessment of BED (32)

The DSM's definition of BED validates the disorder, providing helpful guidelines both for the clinician and for insurance purposes. But it is important to continue to refine the definitions and boundaries (33) of an eating binge, one of the most difficult areas to establish in the treatment of eating disorders (34). For example, how do we quantify the amount of food intake that constitutes a binge? Terminology such as "large quantities" does not easily lend itself to measurement. In clinical situations, the term is assessed by the clinician, based on reports from the client, making such assessment vulnerable to detection bias. In addition, research has suggested that client reports of food amounts are often subject to overestimation (35–37). This lack of clarity can become compounded later in the assessment. Thus, an unreliable measurement of "large quantities" makes it more difficult to accurately assess how many binge eating episodes have occurred in a given period of time.

The subjective nature of some criteria such as "eating until uncomfortably full without compensation" (38,39) or having a "sense of loss of control and distress" (40–42) only adds to diagnostic difficulties.

Apart from reducing selection bias (women, small samples, high dropout rate, and placebo response) that hinders the ability to identify who qualifies for BED (43), the maturing field of BED treatment could benefit from more basic scientific developments. One need is a unifying

Table 12.2 Binge Eating Disorder DSM-V Diagnostic Criteria[a]

- Recurrent episodes of binge eating.
- The binge eating episodes are associated with three or more of the following:
  - Eating much more rapidly than normal
  - Eating until feeling uncomfortably full
  - Eating large amounts of food when not hungry
  - Eating alone because of embarrassment
  - Feeling disgusted, depressed, or guilty after episode
- Marked distress regarding binge eating.
- The binge eating occurs, on average, at least once per week for 3 months.
- The binge eating is not associated with recurrent use of inappropriate compensatory behaviors and does not occur exclusively during the course of bulimia nervosa or anorexia nervosa.

[a] American Psychiatric Association. *Diagnostic and Statistical Manual of Mental Disorders*, 5th ed. Washington, DC: American Psychiatric Association; 2013.

theory that would help interpret the neural correlates playing a role in BED origin and treatment. There also is need for an animal model to help test and interpret questions concerning the impact of arousal, stress, and mood on binge eating behavior.

Loss of control

From the binge eater's perspective, identifying an episode of binge eating has less to do with food quantity than with issues about loss of control (LOC). When asked to quantify binge eating episodes, their responses focus on the sense of being out of control or of transgressing dietary standards when eating (44–47).

An objective binge episode, as classified by the Eating Disorder Exam, occurs when an objective interviewer determines that the amount eaten is relatively large, but it also includes the patient reporting LOC during the episode (48,49).

Although there is no consistent definition of LOC, and the reporting of LOC during a binge episode is inordinately subjective (50), the important takeaway for the treatment field is the psychological distress brought on by LOC (47). This LOC demonstrates a valuable point of entry for clinical intervention, even if clinical binge eating is not present, according to strict definition. Take, for example, the individual who may be driven by LOC stresses to seek bariatric surgery to assert some measure of control. Studies showing that up to 25% of postbariatric patients report LOC eating (51,52) suggest that, for a quarter of patients, the psychological distress is not resolved by the surgery.

DISTINGUISHING BED FROM OTHER DIAGNOSES

Obesity versus BED

When treating obesity, it is important to identify persons who are suffering from BED because research shows that symptoms across many areas of behavior are consistently heightened in cases of BED. In addition to more medical morbidity among the BED population, there is an increased likelihood of psychiatric morbidity, including depression, anxiety, and personality disorders (85). Furthermore, studies verify that a host of issues such as negative body image and weight fluctuations are more severe in those with BED (86,87).

Binge eating versus BED

Episodes of binge eating can exist apart from BED, but binge eating behavior certainly is a central symptom of BED. In both binge eating and BED, shame responses can be exhibited through behaviors such as isolation and hiding food stashes, particularly when the food is highly palatable and deemed to be junk food or bad. The binge eater's desire to keep the eating behavior inconspicuous results in characteristic behaviors such as eating at odd times (late at night, early mornings) or in isolated spaces (at a fast-food drive through or in a car while driving alone). The fear of being caught also encourages faster eating.

Beyond this shame-related behavior, two characteristics signal a shift from episodes of binge eating to a diagnosis of BED. The first characteristic is the associated LOC. There is a constant internal battle between the behavior, which seems driven by overwhelming impulses, and despair, on one hand, and the disgust at the inability to exert control over the behavior on the other hand. Attempts to stop the behavior, go on a diet, or swear off binging habits fail. In these eating episodes, the eater is more likely to continue eating to the point of physical discomfort or some other external limit, such as falling asleep or running out of food. With these distinctions in place to help define BED, the DSM definition becomes a useful tool for distinguishing between the two conditions: in the person with BED, this uncontrollable eating scenario will repeat itself at least once a week for 3 months or more.

BED versus bulimia nervosa and night eating syndrome

Since part of the definition of BED requires that purging behaviors such as inducing vomiting or taking laxatives *not* to be present, the boundary is clear between BED and the purging type of bulimia nervosa (BN). However, the boundary becomes less clear in the case of nonpurging BN. In both cases, large quantities of food are consumed, and determining methods for more clearly distinguishing the two conditions is a possible area for future attention. From several key studies, differences between the BED and BN profiles can be inferred. Barry et al. (88) concluded that, all other things being equal, the presence of obesity distinguishes BED (obesity present) from bulimia (obesity absent). In contrast, those with BED have been distinct in their rate of dropout from programs and studies show that body dissatisfaction (89) issues are a big reason.

Comparisons between BED and night eating syndrome (NES) show higher hunger scores in BED subjects than among those with non-BED and NES. Moreover, Stunkard and Allison (90) concluded, after reviewing the literature on BED and NES through 2002, that BED and NES are two different eating disorders. They observed that NES involves behaviors and neuroendocrine characteristics with distinct markers in patterns of eating, sleep, and mood.

Compulsive overeating versus BED

BED is quite similar to compulsive overeating in that the latter also involves eating excessive amounts of food frequently, and an inability to stop or self-manage, regardless of consequences. However, in compulsive overeating, food ideation is present, and an episode can be preceded by food fantasies or triggered or accompanied by cravings. By contrast, binge eating is more likely to involve indiscriminant eating and less likely to involve food fantasies. In BED, where the individual is eating large amounts in a short time frame, the experience of LOC is a dominant part of the picture. Because BED can overlay much deeper psychological problems, it is important to consider BED whenever compulsive overeating is suspected.

Compulsive eating is perpetuated in spite of negative consequences and this does not have to be present in the binge eater—they just eat unconsciously and the main negativity is shame and guilt stemming from their lack of control ideation. The compulsive eater may be focused on such issues as why they should not eat because it could trigger diabetic symptomology, a recurrence of a heart attack, gastroesophageal reflux disorder, or gastric reflux. All compulsive eaters binge eat; all BED episodes are not perceived as causing negative consequences. Overeating can appear like binge eating, but there is usually not a feeling of LOC followed by guilt or embarrassment. Furthermore, such an episode in the overeater will typically involve highly palatable food, but the binge eater will consume mass quantities of whatever is available, without necessarily regarding taste and pleasure.

BED: Addiction or compulsive disorder?

The desire to eat can feel like an addiction when the food is something forbidden, especially when eating for short-term comfort or fulfillment becomes a priority over long-term harm to health and weight. Studies looking at changes in brain chemistry or behaviors in relation to foods, sugar, or palatable foods show correlations between drug addiction and compulsive eating. Well-documented key correlations are the presence of LOC, powerlessness to control the eating (or drug-taking) behavior, and also the similar alterations in brain chemistry, particularly with respect to dopamine.

Subjectively, both addicts and overeaters experience preoccupation with and cravings for their substance of choice. In both cases, they engage in impulsive eating or drug-taking responses (91), and they engage in spite of resolutions to the contrary, attendant guilt, shame, remorse (40), and consequences to life and health.

Psychiatrist Nora Volkow and colleagues found neurological evidence suggesting a kinship between compulsive overeaters and drug addicts. Volkow found that the anomaly of lower dopamine receptor availability, common to drug addicts, also occurred in overeaters (92–94).

Taking in palatable foods activates dopaminergic enzymes in the nucleus accumbens and other reward centers (95–97). Not only is this intake associated with reward but also repeating the intake, as seen in the development of binge eating, is associated with relief of physiological and psychological stress (98). In those with BED, binge eating is perpetuated—and recovery can even be derailed—by this desire to escape aversive emotional states (99–101). Moreover, rats with a dopamine deficit (due to a lentivirus-mediated knockdown of striatal D2 receptors [D2Rs]) that are given access to palatable, high-fat food quickly developed addiction-like reward deficits that initiated compulsive food seeking. This research is corroborated in a study by Epstein and Shaham (102) who gave rats extended access to high-fat, high-sugar food and observed the development of behavioral and physiological changes similar to those caused by drugs of abuse. Casseus et al. (103) found that binge eating on highly palatable diets can self-perpetuate binge eating by enhancing endogenous opioids.

In obese binge eaters, D2DR deficiency produces a blunted reward response (93,94,104–107). The resulting altered evaluation of food reward leads to a manic search for satisfaction (108,109). These activities are neuroadaptations that may also be self-perpetuating; for example, reduced activity in the dopaminergic system is involved in impulsivity and lack of self-control. It is interesting to note that brain activity increases with anticipation (opioid response in the visceral adipose tissue) and is less during the actual consumption.

Many studies have established similarities between neurochemical pathways activated in compulsive eating and those activated during addictive behavior (95–97,102,110–117). The similarities include LOC, impulsivity (91); priming and intermittent exposure that triggers binging (118,119); and compulsivity, with continued food seeking and intake despite negative consequences (120).

There is some evidence of other similarities between compulsive eating behavior and drug addiction, for example, the process of developing tolerance (108) and the experience of withdrawal (91,95,96,98,109,110,113,117,121–124), and reward deficiency syndrome itself (121,122,125–128).

Physical symptoms of compulsive-eating withdrawal are seen in rats, including teeth chattering, tremors, and head shaking. (98,113,122). Palatable foods release dopamine and endogenous opioid peptides (110,126) similar to gambling and substance abuse (91,121,123). In terms of treatment, a study that observed animals in response to chocolate withdrawal showed that food deprivation increased harmful food seeking that could then be prevented by selective norepinephrine inactivation, connecting prefrontal cortical norepinephrine in a critical way with maladaptive food-related behavior. These findings suggest possible new therapies, top-down approaches, for aberrant eating behaviors (120).

From a survival perspective, it is in the best interest of humans to have an inherent desire for food. However, this desire may go awry, and certain people, including some obese, compulsive eaters, and binge eaters, may develop an unhealthy dependence on palatable food that interferes with well-being. The concept of *food addiction* materialized in the diet industry on the basis of subjective reports, clinical accounts, and case studies described in self-help books. The rise in obesity, coupled with the emergence of scientific findings of parallels between drugs of abuse and palatable foods, has given credibility to this idea. The reviewed evidence supports the theory that, in some circumstances, intermittent access to sugar can lead to behavior and neurochemical changes that resemble the effects of a substance of abuse. According to the evidence in rats, intermittent access to sugar and chow is capable of producing a "dependency." This was operationally defined by tests for binging, withdrawal, craving, and cross-sensitization to amphetamine and alcohol. The correspondence to some people with BED is striking, but whether it is a good idea to call this a food addiction in people is both a scientific and societal question that has yet to be answered. Rats with intermittent access to food and a sugar solution can show both a constellation of behaviors and parallel brain changes that are characteristic of rats that voluntarily self-administer addictive drugs (114,115).

Addictions and binge eating share some features in terms of brain chemistry and circuitry. But in distinguishing compulsion from addiction, it is more important to determine what drives treatment. When we look at the clinical repercussions of these labels, we should be cautioned against applying addictive models too widely. Unlike alcohol or painkillers, abstaining from food is not an option. To treat sugar as an addictive substance would assume our control over it is unmanageable and necessitates total abstinence. With this lifetime of restriction and deprivation comes a need to elucidate exactly what one is abstaining from anything with glucose, any product with sugar listed in the first five ingredients, for example, refined carbohydrates, sweets, deserts, and trigger foods. It could also lead to obsessions and fears regarding foods and evolve into possible orthorexia or eating disorder behavior (anorexia nervosa, bulimia, or upgrading one's BED). Life becomes challenging and unpleasant so much that the restrictions may be nothing more than "changing seats on the Titanic." However, sugar (glucose) is contained in all carbohydrates and is necessary for the growth, maintenance, and repair that are needed for survival. The cravings for specific trigger foods (highly palatable foods containing large quantities of sugar, fat, and salt) can be reduced and managed through behavioral interventions that condition the brain to form new habits.

Further studies are needed to better understand factors that serve as binge triggers (i.e., food cravings and moods) (126). The research in this area is somewhat confusing and makes it difficult to reach a coherent conclusion as to whether the disorder is more compulsive or addictive in nature. Studies use different inclusion criteria; some focus on compulsive overeaters, whereas others center on the obese or those who are chronic overeaters. Although this confusion remains, it is probably prudent to use a "compulsive" model when approaching treatment. This assumes that, through habit and behavioral change, one can reintroduce trigger foods back into the diet, whereas an addiction model would assume that patients are addicted to certain foods and must commit to a lifetime of abstinence from them. This introduces an element of anxiety over ever consuming their "substance" for fear it will pull them back into their disorder. This issue is discussed in more detail later in this chapter.

BED IN CHILDREN

Compared to the many tools for assessing BED in adults, there is an amazing lack of tools taking children, with their growing bodies and brains, into consideration. And yet, obese children are reporting binge eating episodes at a rate of 35% to 57%. Bulik et al. (48) recognized that BED occurs in adolescents and children.

We have to take stock of the assessment measures we have for this population.

- Eating Disorders Examination adapted for children (129)
- Questionnaire of Eating and Weight Patterns—adolescent version (130)
- Children's BED Scale, interviewer-administrated for children aged 5 to 13 years (131)
- Current provisional research criteria for diagnosing BED in children (132):
  - Recurrent episodes of binge eating in which an episode of binge eating is characterized by both of the following:
    - Food seeking in the absence of hunger (e.g., after a full meal)
    - A sense of lack of control over eating (e.g., endorses that "When I start to eat, I just can't stop")
  - Binge episodes are associated with one or more of the following:
    - Food seeking in response to negative affect (e.g., sadness, boredom, restlessness)
    - Food seeking as a reward
    - Sneaking or hiding food
  - Symptoms persist over a period of 3 months
  - Eating is not associated with the regular use of inappropriate compensatory behaviors (purging, fasting, excessive exercise) and does not occur exclusively during the course of anorexia nervosa or BN

There is a lot to learn in the field of treating children with signs of BED, which has distinct differences from treating BED in adults. For example, children may not as easily remember how much food they consume. Also, their access to food is often controlled by parents, making it more difficult to identify the triggering of BED qualifying experiences. In spite of our lack of models for defining or treating child BED, it has serious ramifications. Not only do many of these children grow up to be adult binge eaters, but 32% of children in a recent study who were at risk for adult obesity reported at least one episode of binge eating in the past 6 months (133). In these cases, family-based therapy and parent training may be useful in the treatment of LOC in children, as it has had success with other eating disorders, such as BN. These issues could benefit from further study.

CAUSES OF BED

The way we characterize the causes of BED is important for treatment. Again, the research shows many causative factors present, and some better lend themselves for treatment purposes than others. Is BED

- A dieting disorder
- A food addiction
- A bad habit (134)
- Lack of willpower
- Comfort eating to manage difficult and troublesome feelings
- A stress disorder
- A sign of a deeper emotional problem
- A body-image problem
- A genetic mutation

Next is a discussion of many factors involved in the etiology of BED.

Stress

Stress is commonly present in BED, both as an etiological factor (14,99,135–138) and as a precipitating factor (99,100,139–143). Along with stress, depression accounts for as much as 50% of those with BED (144,145), although Waller and Barter (146) determined that anxiety triggers binging more than depression. Additional research has demonstrated a host of other factors at play in BED, including dietary restraint and being female and obese (139,147–149). Still, it is safe to say that where there is binge eating, there is likely to be stress, depression, or both.

Research indicates that both life stressors and perceived stress link to binge eating (140,141), and that, whatever the stressor may be, it is amplified for the person with BED. Female binge eaters have been shown to score various mundane challenges significantly more stressful than their nonbinging counterparts. According to Adami et al. (150) and Adami (151), individuals vary in their perception of or response to stressors, depending on whether they are harm avoidant or resilient.

Nevertheless, those psychological factors will elicit multiple physical responses. As we have seen, one response to stress is the intake of palatable foods, typically high in glucose, fat, or salt. Fat intake reduces stress, and conversely, stress begins to climb as fat is taken away (148). Studies looking into variants of this formula consistently show a connection between palatable food intake and reduced stress. O'Connor et al. (139) documented the increase of high-fat/high-sugar snack intake with stress. Treasure et al. (152) used images to find that pictures of food calmed the amygdala, and Van Oudenhove et al. (153) used a fatty acid infusion into the gut to reduce the neural response to negative emotions elicited by offensive visual cueing.

Where binge eating is the coping mechanism, fats and/or carbohydrates are sought externally and eating palatable food (143,154,155) can lead, in turn, to the production of fats by internal mechanisms. For example, repeated exposure to stressors leads to the secretion of neuropeptide Y (NPY) that, in turn, acts on preadipocytes to promote fat proliferation and maturation for increased abdominal fat mass (156–159). The studies also showed that abdominal obesity could be prevented in rats simply by blocking the NPY receptors or glucocorticoid receptors with an antagonist (156–159).

Tomiyama et al. (160) worked with chronically stressed rodents eating calorically dense comfort food. The results of this intake among rodents correlated, in humans, to lowering levels of the stress hormone cortisol. There is also a link between overproduction of cortisol and overeating of carbohydrates.

Looking at neurotransmitters, we find that binge eaters experience low levels of serotonin, a calming neurotransmitter, prior to a binge (161,162). Interestingly, serotonin levels will rise *during* the binge since serotonin is involved in the instructions for many processes of our life and health, including appetite, mood, sleep, memory, learning, and temperature regulation. A serotonin shortage or imbalance has been linked to depression, anxiety, panic, obsessive–compulsive disorder, and anger issues. Although causality between low serotonin and depression has yet to be determined, the presence of low levels of serotonin in individuals suffering from depression is well documented (99,100,139,140,142,143,154,161–164).

Both low serotonin and low dopamine have been noted in binge eating behavioral studies. As a key player in the reward centers of the brain, dopamine or dopamine-type reactions can also be activated by eating palatable foods, as discussed above. Studies repeatedly show that in responding to stress, the drive to eat palatable foods is not a hunger response or a metabolic response: it is a drive to stimulate the reward centers of the brain (139,141,154,165,166).

The drive to eat palatable food is also dictated by levels of cortisol. Chronic unresolved stress induces the secretion of glucocorticoids (cortisol) that increases the drive for food (appetite, cravings). The release of excess insulin promotes food intake and hastens fat storage, leading to obesity. The calming produced by consuming pleasurable food will temporarily reduce the stress response network and thereby reinforce the feeding habit (158). There is no appropriate cognitive appraisal. Basically, the dorsolateral prefrontal cortex, or the "wise-advocate" area of the brain, is not engaged to inhibit impulsivity, so the combination of stress and the production of a heightened mesolimbic dopaminergic reward response can result in a feeding frenzy (167). First the chronic stress stimulates the amygdala (center of arousal); the resulting cortisol increases the salience (value) of the pleasurable food (sugar, fat comfort food); and eventually there is the production of abdominal fat (168).

Clinically, we see that people with BED often have trouble managing anxiety and depression appropriately. But the research points more to correlation than causality. Does the stress of life cause binge eating or does the disorder itself cause the stress? Do the blame, shame, guilt, and aggravation of binging exacerbate or elicit negative emotions? The act of overeating can be a self-soothing strategy and a short-term remedy for coping with life's ups and downs. Binging on palatable food can also be an escape when one's world becomes overwhelming. Overeating can be a way to console oneself or the opposite, which would be beating one's self up for not being as perfect as desired. In addition, the findings of the research leave us little ability to predict the occurrence of a binge consistently. Neither stress nor restriction nor palatable food availability alone is consistently responsible for increasing the odds of a binge or for explaining binge eating behavior.

A useful treatment for those who resort to binging as a stress coping mechanism would be to teach them how to process negative thoughts and engage in positive reappraisal. In cases where the individual's response to stress is to release greater amounts of cortisol, the reprocessing of negative thoughts—and there are countless cognitive therapies that could serve—might ultimately help by reducing cortisol levels. There is good news in terms of serotonin balances. Research shows that once we successfully treat binge eating, and the individual is in recovery, both serotonin levels and serotonin binding return to normal (161,162,164,169,170).

Attachment disorder

The seeds for BED can be sown very early in life. In normal nurturing situations, an infant will learn self-soothing from a comforting adult. A lot of this occurs in the right hemisphere, the site of nonverbal communication. If appropriate attachment occurs early, it lays the groundwork through those first connections, so that the orbitofrontal cortex (OfC) will function to calm the amygdala, or the center of arousal (171–174). This is an extremely important function when sensory and emotional input activates the amygdala, which is also responsible for triggering the sympathetic nervous system (energizing or fight-or-flight response) and the parasympathetic nervous system (calming or freeze reaction). Insecure attachment styles in this formative period can result in impaired emotional regulation. A likely outcome might be avoidance and anxiety that could lead to emotional eating, compulsive overeating, and binge eating (175).

Dysfunctional early attachment relationships leave the individual with insufficient self-regulation capabilities, without which the person will have trouble modulating arousal. The BED individual relies on external regulators, often seeking food for comfort. So, binge eating would be one faulty strategy for modulating arousal. Since food is only a temporary solution at best, the binge eater resorts to binging or compulsive overeating to numb painful emotions (self-soothing) in a futile attempt to obtain enough pleasure from what the food can offer.

To some extent, we all probably eat to change our emotional state. We might reward ourselves with food at times, eat to share a social occasion, nibble in response to anxiety, eat to fill the time when we are bored, or fix a special meal to calm ourselves down after a rough day. And we learned these strategies very early in life. However, research clearly shows that a mood change, good or bad, can, in turn, become a trigger for more eating in someone who eats emotionally or compulsively. So feelings such as anger, guilt, sadness, and anxiety can often trigger episodes of overeating.

In the current view, psychologists look at comfort eating as a way to avoid or manage emotions that might lead to shame or emotional discomfort rather than a way to feel better. The proof would be in seeing successful treatment outcomes devised to address the issue based on this view.

Trauma

It is widely believed that compulsive eating and binge eating are signs of deeper psychological issues (176,177). Physically, sexually, or emotionally abused children are 36% more likely to be obese as adults. It has also been observed that one out of every nine women who experience some form of trauma in their lifetimes have an increased risk of experiencing weight gain and gain weight 2 times faster than other women (177,178).

Another response to trauma is depression, also connected with obesity (179). In fact, many of the long-term symptoms of abuse are similar to symptoms seen in those with BED, such as avoidance behaviors involving places, people, and things that remind a person of past traumatic experience (178). Another common symptom is hyperarousal that may take the form of edginess, startle behavior, anxiety, lack of concentration, or sleep irregularities.

The physical impacts of trauma come as a result of stress and the results of cortisol in the system. Long-term exposure to stress continually thwarts the system's return to a natural state of homeostasis and eventually inhibits the natural feedback mechanism that keeps high cortisol levels in check (178,180). Damage to the hippocampus, the memory area of the brain, causes the excess norepinephrine and cortisol response (181–184).

Adding sustained levels of stress during childhood to the fact that even after the period of trauma there may be unwanted flashbacks or recurrences of old symptoms (185), the individual with a traumatic history may have only limited means of self-regulation. Eating food may be one means for a person to control, escape from, reduce awareness of, or block negative emotions such as anger, sadness, or guilt (186,187). Using food for these purposes produces rapid and mindless eating without the ability to stop or exhibit any control. In some way, this binging behavior may help to purge the experience, refocus attention, or offer a feeling of control in the moment (188). For someone with frayed coping skills, binging can become a predictable way of coping with the pain, a self-controlled medication that can numb and soothe.

In other areas of life, severe binge eaters may be so overwhelmed by previous stressful events that their inability to self-regulate prevents them from connecting with their own emotions, possibly resulting in alexithymia (189), the failure to identify, label, or describe their feelings. They may also have difficulty recognizing the emotions of others (190) or may exhibit a mindsight deficit, an impaired ability to understand the emotional experiences of others (191).

Several forms of behavioral treatment are shown to be effective in improving the capacity to self-regulate. Cognitive strategies can encourage reappraisal of trigger stimuli that are intrusive and threatening. One of the best documented is cognitive behavioral therapy (CBT) (192,193). Through education and techniques such as self-monitoring, dietary records, and verbal assessments, CBT can help people become aware of the maladaptive thought processes fueling their eating behaviors. Other treatment regimens that have shown some success include eye movement desensitization and reprocessing therapy that attempts to resolve past traumas by calling them up in the present and adding some sort of interruptive rhythmic stimulus (e.g., eye movement, tapping). The ideal outcome is to disarm the emotional memory and to eventually replace that emotional memory with another emotion. Another type of practice, directed mindfulness, can be useful in working through negative thoughts by keeping them in the present and coming from a nonjudgmental place. Exposure and response prevention can also help individuals learn to face their fears. With internal family systems therapy, trauma survivors can learn to cope through compassion for their "parts" and thereby heal the painful memories.

Body image

Fairly consistently, binge eaters hate the way they look. They not only have a poor body image but also feel that they should be eating less. Bingers and compulsive eaters experience horrible feelings of fatness, especially after eating "forbidden" foods, and they do not have to be fat to feel fat. This means that when they do resort to a comfort food, they can't enjoy it properly. Unfortunately, they cannot always do much to stop themselves. Poor body image has many effects that start with poor self-care and continue through avoiding social situations. It is not unusual for these individuals to dread holidays, or at best, to be very uncomfortable during them.

Issues around weight, particularly in BED, become a self-perpetuating loop. Weight gain leads to depression (194), and the fear of weight gain leads to compensatory strategies such as dieting, calorie counting, starving, or consuming diet pills. All of these routes exacerbate the problem and accelerate the loop. Binge eating as an antidepressant, or attempt to alleviate low self-esteem, leads to more weight gain and back to depression or more dire starvation. This loop can perpetuate indefinitely. Studies show that food deprivation, restriction, and dieting are likely to increase and prolong a binge (104,141,195–197).

In the Minnesota semistarvation experiment, volunteers ranged from tolerating the pseudostarvation diet to finding it intolerable. Some men failed to stick to their diet, reporting episodes of binge eating, followed by self-reproach (198). Within similar starvation parameters, the same binging behavior can be elicited from rats (141,143,155). Although most binge eating is *not* driven by physical hunger or metabolic need (139,166), when stressful stimuli are added and the poststarvation reward is palatable food, significant binge-like behavior can be induced (136,141,154,165,199–201). The binge eating patterns created in the Minnesota semistarvation experiment endured for decades (202).

Furthermore, consider in this discussion about the impact of emotional stressors as antecedents for binging the fact that obese women have higher rates of anxiety (203) and depression (204,205). There are even increased occurrences of somatoform disorders, that is, bodily symptoms, such as pain, purely rooted in mental illness (206). Although Friedman and Brownell (207) reported no added risk for depression as a result of obesity, Simon et al. (208), using more than 9000 adults, found that mood and anxiety disorders, including depression, were about 25% more common in the obese than in the nonobese.

Satiety or satisfaction? How deprivation, restriction, and dieting influence binge eating

Dieting and food restraint have been shown to provoke cravings, impulsive eating, mood swings, and the inability to stop eating when satiated. These symptoms persist well after someone has stopped dieting, and even if they are eating normally. Studies on restraint conclude that it is deprivation, not obesity, that is the critical determinant of human eating behavior (73,137,201,209–212).

Another important finding is that to feel satisfied after fasting, people turn to high-calorie foods first. In general, they will be most drawn to starches and will eat them instead of nutrient-dense vegetables. In addition, no matter what foods they choose to consume, they then end up eating more than needed (213). Even relatively mild food deprivation can alter the foods people choose to eat, potentially leading them to eat starches preferentially, often in excess. Hospitals and cafeterias that deal with food-deprived individuals should make an effort to ensure the convenience and visibility of healthier foods such as vegetables, salads, and fruit. Making healthy foods more enticing and accessible than starches can help prevent many poorer, potentially less healthy food choices.

Binge eaters exhibit some distinct characteristics when it comes to food satiety. For example, binge eaters typically do not feel as full as nonbinge eaters after the same-sized meal, and they will require more food before reporting equal levels of fullness (214). Smith et al. (164) believe this indicates a defect in the satiating process and anorexigenic pathways of the brain and gut. Smith and Geary (215) looked specifically at food feedback in binge eaters, and they maintain that eating continues as long as positive feedback exceeds negative feedback; eating stops and the meal ends when negative feedback exceeds positive feedback for a considerable time.

Perhaps a limited response to negative feedback that occurs in those with BED dictates the need for a stronger response from carbohydrates or fat stimuli (216). In other words, where the average eater will recognize diminishing pleasure after the first few bites and eventually reach a satisfaction threshold, eating stimulates more eating in the binge eater. Rather than recognizing a saturation point, the individual instead feels a continued impulse to eat more.

There is no shortage of theories as to why binge eaters should exhibit these differences. Theories range from positing the existence of a large stomach capacity in binge eaters (217) to a decrease in release of the gut hormone CCK (218,219). Another theory suggests a defect in central processing of gut hormones (leptin resistance) or neurotransmitters such as serotonin (220).

Other pathology constructs look at similarities between overeaters and individuals with structural brain abnormalities such as frontotemporal dementia. These individuals have been reported to overeat far beyond satiety. The group of neural circuits showing brain tissue loss in these individuals (loss of gray matter volume as shown by voxel-based morphometry) included the right ventral insula, striatum, and medial orbital frontal cortex (mOfC). Alterations in these three circuits are also observed in overeaters with obsessive–compulsive disorder, bulimia, and BED. This was considered significant, since the three circuits govern feeding and food choices. In the binge eater, these choices fail to respond appropriately to satiety or fullness (221–223).

The preponderance of studies focuses on the fact that binge eaters continue to consume large quantities of food after reporting fullness. Since these three key neural circuits compose higher order gustatory regions (224), one can infer some kind of alteration with a resulting dysfunction in food reward processing in addition to poor self-regulation. In other words, the dysfunctional design of these "satisfaction areas" gives the brain a skewed message, or there is a misinterpretation ("I am not satisfied and I am determined to be satisfied") with the imperative to keep eating. Analysis by means of voxel-based morphometry supports that there are alterations in ventral striatum and mOfC in BED individuals. The mOfC is engaged in real and imaginary rewards (225). By acting as a stimulus for learning and future rewards, the mOfC can influence future decision making. Thus, the OfC determines the salience or reinforcing value of food (taste, gustatory, auditory, visual, and texture). Activation of the mOfC correlates with subjective emotions (226).

This research shows interesting markers for binge eating, and perhaps indicates directions for future medical research. It also supports the idea that eating patterns are, at the very least, learned behaviors. How much food we consume and the choices we make involve learning and memory, more than being governed solely by the body's need for energy homeostasis (164,215,227). Smith and colleagues' paradigm poses a problem for behavioral neuroscience, along with so much of the research focusing on hunger and fullness. This approach sees the inability to perceive fullness as the main problem of binge eating. The treatments resulting from the "fullness" approaches are based on the idea that if you can make binge eaters aware of physical and mental fullness signals, they will stop mindless overconsumption. This is probably a mistake. For example, evidence of alterations in the ventral striatum and mOfC suggest that the binge eater may be incapable of stopping in response to fullness because hedonistic drive (pleasure) has overridden homeostatic drive (hunger and fullness).

In considering physiological versus psychological hunger, neuroscience research demonstrates a third hunger system operating across, or at the root of these two: the neurophysiological system. In the brain, hunger is the interplay of two operating systems, the homeostatic system, activated by energy deficits; and the hedonic system, activated by the presence of palatable food. Research is continually discovering and documenting the strength of the hedonic system. It seems that regardless of how full a person may feel, the body is hardwired to chemically reward itself by overeating when tempted with highly palatable foods.

When restriction occurs and energy intake goes below homeostatic needs, the result is physiological deprivation. Given the strength of the hedonic system, it is possible that restricting intake of palatable foods produces "perceived deprivation" despite a state of energy balance. Our plentiful and palatable food environment has dramatically changed since periods in our history when food sources were highly constrained. This has strongly underscored the differences between the homeostatic and the hedonic regulation of food intake, with the latter being largely responsible for the pronounced increase in obesity in the past few decades. The motivation to eat more than one needs appears to be every bit as real, and perhaps every bit as powerful (120,228–233), as the motivation to eat when energy deprived (233). In this view of the hunger response, it is possible that the omnipresence of highly palatable food in the environment chronically activates the hedonic system, in turn, producing a need to actively restrain eating, not just to lose weight, but to avoid gaining it (231,232).

The hedonic system may also be reinforced through the workings of digestive chemistry. Two compounds in the gut contribute to our indulgence in "goodies," well beyond the point of caloric need. One of these is a stomach hormone called ghrelin that helps regulate the motivation and drive to eat as well as the capacity to experience reward or pleasure. The other is the endocannabinoid 2-arachindonylglycerol (2-AG) that is involved with appetite and drive to eat as well. These chemicals combine to override fullness when a person wants a particular kind of food.

In other words, we are programmed to stuff ourselves for a rainy day when food may not be as available. Another study suggested that despite the feeling of being satiated, the original amount individuals planned to eat was significantly higher when eating their favorite food as compared to a bland or unappetizing selection (234). When participants ate their favorite food, their blood levels of ghrelin increased significantly and stayed high for as much as 2 hours postingestion. After eating an unappetizing nutritionally equivalent item, the ghrelin levels went progressively down. Levels of 2-AG decreased after eating both the favorite and the unappetizing food. However, exposure to and consumption of a favorite food allowed 2-AG levels to remain higher for up to 2 hours compared to the nonfavorite food.

Taking these findings into consideration, palatable substances and the hedonic system may be more powerful than considered in earlier research. In terms of treatment, this means that a more useful tool for binge eaters might be to direct them toward an awareness of satisfaction rather than fullness. The technique of attuned eating can be a valuable tool because it is designed to address satisfaction as an indicator of bringing the meal to an end, as opposed to using the fullness rating scale (234,235).

As previously discussed, there is also increasing agreement that compulsive overeating shares many characteristics with addiction disorders such as drug abuse. These factors have also fostered a renewed interest in identifying individual differences in personality and motivational systems that increase the risk for overeating and weight gain in our population. Reward sensitivity has been the focus of a recent body of compelling research, with evidence favoring two seemingly opposite points of view. On one hand, studies have found support for a link between low reward sensitivity and obesity, whereas other evidence suggests that a strong appetitive motivation leads to overeating and weight gain (228,229).

Genetics

Genetic factors account for 41% of the occurrence of BED, and environment makes up the rest. A list of possible gene mutations currently thought to be responsible for some of the phenotypic characteristics of subjects with BED is shown in Table 12.3.

Bad habits

To put BED in context, it is important to remember that we are all creatures of habit, and many of our habits originate in childhood. This is especially true of food. Our food favorites, particularly our indulgences, have probably not changed much over the years. Change usually comes from conscious effort. Although our habits are predictable, we probably are not aware of many of them. For example, as a whole we eat more food on weekends. We eat less during the beginning of the week. In these ways, we are no different from someone with BED.

TREATMENT APPROACHES

To give the best care, possible treatments for BED must be somewhat individualized from an array of treatment interventions: psychological, behavioral, and pharmacological treatments. Psychological symptoms related to disordered eating, such as disinhibition, hunger, and depressed mood, respond well to second-generation antidepressants as well as CBT. These are the most widely studied treatments.

Table 12.3 Gene mutations associated with certain factors associated with binge eating disorder

- BN; BED, obese: (*MC4R*) gene melanocortin 4 receptor (236–241)
- BN, BED: 7 repeat allele of *D4R* gene involved with weight gain and distorted body image (242–244)
- BN: Chromosomes 1, 3, 10p (obese) (242–244)
- Obese: Taq A1 allele (*D2R*) genetic variation; reward deficiency syndrome (125)
- Obese: (*LEPR*) gene leptin resistance (245,246)
- Obese: GLUT4; *Cd36; AKT2; IRS1; CAPN10; NR4A3* and *NR4A1:* insulin resistance (247–249)
- Obese: *B3825TT* Thrifty "drifty" gene (250–252)

Note: BED, binge eating disorder; BN, bulimia nervosa.

Unfortunately, treatment that can bring about dramatic weight loss is still elusive, and this is a source of frustration, if not dropout, for many overweight BED sufferers. Although specialty care—or treating these individuals' total lifestyle, produces better outcomes, not all BED sufferers can access such programs. Not only do dieting and limited treatment exacerbate the shame, denial, and interpersonal deficits of this population, randomized controlled trials (RCTs) have been plagued by high dropout rates. In addition, studies have often had high placebo response rates and insufficient follow-up after active treatment ends to determine long-term outcomes.

Furthermore, data suggest that BED is an unstable disorder that may spontaneously remit (253). Cachelin had found that half of the women in a community-based sample no longer had the disorder when they were reassessed after 6 months (254).

Pharmacological treatments

The most effective pharmacological treatments for binge eating involve the antidepressant family of drugs. A review of seven studies on treating binge eating with antidepressants versus a placebo showed that 41% of people taking antidepressants stopped binging after an average of 8 weeks, compared with just 22% of those taking placebo (255).

Among successful pharmacological treatments, second-generation antidepressants, tricyclic antidepressants, and anticonvulsants have been the most widely studied in RCTs. The majority of these trials have been limited in scope; trial samples are typically fewer than 500 total participants. In many medication RCTs, volunteers were primarily Caucasian women over age 18 years. The studies have also been hampered by high dropout rates, high placebo response rates, and by the failure to measure abstinence as a primary outcome (85).

Among the selective serotonin reuptake inhibitors (SSRIs), fluoxetine and fluvoxamine have received the most attention. After 12 weeks, both fluoxetine (average dose 71.3 mg per day) (256) and fluvoxamine (average dose 239 mg per day) (257) showed positive outcomes in reducing binge frequency and depressed mood. Hudson et al. (258), using 50 to 100 mg per day of fluvoxamine over 9 weeks, showed a greater rate of reduction in binge frequency and BMI as well as greater improvement in illness severity. However, in spite of those results, fluvoxamine did not demonstrate superiority over placebo in terms of remission rate. Nor did the changes appear to yield clinically significant effects with respect to binge abstinence or weight loss.

In the SSRI trials, fluoxetine (60 mg per day) combined with therapy was superior to fluoxetine alone and to placebo. This study looked at remission rate and reducing binge frequency, eating and shape concerns, disinhibition, and depression. The findings support the idea that BED may benefit best from a multipronged approach. However, once again, there was no significant difference in weight loss across the groups. There are also side effects of SSRIs that should be noted: sedation, dry mouth, headache, sexual dysfunction and decreased libido, constipation, nausea, sweating, fatigue, blurred vision, and gastrointestinal upset (259,260).

Approaches using serotonin–norepinephrine reuptake inhibitors and other drug families are summarized in Table 12.4.

Thus far, the challenge of achieving weight loss has not been adequately addressed by medication. Medications specifically targeting weight loss generally exert their effects only during active treatment. For this reason, questions remain about pharmacotherapy duration and its relation to remission of behavioral and psychological symptoms and to long-term weight outcomes (296). Also, longevity of positive outcomes may be more likely when pairing medication with behavioral therapy.

Table 12.4 Pharmacological treatments for BED

- Venlafaxine: A study of venlafaxine (serotonin–norepinephrine reuptake inhibitor) displayed a 50% or more reduction in number of binge eating episodes. Of the 29 patients in this study, 15 lost 5% or more of their baseline weight (261).
- Sertraline and citalopram: Sertraline (187 mg per day) (262) and citalopram (40–60 mg per day) (263) also show promise in treatment of BED. In two 6-week treatment trials, sertraline was associated with reduced binge eating and illness severity ratings, as well as positive weight loss. Tricyclic antidepressants (e.g., imipramine) were also helpful in reducing binging episodes, body weight, and depression over an 8- to 32-week period (abstinence rates for binge eating were not reported) (264). Traditional weight loss therapy was compared to CBT supplemented with desipramine (300 mg per day) for 12 weeks, with an outcome of significant reduction in binge eating after 12 weeks. The effect did not persist at 36 weeks of treatment.
- Atomoxetine: It is a highly selective norepinephrine reuptake inhibitor used for short-term treatment of BED and obsessive–compulsive disorder and associated with weight loss (265). It also showed significant reduction in binging frequency (266). In addition, a preliminary trial has demonstrated that atomoxetine may help obese individuals with a minor amount of weight loss and produce a significant reduction in binging frequency (266).
- Topiramate: Eight patients treated with the anticonvulsant topiramate (150 mg) over 16 weeks had a marked reduction of days with binge eating episodes (267). Topiramate (212 mg per day) administered for 14 weeks to obese individuals with BED yielded a significantly greater percentage reduction in binge episodes, binge days per week, illness severity, and depression (268).
- Orlistat plus CBT: A study in which CBT is paired with the lipase inhibitor orlistat (120 mg three times per day) was associated with greater initial weight loss and a greater remission rate after 12 weeks of treatment. The behavioral and psychological components of BED make CBT a good candidate for treating BED, either alone or in combination. However, these potential benefits were not accompanied by any measures of depression, and they were not maintained at 2-month follow-up (23).
- Sibutramine (discontinued): Twelve weeks of sibutramine (15 mg per day), which was marketed for weight loss (but no longer on the market in the United States), produced significantly greater decreases in binge days per weeks and self-reported depression scores (267).
- Lorcaserin (Belviq®) (269–273): Selective serotonin 5-HT2C (receptor agonist). Structurally similar to fenfluramine, but works selectively and is not destructive to heart tissue. Activates one and only one specific serotonin receptor: lorcaserin → 5-HT2C receptor (arcuate nucleus) → α-melanocyte stimulating hormone → melanocortin 4 receptor (paraventricular nucleus of hypothalamus) → satiety.
- Fenfluramine: Discontinued (1997). Heart valve disease (275,276). Activates 5-hydroxytryptamine 2B receptors causing thickening of cardiac valves, resulting in regurgitation pulmonary hypertension or cardiac fibrosis. Fenfluramine gets transported into pulmonary cells, causing toxicity (277).

(Continued)

Table 12.4 *(Continued)* Pharmacological treatments for BED

- Lisdextroamphetamine (Vyvanse®): It is a nonstimulating selective serotonin reuptake inhibitor that has previously been approved for attention deficit hyperactivity disorder. Research reported a significant decrease in binge eating day and episodes per week. After the 12-week study, there was a significant improvement in Yale–Brown–Obsessive Compulsive Scale for Binge Eating and the Three-Factor Eating Scale (278).
- Bupropion/naltrexone (Contrave®): A combination treatment that blunts the hypothalamic reactivity to food cues while enhancing regions involved in self-control and internal awareness (279). It has not been approved for use in the United States by the Food and Drug Administration as of this writing.
- Vigabatrin (Sabril®): It is an antiepileptic that reduces food cravings, produces weight loss, and reduces severe BED. By blocking dopamine, it is reported to decrease urges and compulsive food seeking (280–282).
- Baclofen reduces cravings and drug seeking and demonstrated a 50% decrease in the frequency of binge eating (283–286). The greatest effect was with fatty foods.
- Forms of naltrexone (ReVia® and Vivitrol®): Blocks naltrexone/naloxone opiate receptors that regulate the release of dopamine reward pathways (287). May be promising for binge eaters (288). To date, its efficacy for BED lacks appropriate controlled trials. No effect on sugar or fat consumption of nonbinging obese (289). 50 to 100 mg per day ineffective in bulimia, but 200 to 300 mg may decrease binging and purging (290). Reduced binging in purging BN and restricting BN (291–295).

Note: 5-HT2C, 5-hydroxytryptamine 2C; BED, binge eating disorder; BN, bulimia nervosa; CBT, cognitive behavioral therapy.

Surgical treatments

Although the short-term outcomes of bariatric surgery in individuals with BED are mixed at this time, we should consider the long-term success of the patient. In long-term studies, there is enough evidence to suggest the possibility that, over time, surgery will not bring about the best outcome for the patient. Some obese patients are denied insurance coverage for surgical treatment because of their BED (297); perhaps insurance companies know something about long-term outcomes. In contrast, because some insurers have denied mental health treatment coverage to individuals with eating disorders (298), we can expect some patients who may look to bariatric surgery as the more affordable (coverable) option.

Regardless, the success rates in studies looking at a 12-month to 3-year postoperative period are in contrast to the success rates in studies looking at a period of 5 years or more after surgery.

The most favorable study for a good long-term prognosis of gastric bypass on patients with BED is a 3-year study that followed 25 patients with the disorder and 26 non-BED obese patients postbiliopancreatic diversion (BPD) for obesity (299). The study concluded that post-BPD, binge eating disappears. Adami et al. state, "The loss of control over food intake is mainly dependent on dieting and on the preoccupation with food and body shape." They go on to say, "The derangement of body image in obese patients with BED is only partly dependent on inner feelings. In fact, the stable weight normalization after BPD is accompanied by a sharp improvement in body image in all cases. It does appear that the complete normalization requires more time on BED patients than their non-BED counterparts."

Claims that the psychological aspects of BE are cured by obesity surgery must be viewed with caution. Many people who binged prior to surgery report continued feelings of LOC, even when eating the small amounts of food after surgery (300).

In fact, postoperative LOC is something we should be looking at more closely, since it significantly predicts poorer postsurgical weight loss and psychosocial outcomes at 12 and 24 months after surgery. Since LOC after bariatric surgery significantly predicts attenuated postsurgical improvements, it may signal a need for clinical attention (301).

Saunders' study of 125 patients who had undergone gastric bypass procedures noted that 33.3% still showed "'severe' binge eating," with 50% engaging in binging or grazing in a frequency of two or more times per week (302). Those with presurgical binge eating are more likely to retain the eating pathology and, if they do, to have poorer weight loss outcome.

If BED does return, that is, if the pattern of LOC returns, if the causes of binging were due to stressors other than body image, if treatment around other coping skills was needed but not afforded, the results could be disastrous. Thus, someone with BED (or compulsive overeating) having bariatric surgery should be treated very differently from someone suffering from "simple" obesity.

Clinical observation has recorded some of the maladaptive practices of binge eaters postoperatively. For example, there are several methods binge eaters use to "out eat" the pouch. This postsurgery pouch has limited capacity, but patients have out eaten the pouch by grazing or frequent and continuous feeding (303,304). They have "binged" on soft, semisoft, and liquid high-calorie selections (305). These tactics are unhealthy, and, as a result of them, up to 20% to 30% of BPD patients regain significant weight and as many as 3% to 13% of surgeries are revised yearly (306–310).

Furthermore, several studies have shown that binge eating persists after surgery. As a population, binge eaters were more likely to regain weight after bariatric surgery through overeating. The discrepancy in findings between these and studies such as Adami et al. (299) is due to the duration of the study. Although most patients have reported a drastic decrease in the urge to binge at 12 to 18 months postsurgery, studies reported a recurrence of BED *after* 12 to 18 months (311–317). The excess weight has been shown to return progressively over the 5 years after surgery. Along with the weight regain, issues of body disparagement, body dissatisfaction, or both return. At that point, the patient is prone to lapse back into poor self-efficacy and low self-esteem (318–323). With findings like these in mind, there is an outcry from those in the field who insist that the future generation of obesity treatments is to incorporate procedures to improve body image (300,324–328).

The length of a study is especially critical when it includes self-reporting of binging episodes. Some studies (7,329,330) show approximately 49% to 68% of bariatric surgery patients admitted binge eating prior to surgery. Although their numbers show that only 6.9% admitted binging postsurgery, longer studies showed that at 1 to 2 years, these numbers may rise to 15% to 18% (52,300,331–335).

Other reports, which specifically looked at LOC, contend that presurgery binge eating is likely to be retained postsurgery because LOC persists despite the fact that the actual amounts of food eaten are small. Furthermore, objective results from a 24-hour feeding paradigm showed that patients with BED consumed significantly more liquid meal than those without BED.

Note that these objective results call into question the "no significant difference" (between with and without BED) results of a study conducted by interview. In that study, BED participants were clinically assessed through the Structured Clinical Interview for the Diagnosis of DSM Disorder (SCID) (325). There were no significant differences between participants with BED and those without BED on the SCID (325).

In addition to problems inherent in self-reporting mentioned, another definitional challenge makes the findings of postoperative studies unreliable unless close attention is paid to detail. In postbariatric surgery patients, BED criteria cannot be met technically because their limited stomach capacity negates the possibility of consuming amounts of food that are "objectively large." This abrogates any reliable diagnostic criteria for BED. This challenge makes another case, perhaps, for defining a binge by "LOC" rather than "quantity consumed" when studying the BED postoperative population (336).

The lack of consensus on diagnostic criteria for BED or for its clinical assessment in bariatric surgery patients certainly makes comparing studies of binge eating within surgical outcomes unreliable at best. As long as there is no universally accepted definition for BED or standardized measure for its diagnosis, the effect of this pathological eating pattern on surgical weight loss outcomes will remain unclear. The bariatric community should be aware of the discrepancies in current research and exercise caution when interpreting research results surrounding this topic (331,337,338).

Psychological and behavioral therapy

In 2006, the American Psychiatric Association (APA) published guidelines for the treatment of patients with BED (339–342). The APA uses a 3-point scale for its clinical recommendations: I, recommended with substantial clinical confidence; II, recommended with moderate clinical confidence; and III, may be recommended on the basis of individual circumstances.

The APA general treatment guidelines for BED support a team approach as the recommended model of care (level I). The team model incorporates psychiatrists (and other physicians, as needed), psychologists, registered dietitians, and social workers who assess and treat the primary psychological and behavioral problems and monitor the patient's general medical condition. For the prevention of chronicity, early intervention is recommended (level I).

For treatment effects on binge eating, behavior level I recommendations were made for CBT in various formats, including individual, group, and self-help; antidepressant medications (particularly SSRIs); and behavioral weight control programs incorporating low- or very-low-calorie diets. For weight loss effects, behavioral weight control and antidepressants, but not CBT, received level I recommendations (CBT has not been shown to lead to significant changes in body weight). Interpersonal psychotherapy (IPT), dialectical behavior therapy (DBT), topiramate, and sibutramine received level II recommendations.

Approaches that fall into the level III category include a combination of nutritional and psychological approaches as well as any nonweight-directed psychosocial approaches (e.g., Health at Every Size [HAES], 12-Step, and other nondiet approaches). The pharmacological agent zonisamide (an anticonvulsant) received level III recommendation.

No behavioral interventions have been shown to offer demonstrable efficacy in driving weight loss, which can be a deal breaker for those who are overweight with BED (48). Although nonweight-focused behavioral strategies may not promote significant weight loss in individuals with BED, they may be associated with less weight gain over time.

CBT has been the most commonly tested behavioral therapeutic approach for BED (343–354). CBT for BED is rooted in the idea that inaccurate thoughts (e.g., about body image) lead to inappropriate food consumption (344). The belief is that one can learn to control, adjust, and restructure the destructive trigger thoughts that contribute to binge eating behavior, thus reducing the behavior. CBT seeks to change binge eating habits by understanding the reasons for overeating and the emotions that may trigger a binge. Patients learn to track their food consumption and develop alternative ways of managing stress. CBT seems to increase effectiveness when used in combination with other manipulations such as drug therapy, as documented in several studies, including the following:

- Fluoxetine at 60 mg per day (23)
- Desipramine at 300 mg per day (355)
- Orlistat at 120 mg three times per day (356)
- Exposure therapy
- Family therapy (345)

In terms of behavioral interventions, CBT is effective in reducing binge frequency (whether reported as binge days or binge episodes) and in improving the psychological features of BED such as restraint, hunger, and disinhibition. CBT's effect on binge frequency, in particular, leads to apparently greater rates of sustained abstinence.

CBT offers many techniques that work very well to help clients understand and manage BED. Although not formally considered an obsessive–compulsive spectrum disorder, compulsive overeating often responds extremely well to some of the same CBT techniques used to treat OCD and related conditions.

First, CBT helps clients learn to identify their personal binge-eating triggers better and more quickly. Since binge eaters frequently suffer from low self-esteem or high sensitivity, the common CBT technique known as cognitive restructuring is effective in helping binge eaters learn to challenge the distorted beliefs and thoughts they have about themselves, food, and eating that often precede or accompany a binge. Using other CBT techniques, compulsive overeaters can learn to replace their urges to overeat with new, healthier eating behaviors. In addition, since stress is a large factor in binge eating, CBT can be very effective in providing behavioral tools that help to reduce their stress.

Behavioral approaches can offer several tools that empower the individual to extend his or her own treatment, merging client and cure. When the client understands the disorder and himself or herself better, he or she can contribute to the goal of lessening, and eventually abstaining from, binge eating behavior. The following are behavioral tools that can be highly effective:

- Structured meal and exercise plan
- Exposure response prevention skills
- Problem-solving techniques
- General mindfulness
- Mindful eating
- Cue elimination
- Coping skills (alternatives and relaxation practices)

It is also useful to address weight and size issues with body-image therapy and size acceptance.

Treatment of binge eating and compulsive overeating is more than establishing a positive relationship with food. There is a need to address the whole person and to find solutions to a wide array of challenges:

- Eating comfortably in a wide variety of situations
- Managing problem situations such as parties and holidays effectively

- Sleeping well and feeling healthy
- Managing stress and being happier
- Handling personal relationships well
- Building self-worth
- Being able to say "no" to food and people when you need to

Like CBT, in that it empowers BED sufferers to become part of the solution, DBT adds a self-reflective, observational element to treatment and fosters the development of mindfulness, emotion regulation, interpersonal effectiveness, and distress tolerance (357–359).

IPT helps those with BED to examine their relationships to help identify possible causes of overeating and to resolve interpersonal problems that may contribute to their eating disorder (343,360,361).

Self-help, both with and without a facilitator, has been studied for application to BED. It has been documented to lead to greater reductions in the mean number of binge days and in clinical severity, while also improving abstinence, cessation rates, and Eating Disorder Examination scores (2,41,346,347,359,362–366).

Of course, individuals differ in their responses to therapies. CBT, DBT, IPT, and self-help methodology may not be equally effective for a given individual (367–369). In addition, these behavioral technologies do not necessarily engage all of the underlying mechanisms at work in a given case of BED. The more experienced a professional is within the field of BED, the better the chances for a good assessment of needs.

There is current, on-going investigation with other "alternative" approaches in the treatment of BED, such as exercise (364,370) and virtual reality therapy (371), but currently the data are insufficient for any recommendations.

Mindfulness

For those with BED, it can be difficult to control responses to varying emotional states. Additional stress comes from a lack of self-acceptance. These form the core issues at the heart of BED, along with an inability to make conscious food choices and to recognize hunger and satiety cues (372).

Mindfulness-based eating disorder training (MB-EAT) involves training in mindfulness meditation and guided mindfulness practices that are designed to address these core issues. Evidence to date supports the value of MB-EAT in decreasing binge episodes, improving the sense of self-control with regard to eating, and diminishing depressive symptoms. Mindfulness-based interventions cultivate awareness of the internal experience, interrupt highly conditioned patterns, integrate high-level processes, decrease stress reactivity, and empower through a sense of control and self-acceptance (373–376). Such mechanisms are clearly applicable to addressing the dysregulation of affect, cognition, physiology, and behavior observed in binge eating (377,378). It can take some time to perfect, and engaging in the techniques calls for a degree of commitment to practice.

The MB-EAT program incorporates traditional mindfulness meditation techniques, as well as guided meditation practices, to address eating-related self-regulatory processes such as emotional versus physical hunger triggers, gastric and sensory-specific satiety, food choice, and emotional regulation pertinent to self-concept and stress management. In particular, the MB-EAT program is based on models of self-regulation that emphasize the value of helping the individual re-engage natural processes by cultivating awareness of internal physical signals (379) and innate appetite regulatory processes, and psychological distinctions, such as "liking" versus "wanting" (380). It also helps the patient learn to choose higher level cortical processes over emotionally driven or reactive motivational systems (381). It is a tall order, but small successes can lead to big changes.

MB-EAT appears to have value as an intervention for binge eating and warrants further investigation as an approach to weight loss (382). The mechanisms for change designed into the MB-EAT program involve reregulation of appetitive and emotional processes by cultivating awareness, increasing sensitivity to the hedonic process, and disengaging habitual reactivity.

In Kristeller and Wolever (372), most participants in the MB-EAT group noted substantial improvement in their ability to identify and use internal awareness of hunger and satiety cues. In particular, many participants noted a substantial decrease in their inclination to overeat sweets and high-fat foods, both in regard to amount eaten and in regard to changes in taste preferences. They found themselves satisfied with far smaller portions than they had previously eaten and that these changes were surprisingly powerful. The key concept is "satisfaction" versus "fullness" (372).

Even though individuals who binge eat tolerate more extreme levels of fullness (383), mindfulness practice may assist in reregulating binge-related processes by increasing appreciation of satisfaction from smaller amounts of food. Mindfulness and the sense of satisfaction can interrupt craving cycles in people's natural settings, both in the presence of food and in response to other triggers.

Craving cycles, central to an addiction model of binge eating (196,384), may possibly be driven by the anxiety associated with abstinence from highly palatable food, as supported by animal models (109). Among the theories as to how MB-EAT works is the idea that it may be intervening at the point of impulsive responses to food cravings (385,386) by regulating the neural systems that process those responses. In addition, mindfulness to eating may help interrupt the emotional struggle associated with strong food cravings (387). This way, small amounts of highly preferred foods can be eaten without triggering either guilt or binge-type episodes. In these studies, even for those individuals who continued to binge, did so at lesser frequency over time.

Research supports that MB-EAT is one of the most effective CBT tools in mindfulness-based cognitive behavioral therapy (MBCBT). For binge eaters, the overall goal of MBCBT is to learn to be nonjudgmental while in the present moment. Dispelling judgment helps ratchet down the emotional struggle that binge eaters undergo with their compulsion. A second goal of the immediacy of the moment, in MBCBT, is for binge eaters to give themselves permission to experience their uncomfortable psychological and physiological experiences related to food and eating. Using mindfulness, compulsive overeaters can learn to become more aware and accepting of their uncomfortable thoughts, feelings, sensations, and the urges related to food and eating, *without giving in to the desire to overeat*. Combining these and other CBT tools, compulsive overeaters can change their relationship to food and develop the ability to mindfully and healthfully eat rather than using food as a means of coping with uncomfortable thoughts and feelings (388).

Nutritional therapy

Nutritional therapy involves patients with eating disorders working closely with a dietician or nutritionist. The dietician devises a healthy eating plan for the patient, and the two work together to follow the plan, change eating habits, and monitor the plan's progress. The positive aspect of diet-based treatments is that they can positively impact eating patterns as well as weight (389,390). In contrast, it is at odds with the idea behind mindfulness, which is to cultivate an instinctive capacity to register and respond to internal signals (391) and then to eat from that awareness. Perhaps a diet-based practice can be considered an intermediary aid, while the intuitive processes are being fully developed. Intuitive eating practice brings with it several positive cognitive habits that may be useful adjuncts for treatment. One learns to avoid absolutes and to accept that satisfaction can be a "normal" part of healthy eating. One develops a habit of eating for physiological, and not emotional, reasons. One eats without negative self-talk. This puts the therapist in a nurturing rather than coercive position relative to the patient. It can also clear a space for self-love (acceptance regardless of size) to grow (392).

HAES and intuitive eating

The HAES school of thought has developed as an alternative to the conventional focus on weight reduction. The idea of size acceptance is an important part of the HAES approach, along with the concept of intuitive eating. In place of the conventional imperative to diet and undergo draconian exercise regimes, this group supports enjoyable activity. Other goals of HAES, as it evolves, are ending weight discrimination, lessening the cultural obsession with weight loss and thinness, and cultivating respect for the diversity of body shapes and sizes. They base their approach on the poor success rate of diets and weight loss interventions in terms of the subject's ability to sustain weight loss over the long term. They point to the harmful by-products of weight obsession, namely binging, food and body preoccupation, and yo-yo weight cycles. In the name of weight neutrality, they underplay the connection between health and weight in the treatment of BED. They also eschew the prevalent assumption that anyone who is determined can lose weight and keep it off. Studies that support this school of thought show that attention to weight loss and dieting reduces self-esteem and perpetuates weight stigmatization and discrimination (393–399).

As an alternative to cognitively imposed dietary restriction, promoters of intuitive eating support reliance on internal regulatory processes and trusting the body to make nourishing food choices. Intuitive eating is based on the following principles: (1) reject the diet mentality; (2) honor your hunger; (3) unconditional permission to eat; (4) challenge the "food police"; (5) feel your fullness; (6) discover the satisfaction factor; (7) cope with your emotions without using food; (8) respect your body and accept your genetic blueprint; (9) exercise and feel the difference; and (10) honor your health with gentle nutrition (388,392,400–403).

OUTCOMES

Traditionally, desirable outcomes of BED treatment are reduction in binge eating with the goal of achieving binge abstinence; reductions in distress; and improvement in psychological functioning, including reduced symptoms of anxiety and depression and increased social engagement. Interestingly, a high initial self-esteem may account for a small difference in outcomes (2).

In overweight or obese individuals with BED, treatment goals often include improvement of metabolic health accompanied by sustainable weight reduction. The recommendations maintain consistently that the major focus of treatment should be on behavior and emotion interventions as opposed to weight management through dietary restriction. Treatment programs that focus on the disturbed eating behavior, with the goal of "fixing it," find only temporary fixes. They appear to be somewhat effective in reducing binge eating frequency and related pathology, but patients tend to relapse after completion of treatment (9). As a key goal of a BED program, abstinence from binge eating should be evaluated on its own, independent of weight loss. However, weight loss must not be overlooked. Early abstinence from binge eating has been linked to significantly higher weight loss (355). Even posttreatment, weight is an unavoidable focus for many binge eaters, however enlightened, and it is therefore a potentially significant moderator of their long-term adherence to the changes as well as to their treatment satisfaction.

Natural remission

Data suggest that BED is an unstable disorder that may spontaneously remit (253). Cachelin et al. (254) found that half of the women in a community-based sample no longer had the disorder when they were reassessed after 6 months.

Future study

The research on BED is in some ways a plentiful, but not a cohesive, body of study. There is little overlap between pharmacological and surgical studies, and taken together the medical studies yield conclusions quite unconnected to those of behavioral studies. To date, it is hard to put together a cohesive evidence-based program, and practitioners still base treatment choices solely on experience and intuition. This is so much the case that the Agency for Healthcare Research and Quality review of treatment for eating disorders was unable to draw definitive conclusions concerning the best treatment choices for BED. Complicating this problem, many of the available treatments have been evaluated only in single studies or by too few studies of sufficient quality (404).

Future studies should control for a placebo response that has been shown to be high (yet possibly transitory) in BED (257,405,406). The metric by which we evaluate treatment success must also be defined and standardized to focus on abstinence from binge eating (not merely reduced binge frequency) as the critical outcome (48).

One interesting question that has not been addressed is whether, after treatment, calorie intake previously consumed as binges is maintained but distributed over nonbinge meals.

Treatment may be indicated if any of the following additional warning signs are present:
- A history of significant weight gain and losses (a person may or may not be overweight).
  - Cessation of binging does not necessarily correlate with weight loss nor does binging predict weight gain.
  - It is not likely that there is an association among basal metabolic rate, BMI, weight, or intra-abdominal fat.
- Frequently feeling out of control with eating and the inability to stop eating when full.
- Frequent eating with distractions (television, computer, and reading).
- Others' needs often or always come before your own.
- Difficult saying "no" and setting limits.
- Powerful inner critic voice; self-criticism, low self-esteem, or feelings of worthlessness.
- History of trauma, grief, or loss.
- Family history of depression, obsessive–compulsive disorder (OCD), anxiety, alcoholism, or other addictions.
- Rapid eating pace.
- Mindless eating.

- Body dissatisfaction, body-image distortion.
- Obsessive thinking or talking about body weight, shape, size, appearance, or food.
  - Significant concern and stress over weight issues.
  - Significant over focus on weight and body image.
  - Rituals around body checking, exercise, or food.
- Loss of interest in activities, relationships, or people.
- Large quantities of money spent on food, restaurants, or at the grocery store.
- Hoarding of food.
- Hiding food or food wrappers.
- Eating at other times:
  - Ate more even when not binge eating.
  - Eating fewer but larger meals.

BED is marked by poor self-esteem (26); eating to handle emotional distress; extreme dysregulation of interoceptive awareness, appetite, and satiety mechanisms (27,28); and overreactivity to food cues (29) in amplified versions of more common patterns of mindless or imbalanced eating (30,31). Compulsive overeaters and binge eaters do not have less willpower than people who eat normally and healthfully. They do however have more cravings for food and stronger cravings—DSM–V (3).

Common Co-Occurring Psychological Conditions: BED*
- Depression
- Panic and anxiety disorders
- Sleep disorders
- Bipolar disorder
- Posttraumatic stress disorder
- Borderline personality disorder
- Obsessive–compulsive personality disorder (OCD)
- Substance abuse or dependence

ASSESSMENT TOOLS: INVENTORIES, QUESTIONNAIRES, SCALES, EXAMINATIONS

As pointed out in this chapter, a set of functionally clear diagnostic criteria for BED is still developing, and work continues to refine the criteria and definitions to be applied to even the most basic of concepts, such as binge episode (48,49). Clinicians can still find great difficulty in assessing what is an unusually large amount of food (50).

And yet, the first part of treatment for any eating disorder is a solid assessment. Assessment professionals should understand eating disorders to the extent that they can identify what kind of binge or compulsive eating is materializing. They should also be versed in the current assessment tools, many of which rely on self-report. They should ensure that any assessment tool based on self-report demonstrates reliability across multiple retests, demonstrates internal consistency, and proves consistent with existing eating pathology scales.

---

* American Psychiatric Association. *Diagnostic and Statistical Manual of Mental Disorders*, 5th ed. Washington, DC: American Psychiatric Association; 2013.

Assessment tools for eating disorders (34)

Binge Eating Scale* (53,54)
Body Shape Questionnaire* (55)
Boredom Proneness Scale (56)
Eating Attitudes Test (EAT-26) (57,58)
Eating Disorder Examination (EDE)* (49)
Eating Disorder Inventory (59)
   Eating Disorder Inventory-2 (EDI-2) (60)
   Eating Disorder Inventory-3 (EDI-3) (61)
Five Facet Mindfulness Questionnaire (62)
   Kentucky Inventory of Mindfulness Skills (63)
Food Craving Inventory (64)
Hassles Scale
   Daily Hassles Scale (DHS) (65)
Intuitive Eating Scale-2 (IES-2) (66)
Mindful Eating Questionnaire (67)
Mindfulness Attention Awareness Scale (MAAS) (68,69)
Multifactorial Assessment of Eating Disorder Symptoms (MAEDS) (35)
Multidimensional Body-Self Relations Questionnaire-Appearance Evaluation subscale
   (MBSRO-AE) (70)
Night Eating Syndrome Questionnaire (71)
Questionnaire of Eating and Weight Patterns (10,72)
Restraint Scale (73)
SCOFF Questionnaire (74,75)
Sociocultural Attitudes Toward Appearance Questionnaire (SATAQ) (76)
State Trait Anxiety Inventory (77)
Structured Clinical Interview for the Diagnosis of DSM Disorder (SCID)* (78)
Three Factor Eating Questionnaire* (79)
Visual Analogue Scales (80,81)
Yale-Brown Obsessive–Compulsive Scale for Binge Eating (YBOCS-BE)* (82)
Yale Food Addiction Scale (YFAS) (83)

Ten Facts about Binge Eating That May Surprise You Binging: 11 Dangerous Myths[†]

1. Not All binge eaters are overweight.
   a. Some binge eaters are average size and use crash diets to maintain a normal weight.
2. Dieting cannot cure binge eating.
   a. Scientists turn rats into binge eaters by taking away food. Restriction can trigger a binge.
3. Binge eaters have willpower.
   a. Binge eaters are successful people with drive and determination. They are compelled to overeat and activate similar brain regions (circuits) as alcohol and drug addicts.
4. Binge eating is not a fad disorder people use as an excuse for binge eating.
   a. Accepting binge eating as a disorder is supported by its inclusion in the DSM-V or the "bible of mental illness."

---

* Assessment specifically designed for BED.
[†] http://www.cbsnews.com/2300-204_162-10007463.html

5. Binge eating is not just a female thing.
   a. 40% of binge eaters are male.
6. Binge eaters know when to stop.
   a. Binge eaters know when to stop and about portion control, but they are compelled to eat beyond the point when they are comfortably full. They eat even if the food is unpalatable veggies, burnt, spoiled, uncooked macaroni, or even dropped on the floor.
7. Small children can become binge eaters.
   a. Clues that the disorder exist in children as young as 6 years as they are known to sneak or hide food.
8. Recovery does not necessarily mean avoiding trigger foods forever.
   a. Many can safely eat trigger foods once they recover. Some may need to cut back on their trigger food for a while during the recovery process.
9. Bariatric surgery is not the key to recovery.
   a. Surgery may eliminate or reduce some health problems related to toxic abdominal fat. Surgery cannot eliminate the psychological issues and coping mechanisms that underlie binge eating. Often individuals who stop binging on food will cross over to drinking, sex, or compulsive shopping.
10. Physicians are not the experts at treating binge eating.
   a. A unified integrated group of professionals, including, for example, a trained eating disorder physician, therapist, dietitian, and exercise physiologist, is the most effective at addressing and treating BED.

REFERENCES

1. Stunkard A. Eating patterns and obesity. *Psychiat Quart* 1957; 33(2): 284–295.
2. Fairburn CG. *Overcoming Binge Eating*. New York: Guilford Press; 1995.
3. American Psychiatric Association. *Diagnostic and Statistical Manual of Mental Disorders*, 5th ed. Washington, DC: American Psychiatric Association; 2013.
4. Hudson JI, et al. The prevalence and correlates of eating disorders in the National Comorbidity Survey Replication. *Biol Psychiatry* 2007; 61: 348–358.
5. Striegel-Moore RH, Franko DL. Epidemiology of binge eating disorder. *Int J Eat Disord* 2003; 34(Suppl): 19–22.
6. Gruza RA, et al. Prevalence and correlates of binge eating disorder in a community sample. *Compr Psychiatry* 2007; 48: 124–131.
7. De Zwaan M, et al. Binge eating disorder and obesity. *Int J Obes Relat Metab Disord* 2001; 25(Suppl 1): S51–S55.
8. Fairburn CG, et al. Risk factors for binge eating disorder: A community-based, case-control study. *Arch Gen Psychiatry* 1998; 55: 425–432.
9. De Zwaan M, et al. Binge eating disorder: Clinical features and treatment of a new diagnosis. *Harv Rev Psychiatry* 1994; 1: 310–325.
10. Yanovski SZ. Binge eating disorder: Current knowledge and future directions. *Obes Res* 1993; 1: 306–324.
11. Marcus MDD, et al. Characterization of eating disordered behavior in obese binge eaters. *Int J Eat Disord* 1992; 9: 69–70.
12. Fassino S, et al. Temperament and character in obese women with and without binge eating disorder. *Compr Psychiatry* 2002; 43: 431–437.

13. Guss JL, et al. Binge size increases with body mass index in women with binge-eating disorder. *Obes Res* 2002; 10: 1021–1029.
14. Grilo GM, Masheb RM. Childhood psychological, physical, and sexual maltreatment in outpatients with binge eating disorder: Frequency and associations with gender, obesity, and eating-related psychopathology. *Obes Res* 2001; 9: 320–325.
15. Striegel-Moore RFA, et al. Abuse, bullying and discrimination as risk factors for binge eating disorder. *Am J Psychiatry* 2002; 159: 1902–1907.
16. Striegel-Moore RH, et al. Binge eating in an obese community sample. *Int J Eat Disord* 1998; 23(1): 27–37.
17. Ross CC. *The Binge Eating and Compulsive Overeating Workbook: An Integrated Approach to Overcoming Disordered Eating.* Oakland, CA: New Harbinger Publications; 2009.
18. Stice E, et al. Subtyping binge eating-disordered women along dieting and negative affect dimensions. *Int J Eat Disord* 2001; 30: 11–27.
19. Reas DL, Grilo CM. Timing and sequence of the onset of overweight, dieting, and binge eating in overweight patients with binge eating disorder. *Int J Eat Disord* 2007; 40: 165–170.
20. National Task Force on the Prevention and Treatment of Obesity. Dieting and the development of eating disorders in overweight and obese adults. *Arch Intern Med* 2000; 160: 2581–2589.
21. Ricca V, et al. Screening for binge eating disorder in obese outpatients. *Comp Psychiatry* 2000; 41: 111–115.
22. Grilo CM, et al. Efficacy of cognitive behavioral therapy and fluoxetine for the treatment of binge eating disorder: A randomized double-blind placebo-controlled comparison. *Biol Psychiatry* 2005; 57: 301–309.
23. Grilo CM, et al. Cognitive behavioral therapy guided self-help and orlistat for the treatment of binge eating disorder: A randomized, double-blind, placebo-controlled trial. *Biol Psychiatry* 2005; 57: 1193–1201.
24. Westerburg DP, et al. Binge eating disorder. *Osteopath Fam Physician* 2013; 5: 230–233.
25. Marrazziti D, et al. Latest advancements in the pharmacological treatment of binge eating disorder. *Eur Rev Med Pharmacol Sci* 2012; 16: 2102.
26. Nauta H, et al. Cognitions in obese binge eaters and obese non-binge eaters. *Cognit Ther* 2000; 24: 521–531.
27. Craighead LW, Allen H. Appetite awareness training: A cognitive–behavioral intervention for binge eating. *Cognit Behav Pract* 1995; 2: 249–270.
28. Mcintosh VV, et al. Appetite-focused cognitive–behavioral therapy for binge eating. In: JD Latner, GT Wilson (Eds.), *Self-Help Approaches for Obesity and Eating Disorders: Research and Practice.* New York: Guilford Press; 2007, pp. 325–346.
29. Sobik L, et al. Cue-elicited craving for food: A fresh approach to the study of binge eating. *Appetite* 2005; 44: 253–261.
30. Capaldi ED (Ed.). *Why We Eat What We Eat: The Psychology of Eating.* Washington, DC: American Psychological Association; 1996.
31. Wansink B. *Mindless Eating: Why We Eat More than We Think.* New York: Bantam Books; 2007.
32. Wonderlich SA. The validity and clinical utility of binge eating disorder. *Int J Eat Disord* 2009; 42: 687–705.
33. Bulik C, Sullivan P, Kendler K. Heritability of binge-eating and broadly defined bulimia nervosa. *Biol Psychiatry* 1998; 44: 1210–1218.

34. Anderson DA, et al. Assessment of eating disorders. *Behav Modif* 2004; 28: 763–782.
35. Anderson DA, et al. Development and validation of a multifactorial treatment outcome measure for eating disorder. *Assessment* 1999; 6: 7–20.
36. Hadigan CM, et al. 24-hour dietary recall in patients with bulimia nervosa. *Int J Eat Disord* 1992; 12: 107–111.
37. Schoeller DA. Limitations in the assessment of dietary energy intake by self-report. *Metabolism* 1995; 44(Suppl 2): 18–22.
38. Bruce B, Agras WS. Binge eating in females: A population-based investigation. *Int J Eat Disord* 1992; 12: 365–373.
39. Davis C, et al. Dopamine transporter gene (DAT1) associated with appetite suppression to methylphenidate in a case-control study of binge eating disorder. *Neuropsychopharmacology* 2007; 32: 2199–2206.
40. American Psychiatric Association. *Diagnostic and Statistical Manual of Mental Disorders*, 4th ed. Washington, DC: American Psychiatric Press; 2000.
41. Brownley KA, et al. Binge eating disorder treatment: A systematic review of randomized controlled trials. *Int J Eat Disord* 2007; 40: 337–348.
42. Latner JD, Clyne C. The diagnostic validity of the criteria for binge eating disorder. *Int J Eat Disord* 2008; 41: 1–14.
43. Ramacciotti CE, et al. Therapeutic options for binge eating disorder. *Eat Weight Disord* 2013; 18: 3–9.
44. Belgin SJ, Fairburn CG. What is meant by the term "binge"? *Am J Psychiatry* 1992; 149: 123–124.
45. Johnson WG, et al. What is a binge? The influence of amount, duration and loss of control criteria on judgments of binge eating. *Int J Eat Disorder* 2000; 27: 471–479.
46. Telch CF, et al. Obese women with binge eating disorder define the term binge. *Int J Eat Disord* 1998; 24: 313–317.
47. Goldschmidt AB, et al. Momentary affect surrounding loss of control and overeating in obese adults with and without binge eating disorder. *Obesity* 2012; 20: 1206–1211.
48. Bulik CM, et al. Diagnosis and management of binge eating disorder. *World Psychiatry* 2007; 6: 142–148.
49. Fairburn C, Cooper Z. The eating disorders examination. In: C Fairburn, G Wilson (Eds.), *Binge-Eating: Nature, Assessment and Treatment*, 12th ed. New York: Guilford Press; 1993, pp. 317–360.
50. Cooper Z, Fairburn CG. Refining the definition of binge eating disorder and nonpurging bulimia nervosa. *Int J Eat Disord* 2003; 34(Suppl 1): S89–S95.
51. Trace SE, et al. Effects of reducing the frequency and duration criteria for binge eating on lifetime prevalence of bulimia nervosa and binge eating disorder: Implications for DSM-V. *Int J Eat Disord* 2012; 45: 531–536.
52. Colles SL. Grazing and loss of control related to eating: Two high risk factors following bariatric surgery. *Obesity* 2008; 16: 615–622.
53. Hawkins R, Clement P. Development and construct validation of a self-report measure of binge-eating tendencies. *Addict Behav* 1980; 5: 219–226.
54. Gormally J, et al. The assessment of binge eating severity among obese persons. *Addict Behav* 1982; 7: 47–85.
55. Cooper PJ, et al. The development and validation of the Body Shape Questionnaire. *Int J Eat Disord* 1986; 6: 485–494.
56. Farmer R, Sundberg ND. Boredom proneness: The development and correlates of a new scale. *J Pers Assess* 1986; 50: 4–17.

57. Garner DM, Garfinkel PE. The eating attitudes test: An index of symptoms of anorexia nervosa. *Psychol Med* 1979; 9: 273–279.
58. Garner DM, et al. The eating attitudes test: Psychometric features and clinical correlates. *Psychol Med* 1982; 12: 871–878.
59. Garner DM, et al. Development and validation of a multidimensional eating disorder inventory for anorexia and bulimia. *Int J Eat Disord* 1983; 2: 15–34.
60. Garner DM. *Eating Disorder Inventory—2 Manual.* Odessa, FL: Psychological Assessment Resources; 1991.
61. Clausen L, et al. Validating the Eating Disorder Inventory-3 (EDI-3): A comparison between 561 female eating disorders patients and 878 females from the general population. *J Psychopathol Behav Assess* 2011; 33: 101–110.
62. Baer RA, et al. Using self-report assessment methods to explore facets of mindfulness. *Assessment* 2006; 13: 27–45.
63. Baer RA, et al. Assessment of mindfulness by self-report: The Kentucky inventory of mindfulness skills. *Assessment* 2004; 11: 191–206.
64. White MA, et al. Development and validation of the food-craving inventory. *Obes Res* 2002; 10: 107–114.
65. Holm JE, Holroyd KA. The Daily Hassles Scale (revised): Does it measure stress or symptoms? *Behav Assess* 1992; 14: 465–482.
66. Tylka TL, Kroon Van Diest AM. The Intuitive Eating Scale-2: Item refinement and psychometric evaluation with college women and men. *J Couns Psychol* 2013; 60: 137–153.
67. Framson C, et al. Development and validation of the mindful eating questionnaire. *J Am Diet Assoc* 2009; 109(8): 1439–1444.
68. Brown KW, Ryan RM. The benefits of being present: Mindfulness and its role in psychological well-being. *J Pers Soc Psychol* 2003; 84: 822–848.
69. Van Dam NT, et al. Measuring mindfulness? Item response theory analysis of the mindful attention awareness scale. *Pers Indiv Differ* 2010; 49: 805–810.
70. Brown TA, et al. Attitudinal body-image assessment factor analysis of the body-self relations questionnaire. *J Pers Assess* 1990; 50: 135–144.
71. Allison KC, et al. The night eating questionnaire (NEQ): Psychometric properties of a measure of severity of the Night Eating Syndrome. *Eat Behav* 2008; 9: 62–72.
72. Nangle DW, et al. Binge eating disorder and the proposed DSM-IV criteria: Psychometric analysis of the Questionnaire of Eating and Weight Patterns. *Int J Eat Disord* 1994; 16: 147–157.
73. Herman CP, Polivy J. Restrained eating. In: AJ Stunkard (Ed.), *Obesity.* Philadelphia, PA: Saunders; 1980, pp. 208–225.
74. Morgan JF. The SCOFF questionnaire: Assessment of a new screening tool for eating disorders. *BMJ* 1999; 319: 1467.
75. Morgan JF. The SCOFF questionnaire: a new screening tool for eating disorders. *West J Med* 2000; 172: 164–165.
76. Thompson JK. The sociocultural attitudes towards appearance scale-3 (SATAQ-3): Development and validation. *Int J Eat Disord* 2004; 35: 293–304.
77. Spielberger CD, et al. *Manual for the State-Trait Anxiety Inventory.* Palo Alto, CA: Consulting Psychologists Press; 1983.
78. First MB, et al. *Structured Clinical Interview for Axis I DSM-IV Disorders.* New York: New York State Psychiatric Institute; 2001.

79. Stunkard A, Messick S. Three-factor eating questionnaire to measure dietary restraint, disinhibition, and hunger. *J Psychosom Res* 1985; 29: 71–83.

80. Grant S, et al. A comparison of the reproducibility and sensitivity to change visual analogue scales, Borg scales, and Likert scales in normal subjects during submaximal exercise. *Chest* 1999; 116: 1208–1217.

81. Parker BA, et al. Relation between food intake and visual analogue scale ratings of appetite and other sensations in healthy older and young subjects. *Eur J Clin Nutr* 2004; 58: 212–218.

82. Mazure CM, et al. The Yale-Brown-Cornell eating disorder scale: Development, use, reliability and validity. *J Psychiatr Res* 1994; 28: 425–445.

83. Gearhardt AN, Corbin WR, Brownell KD. Food addiction: An examination of the diagnostic criteria for dependence. *J Addict Med* 2009; 3: 1–7.

84. Gold SS. *Food: The Good Girl's Drug: How to Stop Using Food to Control Your Feelings.* New York: Berkley Trade; 2011.

85. Bulik CM, et al. Medical and psychiatric morbidity in obese women with and without binge eating. *Int J Eat Disord* 2002; 32L: 72–78.

86. Sorbara M, et al. Body image disturbance in obese outpatients before and after weight loss in relation to race, gender, binge eating, and age of onset of obesity. *Int J Eat Disord* 2002; 31: 416–423.

87. Wardle J, et al. Body dissatisfaction and binge eating in obese women: The role of restraint and depression. *Obes Res* 2001; 9: 778–786.

88. Barry DT, et al. Comparison of patients with bulimia nervosa, obese patients with binge eating disorder, and nonobese patients with binge eating disorder. *J Nerv Ment Dis* 2003; 9: 598–595.

89. Aguera Z, et al. Cognitive behaviour therapy response and dropout rate across purging and nonpurging bulimia nervosa and binge eating disorder: DSM-V implications. *BMC Psychiatry* 2013; 13: 285.

90. Stunkard AJ, Allison KC. Two forms of disordered eating in obesity: Binge eating and night eating. *Int J Obesity* 2002; 27: 1–12.

91. Brewer JA, et al. The neurobiology and genetics of impulse control disorders: Relationships to drug addictions. *Biochem Pharmacol* 2008; 75: 63–75.

92. Volkow ND, et al. "Nonhedonic" food motivation in humans involves dopamine in the dorsal striatum and methylphenidate amplifies this effect. *Synapse* 2002; 44: 175.

93. Volkow ND, et al. Dopamine in drug abuse and addiction: Results from imaging studies and treatment implication. *Mol Psychiatry* 2004; 9: 557–569.

94. Volkow N, et al. Overlapping neuron circuits in addiction and obesity: Evidence of system pathology. *Philos Trans R Soc Lond B Biol Sci* 2008; 363: 3191–3200.

95. Kelley AE, et al. Corticostriatal-hypothalmic circuitry and food motivation: Integration of energy, action and reward. *Physiol Behav* 2005; 86: 773–795.

96. Kelley AE, et al. Neural systems recruited by drug—And food-related cues: Studies of gene activation in corticolimbic regions. *Physiol Behav* 2005b; 86: 11–14.

97. Rada P, et al. Daily binging on sugar repeatedly releases dopamine in the accumbens shell. *Neuroscience* 2005; 134: 737–744.

98. Koob GF. Neurobiology of addiction: Toward the development of new therapies. *Ann N Y Acad Sci* 2000; 909: 170–185.

99. Heatherton TF, et al. Binge eating as escape from self-awareness. *Psychol Bull* 1991; 110: 86–108.

100. Heatherton TF, et al. Effects of physical threat and ego threat on eating behavior. *J Pers Soc Psychol* 1991; 60: 138–143.
101. Johnson C, et al. Bulimia: An analysis of moods and behavior. *Psychosom Med* 1982; 44: 341–351.
102. Epstein DH, Shaham DH. Cheesecake-eating rats and the question of food addiction. *Nat Neurosci* 2010; 13: 529–531.
103. Casseus F, et al. High fat, high-sugar foods alter brain receptors in areas that control food intake. From presentation at Annual Meeting of the Society for the Study of Ingestive Behavior, 2009.
104. Stice E, et al. Relation between obesity and blunted striatal response to food is moderated by TaqIA Allele. *Science* 2008; 322: 449–452.
105. Sharot T, et al. Dopamine enhances expectation of pleasure in humans. *Curr Biol* 2009; 19: 1–4.
106. Gold MS. Eating disorders, overeating, and pathological attachment to food: Independent or addictive disorders? *J Addict Disord* 2004; 23: 1–105.
107. Small DM. Weight gain seems to change the brain's response to food. *Paper presented at American College of Neuropsychopharmacology Meeting*, Miami, FL, December 10, 2010.
108. Johnson PM, Kenny PJ. Dopamine D2 receptors in addiction-like reward dysfunction and compulsive eating in obese rats. *Nat Neurosci* 2010; 13: 635–641.
109. Cottone P, et al. BCRF system recruitment mediates dark side of compulsive eating. *Proc Natl Acad Sci U S A* 2009; 106: 20016–20020.
110. Kelley AE, Berridge KC. The neuroscience of natural rewards: Relevance to addictive drugs. *J Neurosci* 2002; 22: 3306–3311.
111. Kelley AE, et al. Restricted daily consumption of a highly palatable food (chocolate Ensure(R)) alters striatal enkephalin gene expression. *Eur J Neurosci* 2003; 19: 2592–2598.
112. Avena NM, et al. Sucrose sham feeding on a binge schedule releases accumbens dopamine repeatedly and eliminates the acetylcholine response. *Neuroscience* 2006; 139: 813–820.
113. Avena NM. Examining the addictive-like properties of binge eating using an animal model of sugar dependence. *Exp Clin Psychopharmacol* 2007; 15: 481–491.
114. Avena NM, et al. After daily binging on a sucrose solution, food deprivation induces anxiety and accumbens dopamine/acetylcholine imbalance. *Physiol Behav* 2008; 94: 309–315.
115. Avena NM, et al. Evidence for sugar addiction: Behavioral and neurochemical effects of intermittent, excessive sugar intake. *Neurosci Biobehav Rev* 2008; 32: 20–39.
116. Colantuoni C, et al. Excessive sugar intake alters binding to dopamine and mu-opioid receptors in the brain. *NeuroReport* 2001; 12: 3549–3552.
117. Colantuoni C, et al. Evidence that intermittent, excessive sugar intake causes endogenous opioid dependence. *Obesity Res* 2002; 10: 478–488.
118. Schmidt HD, et al. Anatomy and pharmacology of cocaine priming-induced reinstatement of drug seeking. *Eur J Pharmacol* 2005; 526: 65–76.
119. Shaham Y, et al. The reinstatement model of drug relapse: History, methodology and major findings. *Psychopharmacology* 2003; 168: 3–20.
120. Latagliata EC, et al. Food seeking in spite of harmful consequences is under prefrontal cortical noradrenergic control. *BMC Neurosci* 2010; 11: 15.
121. Goodman A. Neurobiology of addiction: An integrative review. *Biochem Pharmacol* 2008; 75: 266–322.

122. Koob GF. The neurobiology of addiction: A neuroadaptational view relevant for diagnosis. *Addiction* 2006; 101(Suppl 1): 23–30.
123. Lobo DS, et al. The genetics of gambling and behavioral addictions. *CNS Spectr* 2006; 11: 931–939.
124. Le Magnen J, et al. A role of opiates in food reward and food addiction. In: PT Capaldi (Ed.), *Taste, Experience, and Feeding*. Washington, DC: American Psychological Association; 1990, pp. 241–252.
125. Wang G, et al. Brain dopamine and obesity. *Lancet* 2001; 357: 354–357.
126. Kelley AE, et al. A proposed hypothalamic-thalamic-striatal axis for the integration of energy balance, arousal, and food reward. *J Comp Neurol* 2005; 493: 72–85.
127. Koob GF, Le Moal M. Review. Neurobiological mechanisms for opponent motivational processes in addiction. *Philos Trans R Soc Lond B Biol Sci* 2008; 363: 3113–3123.
128. Stein RI, et al. What's driving the binge in binge eating disorder? A prospective evaluation of precursors and consequences. *Int J Eat Disord* 2007; 40: 195–203.
129. Bryant-Waugh R, et al. The use of the eating disorder examination with children: A pilot study. *Int J Eat Disord* 1996; 19: 391–397.
130. Johnson W, et al. Measuring binge eating in adolescents: Adolescent and parent version of the Questionnaire of Eating and Weight Patterns. *Int J Eat Disord* 1999; 26: 301–314.
131. Shapiro JR, et al. Evaluating binge eating in children: Development of the children's Binge Eating Scale (C-BEDS). *Int J Eat Disord* 2007; 40: 82–89.
132. Marcus MD, Kalarchian MA. Binge eating in children and adolescents. *Int J Eat Disord* 2003; 34(Suppl): S47–S57.
133. Tabifsjt-Kraff M, et al. A prospective study of loss of control eating for body weight gain in children at high risk for adult obesity. *Int J Eat Disord* 2009; 42: 26–30.
134. Hansen K. *Brain over Binge: Why I Was Bulimic, Why Conventional Therapy Didn't Work, and How I Recovered for Good*. Phoenix, AZ: Camellia Publishing; 2011.
135. Grilo CM, et al. Subtyping binge eating disorder. *J Consult Clin Psychol* 2001; 69: 1066–1072.
136. Polivy J, Zeitlin SB, Herman CP, Beal AL. Food restriction and binge eating: A study of former prisoners of war. *J Abnorm Psychol* 1994; 103: 409–411.
137. Polivy J, Herman CP. Distress and eating: Why do dieters overeat? *Int J Eat Disord* 1999; 26: 153–164.
138. Wardle J, et al. Stress, dietary restraint and food intake. *J Psychosom Res* 2000; 48: 195–202.
139. O'Connor DB, et al. Effects of daily hassles and eating style on eating behavior. *Health Psychol* 2008; 27(Suppl 1): S20–S31.
140. Striegel-Moore RH, et al. Risk factors for binge-eating disorders: An exploratory study. *Int J Eat Disord* 2007; 40: 481–487.
141. Hagan MM, et al. The role of palatable food and hunger as trigger factors in an animal model of stress induced binge eating. *Int J Eat Disord* 2003; 34: 183–197.
142. Pike KM, et al. Antecedent life events of binge-eating disorder. *Psychiatry Res* 2006; 142: 19–29.
143. Teegarden SL, Bale TL. Decrease in dietary preference produce increased emotionality and risk for dietary relapse. *Biol Psychiatry* 2007; 61: 1021–1029.
144. Borges MB, et al. Binge-eating disorder in Brazilian women on a weight-loss program. *Obesity* 2002; 10: 1127–1134.

145. Friedman KE, et al. Body image partially mediates the relationship between obesity and psychological distress. *Obes Res* 2002; 10: 33–41.
146. Waller G, Barter G. The impact of subliminal abandonment and unification cues on eating behavior. *Int J Eat Disord* 2005; 37: 156–160.
147. Nieuwenhurizen AG, et al. The hypothalamic-pituitary-adrenal-axis in the regulation of energy balance. *Physiol Behav* 2008; 94: 169–177.
148. Ozier AD, et al. Overweight and obesity are associated with emotion and stress related eating as measured by the eating and appraisal due to emotions and stress questionnaire. *J Am Diet Assoc* 2008; 108: 49–56.
149. Roberts C, et al. The effects of stress on body weight biological and psychological predictors of change in BMI. *Obesity* 2007; 15: 3045–3055.
150. Adami GF, et al. The influence of body weight on food and shape attitudes in severely obese patients. *Int J Obes Relat Metab Disord* 2001; 25(Suppl 1): S56–S59.
151. Adami GF. Binge eating in obesity. *Int J Obes* 1996; 10: 793–794.
152. Treasure J, Tchanturia K, Ulrike S. Developing a model of the treatment for eating disorder: Using neuroscience research to examine the how rather than the what of change. *Couns Psychother Res* 2005; 5: 191–202.
153. Van Oudenhove L, et al. Fatty acid-induced gut-brain signaling attenuates neural and behavioral effects of sad emotion in humans. *J Clin Invest* 2011; 121: 3094–3099.
154. Hagan MM, et al. A new animal model of binge eating: Key synergistic role of past caloric restriction and stress. *Physiol Behav* 2002; 77: 45–54.
155. Goldfield GS, et al. Stress and the relative reinforcing value of food in female binge eaters. *Physiol Behav* 2008; 93: 579–587.
156. Kuo LE, et al. Neuropeptide Y acts directly in the periphery on fat tissue and mediates stress-induced obesity and metabolic syndrome. *Nat Med* 2007; 13: 803–811.
157. Kuo LE, et al. Chronic stress, combined with a high-fat/high-sugar diet, shifts sympathetic signaling toward neuropeptide Y and leads to obesity and the metabolic syndrome. *Ann N Y Acad Sci* 2008; 1148: 232–237.
158. Dallman MF. Stress-induced obesity and the emotional nervous system. *Trends Endocrinol Metab* 2010; 21: 159–165.
159. Abe K, et al. Neuropeptide Y is a mediator of chronic vascular and metabolic maladaptations to stress and hypernutrition. *Exp Biol Med* 2010; 235: 1179–1184.
160. Tomiyama AJ, Dallman MR, Epel ES. Comfort food is comforting to those most stressed: Evidence of the chronic stress response network in high stress women. *Psychoneuroendocrinology* 2011; 36: 1513–1339.
161. Kaye WH, et al. Serotonin alterations in anorexia and bulimia nervosa: New insights from imaging studies. *Physiol Behav* 2005; 19: 73–81.
162. Kaye WH. Brain imaging of serotonin after recovery from anorexia and bulimia nervosa. *Phys Behav* 2005; 86(1–2): 15–17.
163. Singh RP, et al. Posttraumatic stress. *Ophthalmology* 2007; 114: 1238.
164. Smith KA, et al. Symptomatic relapse in bulimia nervosa following acute tryptophan depletion. *Arch Gen Psychiatry* 1999; 56: 171–178.
165. Boggiano MM, et al. Combined dieting and stress evoke exaggerated responses to opioids in binge eating rats. *Behav Neurosci* 2005; 119: 1207–1214.
166. Waters A, et al. Internal and external antecedents of binge eating episodes in a group of women with bulimia nervosa. *Int J Eat Disord* 2001; 29: 17–22.
167. Dallman MF, et al. Glucocorticoids, chronic stress, and obesity. *Prog Brain Res* 2006; 153: 75–105.

168. Dallman MF, et al. Chronic stress and obesity: A new view of "comfort food." *Proc Natl Acad Sci U S A* 2003; 100: 11696–16701.
169. Tammela LI, et al. Treatment improves serotonin transporter binding and reduces binge eating. *Psychopharmacology* 2003; 170: 89–93.
170. Nash JR, et al. Serotonin 5HT1A receptor binding in people with panic disorder positron emission topography study. *Br J Psychiatry* 2009; 193: 229–234.
171. Gillatth O, et al. Attachment style differences in the ability to suppress negative thoughts: Exploring the neural correlates. *Neuroimage* 2005; 28: 835–847.
172. Moll J, et al. Human fronto-mesolimbic networks guide decisions about charitable donation. *Proc Natl Acad Sci U S A* 2006; 103: 15623–15628.
173. Drevets WC, et al. The subgenual anterior cingulate cortex in mood disorders. *CNS Spectr* 2008; 13: 663–681.
174. Rolls ET, et al. Activity of primate subgenual cingulate cortex neurons is related to sleep. *J Neurophysiol* 2003; 90: 134–142.
175. Bowlby J. *Attachment and loss: Vol. 1. Attachment*, 2nd ed. New York: Basic Books; 1969/1982.
176. Tagay S, et al. Eating disorders, trauma, PTSD, and psychosocial resources. *Eat Disord* 2014; 22: 33–49.
177. Backholm K, et al. The prevalence and impact of trauma history in eating disorder patients. *Eur J Psychotraumatol* 2013; 20: 4.
178. Kubzansky LD, et al. The weight of traumatic stress: A prospective study of posttraumatic stress disorder symptoms and weight status in women. *JAMA Psychiatry* 2014; 71: 44–51.
179. Danese A, Tan M. Childhood maltreatment and obesity: Systematic review and meta-analysis. *Mol Psychiatry* 2014; 19(5): 544–554.
180. Van Ast VA, et al. Modulatory mechanisms of cortisol effects on emotional learning and memory: Novel perspectives. *Psychoneuroendocrinology* 2013; 38: 1874–1882.
181. Rainnie DG, et al. Differential actions of corticotropin releasing factor on basolateral and central amygdaloid neurones, in vitro. *J Pharmacol Exp Ther* 1992; 263: 846–858.
182. Scaer R. *The Body Bears the Burden: Trauma, Dissociation and Disease*. Binghamton, NY: The Haworth Press; 2000.
183. Scaer RC. *The Body Bears the Burden: Trauma, Dissociation and Disease*. New York: Routledge; 2007.
184. Van der Kolk B, et al. Inescapable shock, neurotransmitters, and addiction to trauma: Toward a psychobiology of post traumatic stress. *Biol Psychiatry* 1985; 20: 314–325.
185. Brewerton TD. Eating disorders, trauma, and comorbidity: Focus on PTSD. *Eat Disord* 2007; 15: 285–304.
186. Waller G, et al. Somatoform dissociation in eating-disordered patients. *Behav Res Ther* 2003; 41(5): 619–627.
187. Hallings-Pott C, et al. State dissociation in bulimic eating disorders: An experimental study. *Int J Eat Disord* 2005; 38: 37–41.
188. Allison KC, et al. High self-reported rates of neglect and emotional abuse, by persons with binge eating disorder and night eating syndrome. *Behav Res Ther* 2007; 45: 2874–2883.
189. Wheeler K, et al. Exploring alexithymia, depression, and binge eating in self-reported eating disorders in women. *Perspect Psychiatr Care* 2005; 41: 114–123.

190. Fuller-Tyszkiewicz M, et al. The relationship between dissociation and binge eating. *J Trauma Dissociation* 2008; 9: 445–462.
191. Bydlowski S, et al. Emotion-processing deficits in eating disorders. *Int J Eat Disord* 2005; 37: 321–329.
192. Beck AT. *Depression: Causes and Treatment*. Philadelphia, PA: University of Pennsylvania Press; 1972.
193. Beck AT, et al. *Cognitive Therapy of Depression*. New York: The Guilford Press; 1977.
194. Ohzeki T, et al. Specific features of obesity in children and its management. *Nihon Rinsho* 2001; 59: 597–602.
195. Cottone P, et al. Opioid-dependent anticipatory negative contrast and binge-like eating in rats with limited access to limited access to highly preferred food. *Neuropsychopharmacology* 2008; 33: 524–535.
196. Matthes WF, et al. The biology of binge eating. *Appetite* 2009; 52: 545–553.
197. Van Vugt DA. Brain imaging studies of appetite in the context of obesity and the menstrual cycle. *Hum Reprod Update* 2010; 16: 276–292.
198. Tucker T. *The Great Starvation Experiment: Ancel Keys and the Men Who Starved for Science*. New York: Free Press; 2006.
199. Ahima RS, Antwi DA. Brain regulation of appetite and satiety. *Endocrinol Metab Clin North Am* 2008; 37: 811–823.
200. Herman CP, Polivy J. From dietary restraint to binge eating: Attaching causes to effects. *Appetite* 1990; 14: 123–125.
201. Polivy J, Herman CP. Dieting and binging. A causal analysis. *Am Psychol* 1985; 40: 193–201.
202. Keys A, et al. *The Biology of Human Starvation*, 2 Vols. Minneapolis, MN: University of Minnesota Press; 1950.
203. Becker ES, et al. Obesity and mental illness in a representative sample of young women. *Int J Obes Relat Metab Disord* 2001; 25(Suppl 1): S5–S9.
204. Roberts RE, et al. Are the obese at greater risk for depression? *Am J Epidemiol* 2000; 152(2): 163–170.
205. McElroy SL. Obesity in patients with severe mental illness: Overview and management. *J Clin Psychiatry* 2009; 70: 12–21.
206. Britz B, et al. Rates of psychiatric disorders in a clinical study group of adolescents with extreme obesity and in obese adolescents ascertained via a population based study. *Int J Obes Relat Metab Disord* 2000; 24: 1707–1714.
207. Friedman MA, Brownell KD. Psychological correlates of obesity: Moving to the next research generation. *Psycho Bull* 1995; 117: 3–20.
208. Simon GE, et al. Association between obesity and psychiatric disorders in the US adult population. *Arch Gen Psychiatry* 2006; 63: 824–830.
209. Herman CP, Polivy J. A boundary model for the regulation of eating. In: AJ Stunkard, E Stellar (Eds.), *Eating and Its Disorders*. New York: Raven Publishing; 1983, pp. 141–156.
210. Herman CP, Polivy J. Psychological factors in the control of appetite. *Curr Concepts Nutr* 1988; 16: 41–51.
211. Herman CP, Polivy J. Studies of eating in normal dieters. In: BT Walsh (Ed.), *Eating Behavior in Eating Disorders*. Washington, DC: American Psychiatric Association; 1988, pp. 95–112.
212. Polivy J, Herman CP. Undieting: A program to help people stop dieting. *Int J Eat Disorders* 1992; 11: 261–268.

213. Wansink B, et al. First foods most: After 18-hour fast, people drawn to starches first and vegetables last. *Arch Intern Med* 2012; 172: 961–963.

214. Kissileff HR, et al. A direct measure of satiety disturbances in patients with bulimia nervosa. *Physiol Behav* 1996; 60: 1077–1085.

215. Smith GP, Geary N. The behavioral neuroscience of eating. In: KL Davis, D Charney, JT Coyle, C Nemeroff (Eds.), *Neuropsychopharmacology: The Fifth Generation of Progress*. Philadelphia, PA: American College of Neuropsychopharmacology, Lippincott, Williams and Wilkins; 2002.

216. Sunday SR, et al. Relationship of perceived macronutrient and caloric content to affective cognitions about food in eating disordered, restrained and unrestrained subjects. *Am J Clin Nutr* 1992; 55: 362–371.

217. Geliebter A, et al. Gastric capacity, gastric emptying, and test-meal intake in normal and bulimic women. *Am J Clin Nutr* 1992; 56: 656–661.

218. Devlin MJ, et al. Postprandial cholecystokinin release and gastric emptying in patients with bulimia nervosa. *Am J Clin Nutr* 1997; 65: 114–120.

219. Geracioti TD, et al. Impaired cholecystokinin secretion in bulimia nervosa. *N Engl J Med* 1988; 319: 683–688.

220. Weltzin TE, et al. Acute tryptophan depletion and increased food intake and irritability in bulimia nervosa. *Am J Psychiatry* 1995; 152: 1668–1671.

221. Talan J. Why people with frontotemporal dementia overeat: Brain areas implicated in new study. *Neurol Today* 2007; 7: 12–14.

222. Grossman M. The plate is overflowing and it is not enough: Binge eating in frontotemporal lobar degeneration. *Neurology* 2007; 69: 1389–1390.

223. Schafer A. Regional grey matter volume abnormalities in bulimia nervosa and binge-eating disorder. *Neuroimage* 2010; 50: 639–643.

224. Woolley JE, et al. Binge eating is associated with right orbitofrontal insular striatal atrophy in frontotemporal dementia. *Neurology* 2007; 14: 1424–1433.

225. Bray S, et al. Human medial orbitofrontal cortex is recruited during experience of imagined and real rewards. *J Neurophysiol* 2010; 103: 2506–2512.

226. Rolls ET, Grabenhorst F. The orbitofrontal cortex and beyond: From affect to decision-making. *Neurobiology* 2008; 86: 216–244.

227. Smith GP. The controls of eating: A shift from nutritional homeostasis to behavioral neuroscience. *Nutrition* 2000; 17: 10–20.

228. Davis C. Psychobiological traits in the risk profile for overeating and weight gain: Psychobiological risk profile. *Int J Obes* 2009; 33: S49–S53.

229. Davis C, Carter JC. Compulsive overeating as an addiction disorder. A review of theory and evidence. *Appetite* 2009; 53: 1–8.

230. Fedoroff IC, et al. The effect of pre-exposure to food cues on the eating behavior of restrained and unrestrained eaters. *Appetite* 1997; 28: 33–47.

231. Petrovich GD, Gallagher M. Control of food consumption by learned cues: A forebrain-hypothalamic network. *Physiol Behav* 2007; 91: 397–403.

232. Petrovich GD, et al. Learned contextual cue potentiates eating in rats. *Physiol Behav* 2007; 90: 362–367.

233. Lowe MR, Levine AS. Eating motives and the controversy over dieting: Eating less than needed versus less than wanted. *Obes Res* 2005; 13: 797–806.

234. Monteleone P, et al. Hedonic eating is associated with increased peripheral levels of ghrelin and the endocanabinoid 2-arachidonoyl-glycerol in healthy humans: A pilot study. *J Clin Endocrinol Metab* 2012; 97(6): E917–E924.

235. Mozes A. Why you overeat even when you're full: Small study explores how body reacts when aroused by tempting treats. *Health Day*, May 3, 2012.
236. Branson R, et al. Binge eating as a major phenotype of melanocortin 4 receptor gene mutations. *N Engl J Med* 2003; 348: 1096–1103.
237. Yeo GSH, et al. Mutations in the human melanocortin-4 receptor gene associated with severe familial obesity disrupts receptor function through multiple molecular mechanisms. *Hum Mol Genet* 2003; 12: 561–574.
238. Farooqi IS, et al. Clinical spectrum of obesity and mutations in the melanocortin 4 receptor gene. *N Engl J Med* 2003; 348: 1085–1095.
239. Santini F. Genetic screening for melanocortin-4 receptor mutations in a cohort of Italian obese patients: Description and functional characterization of a novel mutation. *J Clin Endocrinol Metab* 2004; 89: 904–908.
240. Vaisse C, et al. Melanocortin-4 receptor mutation are a frequent and heterogeneous cause of morbid obesity. *J Clin Invest* 2000; 106: 253–262.
241. Ho G, et al. Functional characterizations of mutations in melanocortin-4-receptor mutations are a frequent and heterogeneous cause of morbid obesity. *J Biol Chem* 1999; 274: 35816–35822.
242. Scherag S, et al. Eating disorders: The current status of molecular genetic research. *Eur Child Adolesc Psychiatry* 2010; 19: 211–226.
243. Kaye W. Neurobiology of anorexia and bulimia nervosa. *Physiol Behav* 2008; 94: 121–135.
244. Bailer UF, et al. A review of neuropeptides and neuroendocrine dysregulation in anorexia nervosa and bulimia nervosa. *Curr Drug Targets CNS Neurol Disord* 2003; 2: 53–59.
245. Zhang Y, et al. Positional cloning of the mouse obese gene and its human homologue. *Nature* 1994; 372: 425–432.
246. Friedman JM, Halaas JL. Leptin and regulation of body weight in mammals. *Nature* 1998; 395: 763–770.
247. Aitman TJ, et al. Identification of Cd36 (fat) as an insulin-resistance gene causing defective fatty acid and glucose metabolism in hypertensive rats. *Nat Genet* 1999; 21: 76–83.
248. George S, et al. A family with severe insulin resistance and diabetes due to a mutation in AKT2. *Science* 2004; 304: 1325–1328.
249. Rung J, et al. Genetic variant near IRS1 is associated with type 2 diabetes, insulin resistance and hyperinsulinemia. *Nat Genet* 2009; 41(10): 1110–1115.
250. Neel JV. Diabetes mellitus: A thrifty genotype rendered detrimental by progress? *Am J Hum Genet* 1962; 14: 353–362.
251. Neel JV. The "thrifty genotype" in 1998. *Nutr Rev* 1999; 57(5 Pt 2): S2–S9.
252. Speakman JR. Thrifty genes for obesity, an attractive but flawed idea and an alternative perspective: The drifty gene hypothesis. *Int J Obes* 2008; 32: 1611–1617.
253. Fairburn CG, et al. The natural course of bulimia nervosa and binge eating disorder in young women. *Arch Gen Psychiatry* 2000; 57: 659–665.
254. Cachelin FM, et al. Natural course of a community sample of women with binge eating disorder. *Int J Eat Disord* 1997; 25: 45–54.
255. Stefano SC, et al. Antidepressants in short-term treatment of binge eating disorder: Systematic review and meta-analysis. *Eat Behav* 2008; 9: 129–136.

256. Arnold LM, et al. A placebo-controlled randomized trial of fluoxetine in the treatment for binge eating disorder. *J Clin Psychiatry* 2002; 63: 1028–1033.
257. Pearlstein T, et al. A double-blind, placebo-controlled trial of fluvoxamine in binge eating disorder: A high placebo response. *Arch Women Ment Health* 2003; 6: 147–151.
258. Hudson JI, et al. Fluvoxamine in the treatment of binge-eating disorder: A multicenter placebo-controlled, double-blind trial. *Am J Psychiatry* 1998; 155: 1756–1762.
259. Gartlehner G, et al. *Drug Class Review on Second Generation Antidepressants: Final Report*. Portland, OR: Oregon Health & Science University; 2006.
260. Berkman ND, et al. Management of eating disorders. *Evid Rep Technol Assess* 2006; 135: 1–166.
261. Malhotra S, et al. Venlafaxine treatment of binge eating disorder associated with obesity. *J Clin Psychiatry* 2002; 63: 802–806.
262. McElroy SL, et al. Placebo-controlled trial of sertraline in the treatment of binge eating disorder. *Am J Psychiatry* 2000; 157: 1004–1006.
263. McElroy SL, et al. Citalopram in the treatment of binge-eating disorder: A multicenter placebo-controlled, double-blind trial. *J Clin Psychiatry* 2003; 157: 1004–1006.
264. Laederach-Hofmann K, et al. Impiramine and diet counseling with psychological support in the treatment of obese binge eaters: A randomized, placebo-controlled double blind study. *Int J Eat Disord* 1999; 26: 231–244.
265. Gadde KM. Atomoxetine for weight reduction in obese women: A preliminary randomized controlled trial. *Int J Obes* 2006; 30: 1138–1142.
266. McElroy S. Atomoxetine in the treatment of binge eating disorder: A randomized Placebo controlled trial. *J Clin Psychiatry* 2007; 68: 390–398.
267. Appolinario JC, et al. Topiramate use in obese patients with binge eating disorder: An open study. *Can J Psychiatry* 2002; 47: 271–273.
268. McElroy SL, et al. Topiramate in the treatment of binge eating disorder associated with obesity: A Placebo controlled double blind controlled trial. *Am J Psychiatry* 2003; 160: 255–261.
269. Bicherdike MJ. 5-HT2C receptor agonists as potential drugs for the treatment of obesity. *Curr Topics Med Chem* 2003; 3: 885–897.
270. Simansky KJ, et al. A 5-HT2C agonist elicits hyperactivity and oral dyskinesia with hypophagia in rabbits. *Physiol Behav* 2004; 82: 97–107.
271. Smith BM, et al. Discovery and structure-activity relationship of (1R)-8-chloro-2, 3,4,5-tetrahydro-1-methyl-1H-3-benzazepine (Lorcaserin), a selective serotonin 5-HT2C receptor agonist for the treatment of obesity. *J Med Chem* 2008; 51: 305–313.
272. Thomsen WJ, et al. A novel selective human 5-hydroxytryptamine2C agonist: In vitro and in vivo pharmacological characterization. *J Pharmacol Exp Ther* 2008; 325: 577–587.
273. Spreitzer H. Lorcaserin. *Österreichische Apothekerzeitung* 2010; 64: 1083. (in German)
274. Lam DD, et al. Serotonin 5-HT2C receptor agonist promotes hypophagia via downstream activation of melanocortin 4 receptors. *Endocrinology* 2008; 149: 31323–31328.
275. Dahl CF, et al. Valvular regurgitation and surgery associated with fenfluramine use: An analysis of 5743 individuals. *BMC Med* 2008; 6: 34.
276. Rothman RB, Baumann MH. Serotonergic drugs and valvular heart disease. *Expert Opin Drug Saf* 2009; 8: 317–329.

277. Rothman RB, et al. Aminorex, fenfluramine, and chlorphentermine are serotonin transporter substrates implications for primary pulmonary hypertension. *Circulation* 1999; 100: 869–875.
278. McElroy S. Lisdexamfetamine dimesylate safety and efficacy on binge eating days/episodes and behavior in adults with moderate to severe binge eating disorder. *American Psychiatric Association Annual Meeting in San Francisco*, May 19, 2013, APA, 2013. Abstract/Poster #NR4-25.
279. Wang GJ, et al. Effect of combined naltrexone and bupropion therapy on the brain's reactivity to food cues. *Int J Obes* 2013; 38: 682–688.
280. Gerasimov MR, Dewey SL. Gamma-vinyl gamma-aminobutyric acid attenuates the synergistic elevations of nucleus accumbens dopamine produced by a cocaine/heroin (speedball) challenge. *Eur J Pharmacol* 1999; 380: 1–4.
281. Peng XO, et al. Gamma-vinyl GABA inhibits cocaine-triggered reinstatement of drug-seeking behavior in rats by a non-dopaminergic mechanism. *Drug Alcohol Depend* 2008; 97: 216–225.
282. DeMarco A, et al. Subchronic racemic gamma vinyl-GABA produces weight loss in Sprague Dawley and Zucker fatty rats. *Synapse* 2008; 62: 870–872.
283. Berner LA, et al. Baclofen suppresses binge eating of pure fat but not a sugar-rich or sweet-fat diet. *Behav Pharmacol* 2009; 20: 631–634.
284. Corwin RL, et al. Baclofen, raclopride, and naltrexone differentially affect intake of fat and sucrose under limited access conditions. *Behav Pharmacol* 2009; 20: 537–548.
285. Corwin RL, et al. Baclofen reduces binge eating in a double-blind, placebo-controlled, crossover study. *Behav Pharmacol* 2012; 23(5–6): 616–625.
286. Broft AI, et al. Baclofen for binge eating: An open-label trial. *Int J Eat Disorder* 2007; 40: 687–691.
287. Gonzales RA, Weiss F. Suppression of ethanol-reinforced behavior by naltrexone is associated with attenuation of the ethanol-induced increase in dialysate dopamine levels in the nucleus accumbens. *J Neurosci* 1998; 18: 10663–10671.
288. Neumeister A. Addition of naltrexone to fluoxetine in the treatment of binge eating disorder. *Am J Psychiatry* 1999; 156: 797.
289. Drewnowski A, et al. Naloxone, an opiate blocker, reduces the consumption of sweet high fat foods in obese and lean female binge eaters. *Am J Clin Nutr* 1995; 61: 1206–1212.
290. Mitchell JE, et al. A placebo controlled double blind crossover study of naltrexone hydrochloride in outpatients with normal weight bulimia. *J Clin Psychopharmacol* 1989; 9: 94–97.
291. Jonas JM, Gold MS. Naltrexone reverses bulimic symptoms. *Lancet* 1986; 1: 807.
292. Jonas JM, Gold MS. Naltrexone treatment of bulimia clinical and theoretical findings linking eating disorders and substance abuse. *Adv Alcohol Subst Abuse* 1987; 7: 29–37.
293. Jonas JM, Gold MS. The use of opiate antagonists in treating bulimia: A study of low-dose versus high-dose naltrexone. *Psychiatry Res* 1988; 24: 195–199.
294. Marrazzi MA, et al. A detailed longitudinal analysis on the use of naltrexone in the treatment of bulimia. *Int Clin Psychopharmacol* 1995; 10(3): 173–176.
295. Marrazzi MA, et al. ED binge eating disorder: Response to naltrexone. *Int J Obes Relat Metab Disord* 1995; 19(2): 143–145.
296. Yanovski SZ, Yanovski JA. Obesity. *N Engl J Med* 2002; 346: 591–602.

297. Cogan JC. *Essential Health Benefits Bulletin*. Washington, DC: Eating Disorders Coalition; 2012.
298. Hay PP, et al. Psychological treatments for bulimia nervosa and binging. *Cochrane Database Syst Rev* 2009; (4): CD000562.
299. Adami GF, et al. Body image in binge eating disorder. *Obes Surg* 1998; 8: 517–519.
300. Neigo SH, et al. Binge eating in the bariatric surgery population: A review of the literature. *Int J Eat Disord* 2007; 40: 349–359.
301. White MA, et al. Loss of control over eating predicts outcomes in bariatric surgery patients: A prospective, 24-month follow-up study. *J Clin Psychiatry* 2010; 71: 175–184.
302. Saunders R. Binge eating in gastric bypass patients before surgery. *Obes Surg* 1999; 9: 72–76.
303. Saunders R. Grazing: A high risk behavior. *Obes Surg* 2004; 14: 98–102.
304. Colles SL, et al. Loss of control is central to psychological disturbance associated with binge eating disorder. *Obesity* 2008; 16: 608–614.
305. Ames GE, et al. Weight loss surgery: Patients who regain. *Obes Weight Manage* 2009; 5: 154–161.
306. Maine M, et al. *Effective Clinical Practice in the Treatment of Eating Disorders: The Heart of the Matter*. New York: Routledge; 2009.
307. Sarwer DB, et al. Dietary intake and eating behavior after bariatric surgery: Threats to weight loss maintenance and strategies for success. *Surg Obes Relat Dis* 2011; 7: 644–655.
308. Karmali S, et al. Weight recidivism post-bariatric surgery: A systematic review. *Obes Surg* 2013; 23: 1922–1933.
309. Khaitan L, et al. Laparoscopic revision of bariatric procedures: Is it feasible? *Am Surg* 2005; 71: 6–10.
310. Kyzer S, et al. Use of adjustable silicone gastric banding for revision of failed gastric bariatric operations. *Obes Surg* 2001; 11: 66–69.
311. Pekkarinen T. Long term results of gastroplasty for morbid obesity: Binge eating as a predictor of poor outcome. *Obes Surg* 1994; 4: 248–255.
312. Adami GF, et al. Binge eating in massively obese patients undergoing bariatric surgery. *Int J Eat Disord* 1995; 17: 45–50.
313. Hsu LKG, et al. Eating disturbances before and after vertical banded gastroplasty: A pilot study. *Int J Eat Disord* 1996; 19: 23–34.
314. Hsu KG, et al. Eating disturbances and outcome of gastric bypass surgery: A pilot study. *Int J Eat Disord* 1997; 21: 385–390.
315. Hsu LK, et al. Nonsurgical factors that influence the outcome of bariatric surgery: A review. *Psychosom Med* 1998; 60: 338–346.
316. Kalarchian MA, et al. Binge eating in bariatric surgery patients. *Int J Eat Disord* 1998; 23: 89–92.
317. Saunders R, et al. Prevalence of eating disorders among bariatric surgery clients. *Eat Disord* 1998; 6: 309–317.
318. Rotenberg KJ, et al. Selective mood-induced body image disparagement and enhancement effects: Are they due to cognitive priming or subjective mood? *Int J Eat Disord* 2004; 35: 317–332.
319. Thompson K. *Body Image Disturbance: Assessment and Treatment*. Elmsford, NY: Pergamon Press; 1990.
320. Thompson K. *Body Image, Eating Disorders, and Obesity: An Integrative Guide to Assessment and Treatment*. Washington, DC: American Psychological Association; 1996.

321. Thompson K. *Exacting Beauty: Theory, Assessment, and Treatment of Body Image Disturbance*. Washington, DC: American Psychological Association; 1998.
322. Neven K, et al. The effects of Roux en Y gastric bypass surgery on body image. *Obes Surg* 2002; 12: 265–226.
323. Luppino FS, et al. Overweight, obesity and depression: A systematic review and meta-analysis of longitudinal studies. *Arch Gen Psychiatry* 2010; 67: 220–229.
324. Alger-Mayer S, et al. Preoperative binge eating status and gastric bypass surgery: A long-term outcome study. *Obes Surg* 2009; 19: 139–145.
325. Hsu L, et al. Binge eating disorder in extreme obesity. *Int J Obesity* 2002; 26: 1398–1403.
326. Kalarchian MA, et al. Binge eating among gastric bypass patients at long term follow up. *Obes Surg* 2002; 12: 270–275.
327. Fabricatore AN. Self-reported eating behaviors of extremely obese persons seeking bariatric surgery: a factor analytic approach. *Surg Obes Relat Dis.* 2006; 2(2):146–152.
328. Lang T, et al. Impact of gastric banding on eating disorder behavior and weight. *Obes Surg* 2002; 12: 100–107.
329. Mitchell JE. *Binge Eating Disorder: Clinical Foundations of Treatment*. New York: Guilford Press; 2005.
330. Malone M, Alger-Mayer S. Binge status and quality of life after gastric bypass surgery: A one-year study. *Obes Res* 2004; 12: 473–481.
331. Mitchell JE, et al. Eating behavior and eating disorders in adults before bariatric surgery. *Int J Eat Disord* 2015; 48(2): 215–222.
332. Wadden TA, et al. Binge eating disorder and the outcome of bariatric surgery at one year: A prospective, observational study. *Obesity* 2011; 19: 1220–1229.
333. Wadden TA, et al. Psychosocial and behavioral status of patients undergoing bariatric surgery: What to expect before and after surgery. *Med Clin North Am* 2007; 91: 451–469.
334. Wadden TA, et al. Benefits of lifestyle modification in the pharmacologic treatment of obesity: A randomized trial. *Arch Intern Med* 2001; 161: 218–227.
335. Wadden TA, Foster GD. Behavioral treatment of obesity. *Med Clin North Am* 2000; 84: 441–461.
336. Pataky Z, Carrard I, Golay A. Psychological factors and weight loss in bariatric surgery. *Curr Opin Gastroenterol* 2011; 27: 167–173.
337. Mitchell JE, et al. Psychopathology before surgery in the longitudinal assessment of bariatric surgery-3 (LABS-3) psychosocial study. *Surg Obes Relat Dis* 2012; 8: 533–541.
338. Marino JM, et al. The emergence of eating pathology after bariatric surgery: A rare outcome with important clinical implications. *Int J Eat Disord* 2012; 45: 179–184.
339. National Institute for Health and Care Excellence (NICE). *Eating Disorders: Core interventions in the Treatment and Management of Anorexia Nervosa, Bulimia Nervosa and Related Eating Disorders*. National Institute for Health and Clinical Excellence; 2004. http://publications.nice.org.uk/eating-disorders-cg9/guidance#atypical-eating-disorders-including-binge-eating-disorder
340. Yager J, et al. *Practice Guidelines for the Treatment of Patients with Eating Disorders*. American Psychiatric Association; 2012. Accessed at: http://psychiatryonline.org/pb/assets/raw/sitewide/practice_guidelines/guidelines/eatingdisorders-watch.pdf
341. American Psychiatric Association (APA). *Practice Guideline for the Treatment of Patients with Eating Disorders*, 3rd ed. Washington, DC: American Psychiatric Association; 2006.
342. American Psychiatric Association. Treatment of patients with eating disorders, third edition. *Am J Psychiatry* 2006; 163(7 Suppl): 4–54.

343. Wilfley DE, et al. A randomized comparison of group cognitive-behavioral therapy and group interpersonal psychotherapy for the treatment of overweight individuals with binge-eating disorder. *Arch Gen Psychiatry* 2002; 59: 713–721.

344. Hilbert A, et al. Body image interventions in cognitive-behavioral therapy of binge-eating disorder: A component analysis. *Behav Res Ther* 2004; 42: 1325–1339.

345. Gorin A, et al. Effectiveness of spouse involvement in cognitive behavioral therapy for binge eating disorder. *J Eat Disord* 2003; 33: 421–433.

346. Peterson CB, et al. Group cognitive-behavioral treatment of binge eating disorder: A comparison of therapist led versus self-help formats. *Int J Eat Disord* 1998; 24: 125–136.

347. Peterson CB, et al. Self-help versus therapist-led group cognitive-behavioral treatment of binge eating disorder at follow-up. *Int J Eat Disord* 2001; 30: 363–374.

348. Peterson CB, et al. The efficacy of self-help group treatment and therapist-led group treatment for binge eating disorder. *Am J Psychiatry* 2009; 166: 1347–1354.

349. Berkowitz R, et al. Binge eating disorder in obese adolescent girls. *Ann N Y Acad Med* 1993; 699: 200–296.

350. Masheb RM, et al. A randomized controlled trial for obesity and binge eating disorder: Low-energy-density dietary counseling and cognitive-behavioral therapy. *Behav Res Ther* 2011; 49: 821–829.

351. Schlup B, et al. The efficacy of a short version of a cognitive-behavioral treatment followed by booster sessions for binge eating disorder. *Behav Res Ther* 2009; 47: 628–635.

352. Schlup B, et al. A non-randomized direct comparison of cognitive-behavioral short- and long-term treatment for binge eating disorder. *Obes Facts* 2010; 3: 261–266.

353. Munsch S, et al. A randomized comparison of cognitive behavioral therapy and behavioral weight loss treatment for overweight individuals with binge eating disorder. *Int J Eat Disord* 2007; 42: 102–113.

354. Munsch S, et al. Ecological momentary assessment to evaluate cognitive-behavioral treatment for binge eating disorder. *Int J Eat Disord* 2009; 42: 648–657.

355. Agras WS, et al. Weight loss, cognitive-behavioral, and desipramine treatments in binge eating disorder: An additive design. *Behav Ther* 1994; 25: 225–238.

356. Grilo C, Mitchell J. *The Treatment of Eating Disorders*. New York: Guilford Press; 2010.

357. Safter DL, et al. *Dialectical Behavior Therapy for Binge Eating and Bulimia*. New York: Guilford Press; 2009.

358. Safer DL, et al. Outcome from a randomized controlled trial of group therapy for binge eating disorder: Comparing dialectical behavior therapy adapted for binge eating to an active comparison group therapy. *Behav Ther* 2010; 41: 106–120.

359. Telch CF, et al. Dialectical behavior therapy for binge eating disorder. *J Consult Clin Psychol* 2001; 69: 106–165.

360. Hilbert A, et al. Pretreatment and process predictors of outcome in interpersonal and cognitive behavioral psychotherapy for binge eating disorder. *J Consult Clin Psychol* 2007; 75(4): 645–651.

361. Tasca GA, et al. Group psychodynamic interpersonal psychotherapy: Summary of a treatment model and outcomes for depressive symptoms In: ME Abelian (Ed.), *Focus on Psychotherapy Research*. Hauppauge, NY: Nova Science; 2005, pp. 159–188.

362. Carter JC, Fairburn CG. Cognitive-behavioral self-help for binge eating disorder: A controlled effectiveness study. *J Consult Clin Psychol* 1998; 66: 616–623.

363. Carrand I, et al. Randomized controlled trial of a guided self-help treatment on the Internet for binge eating disorder. *Behav Res Ther* 2011; 49: 482–491.
364. Pendleton VR, et al. Exercise augments the effects of cognitive-behavioral therapy in the treatment of binge eating. *Int J Eat Disord* 2002; 31: 172–184.
365. Shapiro JR, et al. Feasibility and acceptability of CD-ROM-based cognitive-behavioural treatment for binge-eating disorder. *Eur Eat Disord Rev* 2007; 15: 175–184.
366. RTI-UNC. *Evidence-Based Practice Center Management of Eating Disorders*. Rockville: Agency for healthcare Research and Quality; 2006.
367. Sysko R, et al. Heterogeneity moderates treatment response among patients with binge eating disorder. *J Consult Clin Psychol* 2010; 78: 661–690.
368. Wilfley DE, et al. Early intervention of eating- and weight-related problems. *J Clin Psychol Med Settings* 2010; 17: 285–300.
369. Wilson GT. Treatment of binge eating disorder. *Psychaitr Clin North Am* 2011; 34: 773–783.
370. Levine MD, et al. Exercise in the treatment of binge eating disorder. *Int J Eat Disord* 1996; 19: 171–177.
371. Riva G, et al. Virtual reality based multidimensional therapy for the treatment of body image disturbances in binge eating disorders: A preliminary controlled study. *IEEE Trans Inf Technol Biomed* 2002; 6: 224–234.
372. Kristeller JL, Wolever RQ. Mindfulness-based eating awareness training for treating binge eating disorder: The conceptual foundation. *Eat Disord* 2011; 19: 49–61.
373. Kristeller JL. Mindfulness meditation. In: P Lehrer, R Wookfolk, WE Simes (Eds.), *Principles and Practices of Stress Management*, 3rd ed. New York: Guilford Press; 2007, pp. 393–427.
374. Siegel D. *Mindsight*. New York: Bantam Books; 2010.
375. Williams JMG. Mindfulness and psychological process. *Emotion* 2010; 10: 1–7.
376. Walsh R, Shapiro SL. The meeting of meditative disciplines and Western psychology: A mutually enriching dialogue. *Am Psychol* 2006; 61: 227–239.
377. Kristeller JL, et al. Mindfulness based approaches to eating disorders. In: RA Baer (Ed.), *Mindfulness-Based Treatment Approaches*. Burlington, MA: Academic Press; 2006.
378. Wolever RQ, Best JL. Mindfulness-based approaches to eating disorders. In: F Didonna (Ed.), *Clinical Handbook of Mindfulness*. New York: Springer; 2009, pp. 259–288.
379. Schwartz GE. Biofeedback, self-regulation, and the patterning of physiological processes. *Am Sci* 1975; 63: 314–324.
380. Finlayson G, et al. Liking vs. wanting food: Importance for human appetite control and weight regulation. *Neurosci Biobehav Rev* 2007; 31: 987–1002.
381. Appelhans BM. Neurobehavioral inhibition of reward-driven feeding: Implications for dieting and obesity. *Obesity* 2009; 17: 640–647.
382. Kristeller J, Wolever R. Mindfulness-based eating awareness training for treating binge eating disorder: the conceptual foundation. *Eat Disord* 2011; 19(1):49–61.
383. Geliebter A, Hashim SA. Gastric capacity in normal, obese, and bulimic women. *Physiol Behav* 2001; 74: 743–746.
384. Cassin SE, von Ranson KM. Is binge eating experienced as an addiction? *Appetite* 2007; 49: 687–690.
385. Batterink L, et al. Body mass correlates inversely with inhibitory control in response to food among adolescent girls: An fMRI study. *NeuroImage* 2007; 52: 1696–1703.

386. Stice E, et al. Relation of obesity to consummatory and anticipatory food reward. *Physiol Behav* 2009; 97: 551–560.

387. Hill AJ. The psychology of food craving. *Proc Natl Acad Sci U S A* 2007; 66: 277–285.

388. Tribole E, Resch E. *Intuitive Eating: A Revolutionary Program That Works*, 2nd ed. New York: St. Martin's Griffin; 2003.

389. Wilfley DE, et al. The clinical significance of binge eating disorder. *Int J Eat Disord* 2003; 34(Suppl): 94–101.

390. Linde JA, et al. Binge eating disorder, weight control self-efficacy, and depression in overweight men and women. *Int J Obesity* 2004; 28: 418–425.

391. Wood W, Neal DT. A new look at habits and the habit–goal interface. *Psychol Rev* 2007; 114: 843–863.

392. Tribole E, Resch E. *Intuitive Eating: A Revolutionary Program that Works*. New York: St. Martin's Griffin; 2012.

393. Bacon L, et al. Size acceptance and intuitive eating improve health for obese, female chronic dieters. *J Am Diet Assoc* 2005; 105: 929–936.

394. Bacon L. Reflections on Fat Acceptance: Lessons Learned from Privilege: An Essay based on a Keynot Speech Delivered at the Conference of the National Association to Advance Fat Acceptance, August 1, 2009.

395. Bacon L. *Eat Well: For Your Self, For the World*. Lulu.com; 2009.

396. Bacon L. Intuitive eating: Enjoy your food, respect your body. *Diabetes Self-Management*, November/December 2010, pp. 44–51.

397. Bacon L. *Health at Every Size: The Surprising Truth about Your Weight*. Dallas, TX: BenBella Books; 2010.

398. Bacon L, Aphramor L. Weight science: Evaluating the evidence for a paradigm shift. *Nutr J* 2011; 10: 9.

399. Bacon L, Aphramor L. *Body Respect*. Dallas, TX: BenBella Books; 2014.

400. Tribole E. Why and how to give yourself permission to eating anything. *Eating Disorders Today*, Fall, 2005.

401. Tribole E. Intuitive eating in the treatment of eating disorders. *Scan Pulse*, Summer 2006, 25(3), p. 12.

402. Tribole E. Intuitive eating: Can you be healthy and eat anything. *Eating Disorders Recovery Today*, Winter 2009, 7(1).

403. Tribole E. Intuitive eating in the treatment of eating disorders: The journey of attunement. *Perspectives*, Winter 2010, pp. 11–14.

404. Berkman ND, et al. Management of eating disorders. *Evid Rep Technol Assess* 2006; 135: 1–166.

405. Jacobs-Pilipski MJ, et al. Placebo response in binge eating disorder. *Int J Eat Disord* 2007; 40: 204–211.

406. Carter WP, et al. Pharmacologic treatment of binge eating disorder. *Int J Eat Disord* 2003; 34: S74–S88.

13

Current research and future hope

FRANK L. GREENWAY AND STEVEN R. SMITH

INTRODUCTION

This chapter reviews some of the current research into treatments for obesity and discusses the future of obesity research. The current research on obesity is divided into diet and lifestyle change, dietary herbal supplements, pharmaceuticals, and surgery and devices. Obesity is the last of the chronic diseases to be defined as such. The future of obesity research can be predicted from the research on other chronic diseases such as hypertension and diabetes. Since the tools available today are more sophisticated than in prior decades, it is likely that obesity treatment will advance faster than what we have seen in the past with other diseases such as hypertension.

A FRESH LOOK AT THE CAUSES OF OBESITY

The last decade of obesity research has identified several new and potentially important discoveries that change our view of why people become obese. Understanding these fundamental causes is needed to develop new therapies. Several examples are reviewed not as a comprehensive account, but rather to highlight the challenges of developing obesity treatments when so little is known about the pathobiology in an individual patient with obesity.

Adenovirus AD-36 (AD-36) was the first reported coincident with the increase in the prevalence of obesity that began about 1980 (1). AD-36 has been shown to cause obesity in chickens, rodents, and marmosets (nonhuman primates) (2). The prevalence of neutralizing antibodies to AD-36 are 30% in obese individuals and only 11% in lean; but even in the lean, the antibody-positive individuals are heavier than antibody-negative individuals (3). When identical twins are discordant for the AD-36 virus, the antibody-positive twin is significantly heavier (3). AD-36 appears to cause obesity in a similar manner to thiazolidinedione drugs that stimulate peroxisome proliferators-activated receptor γ (PPAR-γ). The E4orf-1 gene of the AD-36 virus seems to activate PPAR-γ in human and rodent adipocytes, causing an increase in adipogenesis and an increase in insulin sensitivity characteristic of small fat cells (4). Thus, AD-36 may be one reason for insulin-sensitive obesity.

Alterations in the microbiome

The gut microbiome may play an important role in weight gain in humans. As reviewed in Krajmalnik-Brown et al. (5), the bioenergetics of the gut bacteria may lead to small incremental changes in nutrient absorption and also may change the signaling of the enteroendocrine hormonal signals.

Environmental changes

There are many factors in our environment that are correlated with obesity beyond the typically assumed diet and inactivity (6–8). The evidence for some of these factors is simply epidemiological and not proven. Heating and air conditioning, computer use, antidepressant use, and antibiotic use are all correlated and may be causal; however, caution is needed when ascribing causality to any of these associated factors.

Hypothalamic gliosis

In rodents and potentially in humans, high-fat diets and obesity lead to gliosis in the hypothalamus, a key area for neural control of food intake (9–11). The glial cells expand and reduce the signals for nutrients, leptin, and other hormones from reaching these cells. In other words, once obesity is established there are potentially structural changes in the brain that maintain the obese state.

Metabolic adaptation

In the weight reduced state, energy metabolism decreases by about 10%, even taking into account the reduction in body composition (12). This metabolic adaptation is one of many components, such as reduced fat oxidation (13), seen in the weight reduced state. These and other discoveries will open up new ways of thinking about and developing treatments for obesity.

DIET AND LIFESTYLE

Combined diet and lifestyle research

Promoting diet and lifestyle intervention has been a priority of the National Institutes of Health (NIH). The Diabetes Prevention Trial enrolled 3234 subjects with impaired glucose tolerance into an intensive lifestyle group, a group treated with metformin 850 mg twice a day and a usual care group. The intensive lifestyle group lost 7% of body weight and exercised 150 minutes per week, causing a 58% reduction in the conversion from impaired glucose tolerance to diabetes compared to the usual care group. Metformin reduced the conversion to diabetes by 31%. This first phase of the study was stopped prematurely due to the strength in the results at an average follow-up period of 2.8 years (14). Interestingly, the Finnish Diabetes Prevention Study confirmed that diet and lifestyle reduced the conversion from impaired glucose tolerance to diabetes by 58% compared to control (15). The primary medical concern surrounding obesity is its association with diabetes and other cardiovascular risks. These diabetes prevention studies have emphasized the importance of diet and lifestyle interventions to the treatment of obesity and underscore the recommendations in obesity treatment guidelines that suggest diet and lifestyle should be the basis of any obesity treatment program (16). Weight loss was the strongest predictor of remaining diabetes-free, even in patients who did not exercise (17).

Commercial weight loss programs

Commercial weight loss programs have traditionally been advertisement driven and either unable or reluctant to share results with the scientific community. This is changing. Weight Watchers published a 2-year trial performed at six academic centers that randomized 211 subjects to the Weight Watchers program and 212 subjects to self-help. The subjects had a body mass index (BMI) of 27 to 40 kg/m²; lost 4.3 ± 6.1 kg (4.6% initial body weight) in the Weight Watchers group and 1.3 ± 6.2 kg (2% initial body weight) in the self-help group at 1 year; and at 2 years, the weight losses were 2.9 ± 6.5 and 0.2 ± 6.5 kg, respectively, by intention-to-treat analysis (18). Jenny Craig® performed a similar study, enrolling 442 subjects at four sites into a center-based behavioral intervention or a telephone-based behavioral intervention, both of which included prepackaged food in a planned menu and exercise advice or a usual care group as a control population. At the end of the 2-year intervention, weight loss was 7.4 kg (7.9% of initial body weight), 6.2 kg (6.8% of initial body weight), and 2.0 kg (2.1% of initial body weight) in the center-based, telephone-based, and usual care groups, respectively (19). The difference in the two programs is that Weight Watchers use a group format for delivering behavior change instruction, whereas Jenny Craig uses individual counseling and calorie-controlled portions. These two large commercial weight loss programs are the only ones that have subjected their programs to long-term randomized clinical trials by outside groups, but now that a trend has been set, it would not be unexpected for other programs to follow suit, since this information is essential to referring physicians.

Exercise

Exercise is known to be of help with weight maintenance, but adding exercise to a weight loss program gives at best only a marginal increase in weight loss (20). The reasons for this were obscure, but the Dose–Response to Exercise in Women (DREW) study has shed some light on the issue. The DREW study evaluated exercise in postmenopausal women at 50%, 100%, and 150% of the NIH-recommended levels. Although exercise increased weight loss to the degree expected in the 50% and 100% groups, the 150% group had a compensatory increase in food intake that defeated the increase in physical activity (21). Thus, although more physical activity did increase fitness and seemed to have additional health benefits, exercise in excess of the recommended 8 kcal/kg/week has little incremental benefit for weight loss.

Diet

There has been controversy regarding the best diet for obesity, with some advocating a low-carbohydrate diet and others advocating a low-fat diet (22). There have been proponents and detractors on both sides of the issue, at least since the 1970s when the first Atkins diet book was published. A large study tried to address this question by enrolling 811 overweight adults into a behavior modification program and randomizing them to four diets in which the percentages of fat, protein, and carbohydrate were as follows: 20%, 15%, and 65%; 20%, 25%, and 55%; 40%, 15%, and 45%; and 40%, 25%, and 35%, respectively. All groups lost an average of 6 kg (7% of their initial body weight) at 1 year and maintained a 4 kg weight loss at 2 years. There was no significant difference in weight loss across the diets, and it was concluded that calories, rather than macronutrient distribution, were important (23).

It now appears, as is often the case, that the answer is more complex than a single diet that is best for all obese individuals. Cornier et al. (24) developed two groups of obese nondiabetic women: one with fasting insulin values >15 µU/mL (insulin resistant) and one with fasting insulin values <10 µU/mL (insulin sensitive). Both groups had insulin sensitivity characterized by using a frequently sampled insulin glucose tolerance test and were randomized to a low-carbohydrate (40% carbohydrate and 40% fat) or a low-fat (60% carbohydrate and 20% fat) diet. The insulin-sensitive group lost more weight on the high-carbohydrate diet (13.5 ± 1.2% initial body weight vs. 6.8 ± 1.2%; $P < 0.002$) and the insulin-resistant group lost more weight on the low-carbohydrate diet (13.4 ± 1.3% vs. 8.5 ± 1.4%; $P < 0.04$) (24). Since insulin resistance is more common in obesity, it is not surprising that many studies have found a greater weight loss in obese subjects treated with a low-carbohydrate diet than with a high-carbohydrate diet. It has been observed that weight loss with a low-carbohydrate diet is greater at 3 and 6 months than the conventional diet, but the difference is lost by 12 months. This has been attributed to difficulties in dietary adherence, but it may also be due to reversal of the insulin resistance in the first 3 to 6 months making a higher carbohydrate diet more effective (25). Ebbeling et al. (26) reported a study in which a low-carbohydrate diet was compared to a low-fat diet with an intensive phase during the first 6 months and a maintenance phase from 6 to 18 months. Although there was no difference in weight loss between the two groups, those individuals who had insulin resistance (insulin secretion above the mean on a glucose tolerance test) lost significantly more weight and body fat by dual-energy absorptiometry on the low-carbohydrate diet (26).

Those who treat obesity have observed for some time that any treatment one uses seems to have responders and nonresponders. This has prompted the hypothesis that, like diabetes that is divided into type 1 and type 2, there are also different types of obesity. The differential response to macronutrient composition of the diet, depending on the degree of insulin sensitivity or insulin secretion to an oral glucose tolerance test, is the first example that this hypothesis may indeed be true. This raises the question as to why some obese individuals are insulin sensitive and others are insulin resistant. Research into the obesity virus seems to be shedding some light in this area.

Another interesting dietary intervention is methionine restriction. Methionine restriction increases life span in rats by 30%, similar in magnitude to calorie restriction, but it does so while increasing food intake and metabolic rate and reducing body weight (27,28). Epner et al. (29) treated eight patients with cancer who were not cachectic with a methionine-restricted diet for 8 to 39 weeks (mean 17 weeks). Protein was supplied in the form of a commercial methionine-deficient medical food called Hominex®-2. The diet was not restricted in calories, but methionine was restricted to 2 mg/kg/day. The only side effect appeared to be an average weight loss of 0.5 kg per week that occurred despite a 20% increase in dietary calories. Albumin and prealbumin remained normal, suggesting that the weight loss was not associated with malnutrition. Another trial treated 26 obese subjects with metabolic syndrome with a calorie-unrestricted diet in which protein was restricted to 2 mg/kg/day of methionine by using Hominex-2 for 16 weeks, and demonstrated an increase in fat oxidation and a decrease in liver fat (30). The reason for the lack of an effect on energy expenditure may have been due to cysteine in the Hominex-2, since cysteine-supplemented diets have been demonstrated to reverse the effects of methionine restriction (31). A methionine-deficient diet holds some promise as an intervention that will allow weight loss without calorie restriction and prolong life.

Lifestyle

Clearly, recording of dietary intake, activity, and other eating-related activities are associated with weight loss and are a major component of the success of behavior modification or lifestyle strategies (32). Unfortunately, although recording of dietary intake does help to reduce food intake and induce weight loss, the accuracy of self-recorded intake or physical activity is dismal in obese subjects. In one study, obese subjects ate 50% more than recorded and exercised 50% less (33). Increasing the accuracy of self-reported energy intake and energy expenditure is essential to the study of obesity and in judging the effectiveness of interventions. Doubly labeled water has been the standard to measure energy intake and expenditure in a free-living environment, but it is too expensive for general use (33). There have been attempts to develop new techniques for measuring food intake. One of these methods involves photography of the meal and plate waste by using cellular phones with data transfer capability in a free-living environment (34). The accuracy of this method was shown to be statistically equivalent to doubly labeled water during the 6-day testing period (35). Mathematical modeling of weight loss has not only improved the accuracy of weight loss prediction but also has practical applications to behavior modification by defining what is not physiologically possible for a patient claiming adherence and changes the discussion to *how* the patient got off their diet, from *if* they did so (36,37). A free version of a body-weight mathematical model is now available (38). The software can be used to determine whether a patient is adhering to a calorie-restricted diet and/or exercise program.

Likewise, attempts have been made to quantitate energy expenditure. A sensor to measure movement and posture on various areas of the body is the Intelligent Device for Energy Expenditure and Activity (IDEEA®). This device depends on computer analysis of the data collected and gives estimates of energy expenditure in agreement with metabolic chamber studies at greater than 95% accuracy (39). The IDEEA and activity monitors RT3 and SWA have been compared and show good agreement (40). Some have been validated against the doubly labeled water standard (41). Thus, although these new devices may still be more expensive than self-report, reasonably accurate methods to judge food intake and physical activity that are less expensive than doubly labeled water are being developed. Clearly, more accurate estimates of food intake and energy expenditure will add to our knowledge of these areas and hopefully contribute to progress in lifestyle modification research.

Summary

The importance of diet and lifestyle change in preventing diabetes and causing weight loss gives credence to recommendations that lifestyle and diet be the basis for all weight loss programs. Commercial weight loss programs that use diet and lifestyle change with or without prepackaged foods to treat obesity have been evaluated by independent third parties in randomized clinical trials testing the program's safety and efficacy. This line of research should prove useful to both potential clients and to the physicians who advise them. Exercise to the level of NIH recommendations improves weight loss, but higher levels result in compensatory food intake with improved fitness. The controversy regarding the optimal macronutrient composition for a weight loss diet is probably an artifact of the difference in weight loss response related to insulin sensitivity. Evidence suggests that insulin-sensitive obese individuals lose more weight on a high-carbohydrate diet, whereas those who are insulin resistant lose more weight to a low-carbohydrate diet. A methionine-restricted diet may have value in the future. New devices to quantitate food intake and energy expenditure may advance lifestyle research by increasing accuracy, and mathematical modeling can change a discussion from whether a subject is nonadherent to diet to why they were nonadherent and how to help them become so.

DIETARY HERBAL SUPPLEMENTS

As a consequence of the Dietary Supplement Health and Education Act of 1994, dietary herbal supplements are classified as food in the United States (42). Unlike drugs that need to prove safety and efficacy to the satisfaction of the Food and Drug Administration (FDA) prior to approval for sale, foods are presumed safe, and the FDA must prove them to be unsafe to remove them from the market. This is a much higher bar to meet and difficult to do without controlled trials that rarely exist. The Federal Trade Commission (FTC) controls truth in advertising and is responsible to police the claims made by supplement manufacturers. There are many unsubstantiated claims made regarding dietary supplements. Dr. Mehmet Oz, a popular physician and television personality, was the subject of a congressional hearing on his "miracle" weight-loss claims (43). One of the products he was promoting, green coffee bean extract for weight loss was shown to be inaccurate, the paper was withdrawn by the authors and the company paid $3.5 million in fines to settle with federal authorities (44). Many dietary herbal supplements continue to make false claims, and only a fraction is investigated by the FTC. Thus, the consumer must beware of claims made for dietary herbal supplements. There have been a small number of dietary herbal supplement with studies that support or discourage their use. Some of those supplements are reviewed herein.

Caffeine/ephedrine

Caffeine/ephedrine was a prescription drug in Denmark between 1990 and 2002, but it was taken off the market due to reports that raised safety concerns. Other stimulant anorectics for the treatment of obesity, such as phentermine and diethylpropion, were removed from the European market for safety concerns around the same time, but they were reinstated a year or two later on appeal. Caffeine/ephedrine was not reinstated in Denmark, but it held an 80% market share while it was approved, even when fenfluramine was available (45). Ephedra is an herb used in tea consumed by some ethnic populations. Since ephedra was in the food chain prior to 1994, it was classified as a dietary herbal supplement in the United States and is regulated like a food. Ephedra and ephedra/caffeine were removed from the US market in 2004 by the FDA, which classified it as an adulterant (46). This decision was based on adverse event reports and a review of the literature by Shekelle et al. (47). This report documented the efficacy of ephedrine and ephedra combined with caffeine. There were no serious adverse events in the controlled trials that lasted up to 6 months, and there were approximately 1000 subjects in total in those combined trials. There was a 2.2- to 3.6-fold increase in side effects in the ephedra- or ephedrine-treated groups compared to placebo, consisting of psychiatric, autonomic, and gastrointestinal symptoms and heart palpitations (47). Ephedra exists as four isomers, the most active of which is ephedrine (45). Ephedrine is still available by prescription and although it does not have an indication for the treatment of obesity, it could still be used by a physician in an off-label manner and could also be combined with caffeine. The dose of caffeine and ephedrine used in the combination pill approved for obesity treatment in Denmark was 200 mg caffeine and 20 mg ephedrine (equivalent to 25 mg ephedrine HCl) three times a day (45). The symptoms of stimulation seen initially (in the trial to register caffeine and ephedrine as a prescription obesity drug in Denmark) returned to placebo levels by 8 weeks, similar to the manner one develops tolerance to the stimulation associated with coffee when one drinks it daily (45). Ephedrine is listed in the Drug Enforcement Administration (DEA) Chemical Control Program of the Controlled Substance Act. Since ephedrine has been used as a starting product to make illegal methamphetamine, it can only be sold in limited amounts, and its sale is closely tracked, thereby discouraging its use as an off-label obesity therapy (48). Thus, caffeine and ephedrine are no longer widely used, but they were one of the first, if not the first, truly efficacious dietary herbal supplement.

Fucoxanthin

Fucoxanthin is the major carotenoid in edible seaweed such as *Undaria pinnatifida*. When fed to rodents, fucoxanthin increased uncoupling protein 1 in white adipose tissue and reduced fat accumulation compared to a control (49). Fucoxanthin is effective at a lower dose when combined with lipids in animals and in humans (50–52). Compared to placebo, the combination of fucoxanthin (1.6–2.4 mg) with pomegranate oil (200–300 mg) reduced body weight (5.5 ± 1.4 kg; $P < 0.05$), body fat, and liver fat and increased resting energy expenditure in obese nondiabetic premenopausal women in a single human trial (50). Although more human trials are needed, fucoxanthin holds promise as an effective dietary herbal supplement for the treatment of obesity.

Hoodia gordonii

Hoodia gordonii, a succulent that grows in Africa, has been used by Bushmen to decrease appetite on long treks across the desert. The active ingredient is the steroidal glycoside P57. When P57 is injected into the third ventricle of animals, it increases the ATP content of the hypothalamic tissue by 50% to 150% ($P < 0.05$) and decreases food intake by 40% to 60% over 24 hours ($P < 0.05$) (53). Based on these data, *Hoodia* became a popular dietary herbal supplement for weight loss. In a 15-day study, 49 overweight females were randomized to 1110 mg of *H. gordonii* purified extract or placebo. The *H. gordonii* purified extract gave more nausea, vomiting, and skin sensations, along with increases in blood pressure, pulse rate, bilirubin, and alkaline phosphatase ($P < 0.05$). There was no change in measured food intake or body weight (54). Thus, due to safety and questionable efficacy, the use of *Hoodia* as a dietary supplement for the treatment of obesity should be discouraged.

Cissus quadrangularis

Cissus quadrangularis is a commonly used folk medicine in India, Africa, and Asia for a variety of purposes. Oben et al. (55–57) have published three papers on the use of *C. quadrangularis* for the treatment of obesity in humans. The first study (55) compared *C. quadrangularis* standardized to 2.5% phytosterols and 15% soluble plant fibers combined with green tea extract (22% epigallocatechin gallate and 40% caffeine), niacin-bound chromium, selenium (0.5% L-selenomethionine), pyridoxine, folic acid, and cyanocobalamin compared to placebo in a double-blind trial with 123 subjects. In this 8-week study, obese subjects lost 7.2% of initial body weight compared to 2.5% for placebo and 6.3% for the overweight subjects ($P < 0.05$). Body fat and waist circumference were also reduced ($P < 0.01$). There were significant reductions in low-density lipoprotein (LDL) cholesterol, triglycerides, C-reactive protein, and glucose and a significant increase in high-density lipoprotein cholesterol compared to placebo (55). The second study (56) compared *C. quadrangularis* standardized to 5% ketosteroids to placebo in 64 obese subjects. The placebo group gained 1% of initial body weight over 6 weeks compared to a loss of 4% in the *C. quadrangularis* group. Adverse events were greater in the placebo group. The third study (57), *C. quadrangularis* standardized to 2.5% ketosteroids (150 mg), was compared to *C. quadrangularis* with *Irvingia gabonensis* standardized to 7% albumin (250 mg) or a placebo given twice a day for 10 weeks. At the end of 10 weeks, the placebo group lost 2.1% of initial body weight compared to 8.8% in the *C. quadrangularis* group and 11.9% in the *C. quadrangularis* combined with *I. gabonensis* group. Both treatment groups lost more weight than placebo, and the combination group lost more weight than the group taking *C. quadrangularis*. There were corresponding changes in body fat, waist circumference, total cholesterol, LDL cholesterol, and blood sugar. Thus, *C. quadrangularis* alone or in combination with *I. gabonensis* appears to be effective in the treatment of obesity. These findings await confirmation by an independent group.

Garcinia cambogia

Garcinia cambogia and its active ingredient hydroxycitric acid have been a popular dietary herbal supplement. The original studies in rodents by Roche in the 1960s and 1970s used a sodium salt of hydroxycitrate and saw weight loss (58–61). The monovalent salts, however, are hygroscopic and difficult to make into capsules. Thus, the salt sold as a dietary herbal supplement was largely the calcium salt. The calcium salt was tested by Heymsfield et al. (62) in a well-done clinical trial and showed it to be ineffective for weight loss probably due to its insolubility. Preuss et al. (63) reported a randomized, double-blind, placebo-controlled trial in which 90 subjects were randomized to 2800 mg of a calcium and potassium salt of hydroxycitrate or a placebo. Over 8 weeks, there was a 4.9 kg weight loss in the hydroxycitrate group compared to a 1.5 kg weight loss in the placebo group. Thus, it appears that *G. cambogia* as a monovalent salt may be an effective dietary supplement for the treatment of obesity.

Mixed dietary herbal supplement

A randomized, double-blind, placebo-controlled clinical trial in 60 obese subjects was reported with a mixture of *Sphaeranthus indicus* and *Garcinia mangostana*. After 8 weeks, the group treated with the herbal combination lost 3.74 kg more than the placebo, a loss that was statistically significant (64). Although needing confirmation, this dietary herbal supplement holds promise of efficacy for the treatment of human obesity.

Functional foods

Functional foods are foods that have a specific health function separate from their use as foods. Dietary fiber, also called fermentable fiber or resistant starch, is one example (65). In rats and probably in humans, resistant starch is fermented in the colon to form butyrate that stimulates the colonic L cells to produce the satiety hormones peptide-YY and glucagon-like peptide 1 (66). These hormones mediate the reduction in body fat seen in resistant starch-fed animals, and feeding resistant starch to humans results in elevation of these same hormones (67). Another example of a functional food is 1,3-diacylglycerol that is used as a cooking oil and sold under the trade name Econa™. Although there are small amounts of this diglyceride in all vegetable oils, the product is made enzymatically so the oil contains 70% 1,3-diglyceride. The lack of a free fatty acid at the 2-position makes it impossible for the body to store, and it is oxidized in the liver instead (68). The fatty acids on the 1,3-diglyceride have the same caloric value as the free fatty acids on triglyceride, but 1,3-diacylglyceride decreases appetite in addition to increasing fat oxidation (69,70). One double-blind study randomized 131 overweight and obese subjects to food containing triglyceride or 1,3-diacylglyceride for 24 weeks. The body weight and body fat decreased by

3.6% and 8.3%, respectively, in the 1,3-diacylglyceride group and by 2.5% and 5.6%, respectively, in the triglyceride group ($P < 0.04$) (68). A 5-month study in children between 7 and 17 years of age showed similar results (71). Although these functional foods give between 1% and 2.5% greater weight loss than placebo, using functional foods in combination may give clinically significant weight losses.

Summary

Caffeine combined with ephedrine is no longer available as a dietary herbal supplement. Ephedrine is still a prescription medication, but since it is the starting product to make illegal methamphetamine, it is a controlled chemical substance that has discouraged its off-label use for the treatment of obesity. Human studies of fucoxanthin, *C. quadrangularis*, *G. cambogia*, and a mixture of *S. indicus* and *G. mangostana* suggest the potential for weight loss equivalent to prescription medications, but all await independent confirmation. Although *Hoodia* has been a popular dietary supplement for the treatment of obesity, safety issues have been discovered that should discourage its use. Functional foods are a new category of treatments for obesity that give small weight losses in excess of placebo, but due to their safety it is probable that if used in combination they could result in clinically significant weight losses.

PHARMACEUTICALS

Cannabinoid-1 receptor antagonists

The cannabinoid-1 (CB-1) receptor antagonist rimonabant was removed from the European market and was never approved in the United States due to increased suicidal ideation and a possible increase in seizures. Marijuana, a cannabinoid, increases hunger, so the CB-1 antagonists were developed for the treatment of obesity and were designed for brain penetration with the thought that hunger control was mediated in the central nervous system. New CB-1 antagonist compounds have been synthesized that are specifically excluded from the central nervous system. These compounds have most, if not all, of the desired effects of the brain-penetrant compounds without the adverse effects on mood that were seen with CB-1 compounds that enter the brain. Thus, although brain-penetrant CB-1 antagonist development has been stopped, there is hope for developing the CB-1 antagonist class that is excluded from the central nervous system as treatment for diabetes, liver disease, and obesity (72,73).

Lorcaserin

Lorcaserin is a serotonin agonist specific to the serotonin 5-hydroxytryptamine (5-HT) 2C receptor. Fenfluramine was a nonspecific agonist of this receptor that is metabolized to nor-dexfenfluramine, which has a greater affinity for the 5-HT2B receptor, the receptor associated with heart valve pathology, than serotonin itself (74). Thus, lorcaserin has the potential to replace fenfluramine in the phentermine/fenfluramine combination without the risk of heart valve pathology. Lorcaserin was approved for the treatment of obesity in 2012 and gives 3.6 kg greater weight loss than a placebo (75). A clinical trial testing the efficacy and safety of the lorcaserin/phentermine combination for the treatment of obesity is presently in progress (76).

Cetilistat

Cetilistat is a lipase inhibitor like orlistat and appears to give similar efficacy and similar side effects, although the side effects may be less severe (77). Cetilistat has completed phases I and II in the United States and is now in phase III trials in Japan.

Tesofensine

Tesofensine is a norepinephrine, dopamine, and serotonin reuptake inhibitor that was being developed for the treatment of Parkinson's and Alzheimer's diseases, and weight loss was noted in the clinical trials (78). A 24-week trial randomized 203 obese subjects to 0.25, 0.5, 1, or placebo once a day; weight loss was 6.8%, 11.4%, 12.7%, and 2.3%, respectively (79,80). This efficacy is greater than for presently approved single obesity pharmaceuticals, but the elevations in blood pressure and heart rate are a cause for concern and led to discontinuation of development.

Bupropion/naltrexone

Bupropion (BUP) is known to activate melanocortin pathways, and naltrexone (NAL) is an antagonist of the opioid receptor, a receptor on the proopiomelanocortin (POMC) neurons that inhibit the secretion of POMC. The BUP/NAL combination acts on both the hypothalamus and the reward system, and the phase III clinical trials gave a 4.8% greater weight loss than placebo (81). Although the BUP/NAL met other requirements for approval, a cardiovascular safety study was requested by the FDA prior to approval. That cardiovascular safety trial has met its intermediate goal, and the drug was approved to treat obesity by the FDA in September 2014 (42).

Bupropion/zonisamide

A time-released formulation of BUP and zonisamide is being developed for the treatment of obesity. A phase II clinical trial randomized 226 obese subjects to placebo, 300 mg BUP per day, 400 mg zonisamide per day, or the combination. This 6-month study produced body-weight losses of −0.4%, −3.6%, −6.6%, and −9.2%, respectively. The BUP/zonisamide group lost 12% of initial body weight at 48 weeks. Adverse events with a prevalence greater than 10% included insomnia, nausea, fatigue, upper respiratory infection, headache, and anxiety (82).

Phentermine/topiramate

A combination of phentermine at 7.5 or 15 mg per day and topiramate at 46 or 92 mg per day was approved for the treatment of obesity in 2012. The phase III trial showed a 6.4% and 8.6% greater weight loss than placebo for the 7.5/46 mg and 15/46 mg doses, respectively (83).

Liraglutide

Liraglutide is a glucagon-like peptide 1 agonist approved for the treatment of type 2 diabetes at a dose of 1.8 mg per day. Liraglutide at a dose of 3 mg per day is being developed for the treatment of obesity. At the end of 20 weeks, the 3 mg dose of liraglutide gave 6.4 kg more weight loss than placebo and 3.1 kg more weight loss than orlistat (84). The FDA advisory committee considered the approval of liraglutide at the 3 mg dose for the treatment of obesity in September 2014 and recommended its approval by a 14-to-1 majority. The response of the FDA to their recommendation is still pending (85).

Beloranib

Beloranib is a fumagillin derivative and an inhibitor of methionine aminopeptidase-2 that is being developed for the treatment of obesity. Women treated with intravenous beloranib twice a week at a dose of 0.9 mg/m² lost 3.8 kg over 4 weeks, and the drug was well tolerated, with side effects being headache, nausea, vomiting, and diarrhea. Since beloranib acts through a peripheral mechanism, it should be effective in hypothalamic obesity, a site where medications acting on the hypothalamus have been ineffective. In a phase IIa trial of subjects with Prader–Willi syndrome, a genetic type of hypothalamic obesity, beloranib gave satiety and weight loss in this difficult-to-treat condition (86).

Velneperit (S-2367)

Velneperit is a selective neuropeptide Y receptor Y5 antagonist, also known as S-2367, that is being developed for the treatment of obesity. The drug was in phase II of drug development, but the program has been dormant for almost 10 years. An announcement was made that development will resume as the need for obesity drugs seems to have created a more favorable drug development climate (87).

SURGERY AND DEVICES

Surgery

Surgical treatment is the only obesity treatment that has been shown to decrease mortality, possibly because it is the only obesity therapy that enforces the maintenance of a weight loss for more than a decade of a magnitude necessary to document a decrease in mortality (88). A meta-analysis demonstrated that the mortality rate at 30 days was 0.8% and that the complication rate was 0.31%. Gastric bypass and sleeve gastrectomy seem to have comparable weight losses, and sleeve gastrectomy is gaining in popularity due to its being a simpler operation. The laparoscopically placed gastric band (lap-band) has a lower complication rate and has been approved to treat people with a BMI >30 kg/m² and at least one obesity-related complication. The lap-band is falling out of favor due to its higher reoperation rate and smaller weight loss that is achieved over a longer period with multiple adjustments of the fluid in the band (89). Since there is a need for outpatient procedures that can be done endoscopically entirely through the gastrointestinal tract to decrease cost and morbidity, transoral procedures have been done to reduce the size of the stomach and create a tube similar to the sleeve gastrectomy without resecting tissue (90).

Devices

The development of devices to treat obesity has been an active field with the goal of creating less invasive and less expensive treatments associated with lower morbidity. The FDA advisory committee recently voted to approve a vagal nerve stimulation device to decrease food intake and cause weight loss (91). There are several gastric balloons in development that are designed to take up room in the stomach and decrease food intake, but none are yet approved in the United States. One of these balloons, the Obalon balloon, can be placed by swallowing; the number of balloons can be increased monthly, but the balloons require endoscopy for removal (92). Most other gastric balloons in development need to be both placed and removed through a gastroscope. The transpyloric shuttle is a ball that is inserted and removed through a gastroscope. The ball is connected to a tether to which a smaller ball is attached. The tether passes across the pylorus, and the smaller ball rests into the duodenum. This device causes an intermittent obstruction to the stomach emptying, is placed and removed in less than 15 minutes and led to weight losses of 8.9 and 14.6 kg at 3 and 6 months, respectively, without any evidence of the weight loss starting to plateau (93). The endobarrier is a gastrointestinal liner that is placed and removed through a gastroscope and keeps food from contacting the intestinal wall for 80 cm from the duodenum into the jejunum. Three randomized trials of the endobarrier gave an average of 13% reduction in excess weight loss more than the control condition. A 52-week case series of the endobarrier in 13 type 2 diabetic subjects significantly reduced fasting blood sugar and glycohemoglobin (94). It is likely that there will be several antiobesity devices approved in the near future by the FDA.

FUTURE HOPE

History of obesity and chronic disease research

As physicians, we believe the goal of research into obesity or other chronic diseases is to develop better treatments and ultimately a cure as a means of improving the quality of life for those afflicted with the disease. The bench-to-bedside principle of medical research still applies today as it did in time of William Osler (95). Discoveries in the clinic will stimulate laboratory investigations and laboratory discoveries will stimulate clinical trials.

Obesity is the chronic disease that has been most recently recognized as such. Obesity was considered to be merely the results of bad habits prior to the 1985 NIH Consensus Conference (96). This late recognition of obesity as a chronic disease is the reason that drugs developed prior to 1985 were tested and approved for up to 12 weeks of use. It was believed that one could develop a new habit or extinguish an old habit over that period. Obesity in that era was likened to learning to ride a bicycle, and one should be able to take the training wheels off a bicycle after 12 weeks or less of practice. In fact, the American Medical Association did not recognize obesity as a chronic disease until June 2013 (97). Since obesity is the most recent of the chronic diseases to be recognized, we can learn the probable future of obesity research from observing the progress of research in other chronic diseases that preceded it.

The initial treatments of chronic diseases have been dietary. Diets limited to 10 g of carbohydrate and 2400 kcal per day were typical for the treatment of the type 1 diabetic patient in the era prior to the discovery of insulin (98). The rice diet was the basis for the most successful treatment of hypertension prior to the advent of effective antihypertensive drugs (99). Although the first treatments for chronic diseases were dietary, the first treatments that were effective long term have traditionally been surgical. Malignant hypertension resulted in death within 6 months when treated with dietary therapy alone, but the use of surgical sympathectomy reduced this figure by half (100). Pancreatic islet transplant is still the only cure for type 1 diabetes (101). Coronary artery bypass surgery for coronary atherosclerosis is still used today, as is gastric bypass and other operations for obesity (102,103).

Safe and effective antihypertensive medications have essentially eliminated the need for surgery in the treatment of hypertension. It is the hope and expectation that safe and effective drug treatments for obesity will also eliminate the need for obesity surgery in the future. The first effective medications for hypertension in the 1940s, such as reserpine and ganglionic blockers, worked upstream on the central nervous system or on the sympathetic nerves to control blood pressure. Due to their associated side effects and their mode of action far from the blood vessels that mediate blood pressure, these drugs had side effects and are rarely used today. Ganglionic blocking agents interfered with the ability of the eye to focus, caused impotence and ileus and peptic ulcer disease, whereas reserpine caused depression (104).

Hydrochlorothiazide, which causes the loss of salt into the urine, was introduced in the 1950s and is still in use today (105). As the number of blood pressure medications increased, combination therapy became the norm, and some combinations with component medications affecting different control points in the same pathway gave more than additive reductions in blood pressure (106). With the multiple medication combinations now available to treat hypertension, it is the rare circumstance when good control of blood pressure cannot be obtained with well-tolerated medication combinations. This situation can be anticipated to occur in the future for obesity medication.

The second advance, in addition to combination therapy for hypertension, was the development of drugs that act on the blood vessels themselves. By having a mode of action on the blood vessels, spillover of side effects to other systems becomes less likely. For example, angiotensin receptor blockers act directly on blood vessels and are almost devoid of adverse events.

Presently, there is a limited arsenal of medications with which to treat obesity. In fact, there are only four drugs approved by the FDA for use in the United States without time limitations, based on the indications in the package insert. Approval of these drugs was based on 1- to 2-year trials. Liraglutide is approved for the treatment of diabetes, and its new drug application is presently pending at the FDA at a higher dose for the treatment of obesity. Orlistat, which causes a loss of fat in the stool, can be likened to a thiazide diuretic in the treatment of hypertension that causes a loss of sodium into the urine. As with thiazides, due to their safety and proven efficacy, orlistat is likely to remain an obesity treatment option even as more effective medications are developed. Phentermine/topiramate, lorcaserin, NAL/BUP, and liraglutide act on the central nervous system. Although these medications are effective and reasonably well tolerated, targeting of the central nervous system increases the risks of unintended adverse events in other systems. Symptoms such as headache may be only an annoyance, but teratogenicity has created concern in the medical community. It seems likely that phentermine/topiramate will become relegated to use in unusual circumstances for the treatment of obesity, much as α-methyldopa, an antihypertensive drug with actions in the central nervous system and once a popular treatment for hypertension is now reserved for unusual circumstances.

Developing drugs for the treatment of obesity comes with some special challenges. First, the drugs that have been used for the treatment of obesity have been accompanied by a litany of safety problems. This started with the first drug to be used for the treatment of obesity, thyroid hormone, which caused hyperthyroidism (107,108). Dinitrophenol was associated with cataracts, neuropathy, and even death by hyperthermia (109,110). Amphetamine was addictive, and aminorex, an amphetamine derivative with a noradrenergic mechanism, was removed from the European market for its association with primary pulmonary hypertension that carried 50% mortality (111,112). More recently, fenfluramine was removed from the market due to its association with cardiac valvulopathy, phenylpropanolamine was removed due to the risk of hemorrhagic stroke, and ephedra was removed due to systemic adrenergic stimulation (47,113,114). Most recently, sibutramine was removed from the market for an increase in nonfatal stroke, nonfatal myocardial infarction, resuscitation after cardiac arrest, or cardio-vascular death ($P < 0.02$) in a cardiovascular safety trial (115). This history has raised the bar for ensuring the safety of obesity medications. Adding to the concern about safety is the inadequacy of BMI categorization of obesity risk. The Edmonton Obesity Staging System (EOSS) proposes dividing overweight and obesity into stages: stage 0 that has no medical issues, stage 1 that has predisease risk such as prediabetes, stage 2 that has an established disease such as diabetes, stage 3 that has complications of diseases such diabetic retinopathy, and stage 4 that is end-stage disease (116). The BMI categories approach to assessing obesity risk was evaluated using mortality data from the NHANES and compared to the EOSS. Overweight (BMI 25–30) had mortality data that almost superimposed on Class III obesity (BMI >40) using the BMI risk categories, but the EOSS gave a progressively increasing mortality risk when going from stage 0 to stage 3 (117). Being able to assess obesity risk accurately should be of considerable help to drug development. The use of any drug is a process of weighing risks and benefits. Using the staging system, one could theoretically assign or develop drugs with more risks for those with the stages of obesity associated with higher mortality risks.

Another challenge is cost. Unlike medications for the other chronic diseases, obesity drugs are rarely covered by third-party payers. Thus, the cost of obesity drugs is borne by the patients, and price becomes a much greater constraint to sales than when medical insurance reimburses a large portion of the costs as is the case with diabetes. As safer and more effective drugs are developed for treating obesity, it is possible or even likely that patients will want access to these medications and their demand will prod insurance companies to include obesity drugs in the covered benefits. Coverage of obesity medications for federal workers has just recently been instituted, and if this trend continues, it may be another solution to the problem. Phentermine, a drug that is labeled for short-term use and has the DEA designation of class IV, suggesting addiction potential, albeit low, has consistently outsold the combined sales of the other drugs approved for the treatment of obesity without time limitations on use—lorcaserin, phentermine/topiramate, and orlistat—suggesting the importance of pricing (118).

The ideal obesity drug

Epidemiological studies have shown that weight loss increases mortality despite weight loss being associated with a reduction in cardiovascular risk factors (119,120). This paradox was first explained by the reanalysis of two previously published cohort studies that both measured skinfold thickness as a measure of body fat, in addition to body weight. This reanalysis showed that mortality increased by 30% for every standard deviation of weight loss, but decreased by 15% for every standard deviation of fat loss (121). Thus, a loss of fat seems to confer health while a loss of lean tissue is unhealthy. There is now clinical trial data to support the epidemiological assessments. The Swedish Obese Subjects Study demonstrated a reduction in all-cause mortality and cardiovascular mortality in subjects undergoing bariatric surgery compared to matched obese controls (84,119). Although an increased amount of body fat is a recognized mortality risk, visceral fat, the intra-abdominal fat that drains through the liver, is a greater mortality risk due to its association with insulin resistance (122). Visceral fat, liver fat, and insulin resistance are associated with hypertension, dyslipidemia, and diabetes, the major cardiovascular risks associated with obesity (123). Therefore, the ideal obesity drug would give substantial weight loss that was safe and well tolerated. Also, this ideal drug would give preferential loss of fat tissue and visceral fat in particular. This ideal agent is probably a combination of drugs, due to the redundant nature of control mechanisms for chronic diseases.

Approaches to obesity research

Empirical observations have been the most common impetus for progress in obesity research. Coleman and Hummel (124), for example, discovered a mouse that was massively obese due to a spontaneous mutation. They were able to demonstrate that its obesity was due to the lack of a receptor by parabiosis experiments. These observations eventually lead to the discovery of leptin (125). Progressing from empirical observations to physiological explanations, and then to molecular approaches that define the mechanism, has been the most common pathway of discovery in obesity. Physiological observations leading directly to new treatment has occurred less commonly, but Cone et al. (126) were able to demonstrate that μ-opioid receptors exist on POMC neurons in the arcuate nucleus of the hypothalamus. These μ-opioid receptors were subsequently shown to reduce the secretion of POMC. The cleavage products of POMC are α-melanocyte-stimulating hormone and an opioid. These observations lead to the combining of BUP, a stimulator of POMC, with NAL, an inhibitor of the μ-opioid receptor, and a time-released formulation of BUP and NAL was approved in September 2014 for the treatment of obesity (127). The human genome has now been sequenced and put in the public domain (128). This opens the possibility of moving from genes and the molecular basis of disease to physiology and then to new treatments. Thus, there is potential for much more rapid advances in treatment of obesity than existed when antihypertensive medications were developing.

MOLECULAR APPROACHES

An explosion of new technologies has increased the sensitivity of clinical analyte detection and the numbers of analytes that can be detected in a single biological sample. This is true not only for the measurement of hormones in blood but also for the measurement of metabolites of pathways, vitamins, and the circulating products of cell lysis. These tools can be used to tell whether a drug engages a target and to diagnose subtypes of obesity. These capabilities have the potential to revolutionize the way that we diagnose and therefore treat obesity.

One example of this technology is the bead-based immunoassay. This assay allows for the measurement of dozens of hormones in a single blood sample. In fact, most only require 50 μL or less of blood and are as accurate and precise as the classical enzyme-linked immunosorbent assay or radioimmunoassay. Sensitivity is occasionally a limitation (Table 13.1).

The major advances, however, have been in genome-based molecular approaches and technologies. For example, this kind of technological development is already changing the way in which we view cancer and cancer therapy. Widespread and inexpensive genetic testing leads to improved treatments for breast cancer and the identification of those women at increased risk. The rarity of genes where mutations lead to major effects has stymied the field of obesity research, but new discoveries such as the FTO (fat mass and obesity-associated) gene make it more likely that our genetic knowledge base will develop beyond the random candidate SNP analyses where the results are so often nonreproducible. Sequencing the genome of an individual is not that far away and promises to increase the power to identify genetic variation in genes that influence not only body weight but also other important subphenotypes, such as energy metabolism, propensity to binge eat, and capacity for burning fat. The promise of this kind of research is that treatments might be better tailored toward the specific causes. This field, called pharmacogenomics, should tip the risk–benefit ratio in a favorable direction by enhancing the prospects of a successful treatment and reduce the risk of treating patients with the "wrong" drug. When the

Table 13.1 Molecular approaches in obesity research

Sample type	Analysis	Classical measurement	New technology
Blood	Hormones, cytokines	Radioimmunoassay, enzyme-linked immunosorbent assay	Multiplex bead–based immunoassays
	Metabolites	Enzyme-based assays	Mass spectrometry–based metabolomics
	mRNA	Northern blots	Gene expression level[a]
	Protein, enzyme	Western imunoassay	Proteomics
	Gene variation	DNA single-nucleotide polymorphisms	Whole-genome sequencing, genome-wide association studies
	Genomic modification	None	Epigenome analysis[b]
Tissue	mRNA	None	Gene expression level[a]
	Protein	None	Proteomics, multiplex bead–based immunoassays
	Protein	None	Tissue arrays
	Metabolism	None	Stem cell isolation for metabolic studies

[a] New techniques for gene expression include quantitative reverse transcriptase-polymerase chain reaction and various platforms for near-whole genome "transcriptome" analysis.

[b] See text for a discussion.

genetic science is fully developed, in other words when we know which genes are responsible for what subtypes of obesity, the diagnostic technologies will already be available to roll this into the clinic.

Another example of how a new technology promises to revolutionize is the microarray (transcriptome). Microarray analysis allows for the measurement of essentially every gene that is expressed in a sample. This kind of analysis can be used for peripheral blood mononuclear cells or any tissue to identify which genes are up-regulated and which genes are downregulated in a given condition. The cost of this technology has dropped dramatically, leading to clinical utility in cancer. For example, knowing the pattern of gene expression in biopsy specimens from cancers leads to a more precise diagnosis compared to histopathological analysis alone. Furthermore, the pattern of genes expressed predicts responses to specific kinds of treatments. We are just now beginning to see this kind of analysis in patients with obesity where the promise will lead to better strategies for the diagnosis and treatments that are specific for a person's subtype of obesity (129).

The new field of epigenomics is charging ahead. The epigenome refers to modification of the DNA or the proteins that fold and coil the DNA (130). The best studied is the methylation of cytosines in the DNA backbone. These modifications occur in regions known as CpG islands and modify the expression of genes (i.e., turn them on or off). There is growing evidence that these DNA modifications might predispose persons to the risk of obesity, just like for mutations in the classic ATGC nucleotides (SNPs) (131). When the important regions of the genome are identified, a simple blood sample could identify a specific subtype of obesity—another type of genetic testing—as a means of improving patient care.

Not all new technologies are genetic, however. A few others deserve mention. Metabolome (132–134) and lipidome (135) refer to the overall pattern of metabolites and lipids in the blood. Mass spectrometry methods allow for the simultaneous detection of hundreds to thousands of analytes in blood or urine.

So, how might all of these data points fit together to help us in the treatment of obesity? Will we require genomics, epigenomics, transcriptomics, proteomics, metabolomics, *and* lipidomics? Probably not. We are generally optimistic that the research process will lead us to a small group of analytes that capture the complexity of a person's diagnostic pattern. Alternately, there may be more power and/or precision in measuring multiple analytes simultaneously. New statistical techniques such as advanced principal components analysis, cluster analysis, or FOREL (FORmal ELement) can reduce a multidimensional dataset into two or three dimensions, making the subgrouping of subjects into discrete diagnostic categories much easier (136). Pathway analysis of transcriptome data or metabolome data may identify metabolic pathways where a specific therapy can be applied. At this point, all we can say is that the tools and techniques are in place to move us toward a molecular diagnostic paradigm in obesity. This is the clear trend in most other diseases, such as cancer (137,138).

The major barrier to the adoption of these technologies is cost. Payers seem willing to pay for these kinds of technologies, such as magnetic resonance imaging and positron emission tomography scans, when a patient is diagnosed with cancer. The situation is very different with obesity and metabolic disorders, even though the risk of dying from obesity can be very high for some patients. For example, it is difficult for the average physician to get paid for the measurement of two of the most important metabolic hormones: insulin and adiponectin. Both have strong positive predictive values for disease and can be used to gauge the effectiveness of a therapy such as thiazolidinediones; however, it is difficult to convince payers of the value of these tests when the economics are difficult to quantify. We believe that one likely scenario is that one of these molecular technologies will become cost effective by identifying a subpopulation of obese patients that will be super-responders to a specific drug therapy. If one of these tests could identify even 5% of the population who would lose 25% body weight with a drug that typically produces 5% to 10% body weight loss, it would make the test much more attractive from a cost perspective. Thus, pharmacogenomics, or "personalized medicine" (139), is one way to get payers to reimburse the molecular testing, giving them justification for not paying for pharmacotherapy of obese patients that are unlikely to respond, and yet paying for pharmacotherapy of obese patients that are likely to respond. This scenario is a double-edged sword because this approach might be used to deny treatment to patients who might benefit from a drug.

New molecular technologies and approaches will revolutionize the diagnosis of obesity and influence pharmacotherapy. Picking the "winning horse" in this race is no easy task, but it is almost certain that one of them will be a winner.

ADVANCED CLINICAL ENDPOINTS

When testing a new drug for obesity, the simplest approach is to see whether the drug causes weight loss. This is a long and expensive process requiring hundreds of participants and months of treatment. An alternate approach is, after confirming that the drug is safe and tolerated in multiple-dose phase I studies, to test for effects on resting or 24-hour energy expenditure (140), hepatic lipid, food intake (141,142), or other behaviors such as binge eating (143). These kinds of advanced clinical endpoints may provide early clues to a drug's efficacy in short-term studies and stimulate the investment in a subsequent classic clinical phase II testing paradigm. The danger in these intermediate proof-of-concept studies is twofold. An ambiguous outcome where a drug gives some positive result, but not a definitive answer, can slow decision making and stall the development of a good drug. Alternately, a negative result for a "noisy" measure, as is often the case for measuring food intake, does not absolutely mean the drug will be ineffective in a longer clinical study. Newer technologies such as whole-body nuclear magnetic resonance (144) may be more precise than existing technologies. This may lead the measurement of changes in body energy stores (body fat) as opposed to the measurement of body weight; measuring body weight is often noisy because of changes in body water. With some caveats, the drug development field has a love–hate relationship with advanced clinical endpoints. The advantages of these measures in developing obesity drugs (justifies the investment, reveals new pharmacodynamic properties of a target) do not always outweigh the disadvantages (slow, often not definitive). A full discussion is beyond the scope of this chapter, but suffice it to say that advanced clinical endpoints can be helpful in drug development if used carefully and judiciously (Table 13.2).

Table 13.2 Clinical approaches in obesity research

Measurement	Technology
Food intake	Single meal or 24-hour inpatient testing
	Telephone- or Internet-based diet intake assessment
Hunger	VAS and/or fMRI (leptin)
Energy expenditure	DLW, hood (indirect) calorimetry[a]
Spontaneous physical activity	Pedometers, accelerometers, or DLW + REE
Body composition	Weight, DEXA, MRI, qNMR
Fat distribution	
Visceral adipose tissue	CT scan or MRI
Intermuscular adipose tissue	CT scan or MRI
Epicardial adipose tissue	CT scan or MRI, also echocardiography
Fat oxidation during a meal	Stable isotope
Gastric emptying	Stable isotope or acetaminophen appearance
Gut peptide secretion	Indwelling IV catheter and special blood specimen–handling procedures
Vascular reactivity	Brachial artery flow–mediated dilatation
	Peripheral arterial tonometry[b]
"Ectopic" lipid	
Intramyocellular or intrahepatic lipid	MRS
Exercise parameters	VO_2
	Maximal oxygen consumption
	^{31}P magnetic resonance spectroscopy
Blood pressure	24-hour ambulatory blood pressure monitoring
Insulin sensitivity	Euglycemic hyperinsulinemic clamp, FSIGTT, oGTT
Tissue effects	Microdialysis of adipose tissue to measure lipolysis
	Adipose tissue, liver, or muscle biopsy

Note: CT, computed tomography; DEXA, dual-energy x-ray absorptiometry; DLW, doubly labeled water; fMRI, functional MRI; FSIGTT, frequently sampled intravenous glucose tolerance test; MRI, magnetic resonance imaging; MRS, magnetic resonance spectroscopy; oGTT, oral glucose tolerance test; qNMR, quantitative nuclear magnetic resonance; REE, resting energy expenditure; VAS, Visual Analog Scales.

[a] Measures resting energy expenditure only.
[b] See text for a discussion.

An alternate view of advanced clinical endpoints is that they can reveal beneficial effects of a drug. For example, magnetic resonance spectroscopy can be used to measure fat in the liver as a surrogate for biopsies. Some obesity drugs may have direct effects on the liver or modulate areas in the brain that control liver metabolism. Many of the newer obesity targets are likely to have weight loss–independent effects on insulin secretion or insulin resistance (145). This makes the measurement of insulin sensitivity particularly important. Many of these measures are not practical in large numbers of subjects. The more invasive studies can often make up for this limitation as they are more precise. It is critical to know in advance the test–retest stability of a measure—that is, precision—before including these measures. This is important not only to reduce sample size and cost but also to be able to trust the negative result.

CONCLUSIONS

We are presently experiencing a proliferation in obesity research. The declaration of obesity as a chronic disease and not just bad habits was not nearly as powerful as the discovery of leptin, a hormone that is genetically absent in a small minority of rodents and humans. The response of leptin-deficient obesity with weight loss to the replacement of leptin, more than anything else, convinced the scientific community that obesity is a chronic physiological problem worthy of study. This interest and scientific exploration have resulted in new discoveries that impact obesity treatment.

This chapter has reviewed some of these advances in diet, lifestyle, and exercise therapy. Dietary herbal supplements have been developed that are more promising than in the past, but these promising trials still require confirmation by independent research groups. Not only are obesity surgeries advancing, but also new devices based on the physiology of obesity surgery are making surgical strategies less invasive. The stimulation of obesity research has resulted in a better understanding of obesity pathophysiology, and several new drugs, many of which are combination pharmaceuticals. We are in a new era of scientific tools and technology. The human genome has been sequenced, and we have sophisticated molecular tools in addition to advanced physiological endpoints that we did not previously have. This places obesity in a situation that predicts much more rapid progress in reaching the goal of a safe and effective treatment than was the case for other chronic diseases such as hypertension. Thus, there is hope for returning those who suffer from the disease to a healthy and socially acceptable weight in the foreseeable future. The safety and efficacy of these various treatment modalities vary. Diets and herbs that are classified by the FDA as foods are the least risky, medications and devices are intermediate in risk, and surgery carries the highest risk, but efficacy is greater for long-term maintenance of weight loss as the risk increases. It is hoped that the expected progress will provide new treatments that increase efficacy and reduce risk for the same degree of efficacy.

REFERENCES

1. Wigand R, Gelderblom H, Wadell G. New human adenovirus (candidate adenovirus 36), a novel member of subgroup D. *Arch Virol*. 1980;64(3):225–33.
2. Atkinson RL. Viruses as an etiology of obesity. *Mayo Clin Proc*. 2007;82(10):1192–8.
3. Atkinson RL, Dhurandhar NV, Allison DB, Bowen RI, Israel BA, Albu JB, et al. Human adenovirus-36 is associated with increased body weight and paradoxical reduction of serum lipids. *Int J Obes (Lond)*. 2005;29(3):281–6.

4. Rogers PM, Fusinski KA, Rathod MA, Loiler SA, Pasarica M, Shaw MK, et al. Human adenovirus Ad-36 induces adipogenesis via its E4 orf-1 gene. *Int J Obes (Lond)*. 2008;32(3):397–406.

5. Krajmalnik-Brown R, Ilhan ZE, Kang DW, Dibaise JK. Effects of gut microbes on nutrient absorption and energy regulation. *Nutr Clin Pract*. 2012;27(2):201–14.

6. Casazza K, Brown A, Astrup A, Bertz F, Baum C, Bohan Brown M, et al. Weighing the evidence of common beliefs in obesity research. *Crit Rev Food Sci Nutr*. 2015;55(14):2014–53.

7. Casazza K, Pate R, Allison DB. Myths, presumptions, and facts about obesity. *N Engl J Med*. 2013;368(23):2236–7.

8. Casazza K, Fontaine KR, Astrup A, Birch LL, Brown AW, Bohan Brown MM, et al. Myths, presumptions, and facts about obesity. *N Engl J Med*. 2013;368(5):446–54.

9. Shefer G, Marcus Y, Stern N. Is obesity a brain disease? *Neurosci Biobehav Rev*. 2013;37(10 Pt 2):2489–503.

10. Thaler JP, Yi CX, Schur EA, Guyenet SJ, Hwang BH, Dietrich MO, et al. Obesity is associated with hypothalamic injury in rodents and humans. *J Clin Invest*. 2012;122(1):153–62.

11. Horvath TL, Sarman B, Garcia-Caceres C, Enriori PJ, Sotonyi P, Shanabrough M, et al. Synaptic input organization of the melanocortin system predicts diet-induced hypothalamic reactive gliosis and obesity. *Proc Natl Acad Sci U S A*. 2010;107(33):14875–80.

12. Heilbronn LK, De Jonge L, Frisard MI, Delany JP, Larson-Meyer DE, Rood J, et al. Effect of 6-month calorie restriction on biomarkers of longevity, metabolic adaptation, and oxidative stress in overweight individuals: A randomized controlled trial. *JAMA*. 2006;295(13):1539–48.

13. Astrup A. Dietary composition, substrate balances and body fat in subjects with a pre-disposition to obesity. *Int J Obes Relat Metab Disord*. 1993;17 Suppl 3:S32–6; Discussion S41–2.

14. Knowler WC, Barrett-Connor E, Fowler SE, Hamman RF, Lachin JM, Walker EA, et al. Reduction in the incidence of type 2 diabetes with lifestyle intervention or metformin. *N Engl J Med*. 2002;346(6):393–403.

15. Tuomilehto J, Lindstrom J, Eriksson JG, Valle TT, Hamalainen H, Ilanne-Parikka P, et al. Prevention of type 2 diabetes mellitus by changes in lifestyle among subjects with impaired glucose tolerance. *N Engl J Med*. 2001;344(18):1343–50.

16. Clinical Guidelines on the identification, evaluation, and treatment of overweight and obesity in adults—The evidence report. National Institutes of Health. *Obes Res*. 1998;6 Suppl 2:51s–209s.

17. Hamman RF, Wing RR, Edelstein SL, Lachin JM, Bray GA, Delahanty L, et al. Effect of weight loss with lifestyle intervention on risk of diabetes. *Diabetes Care*. 2006;29(9):2102–7.

18. Heshka S, Anderson JW, Atkinson RL, Greenway FL, Hill JO, Phinney SD, et al. Weight loss with self-help compared with a structured commercial program: A randomized trial. *JAMA*. 2003;289(14):1792–8.

19. Rock CL, Flatt SW, Sherwood NE, Karanja N, Pakiz B, Thomson CA. Effect of a free prepared meal and incentivized weight loss program on weight loss and weight loss maintenance in obese and overweight women: A randomized controlled trial. *JAMA*. 2010;304(16):1803–10.

20. Pavlou KN, Krey S, Steffee WP. Exercise as an adjunct to weight loss and maintenance in moderately obese subjects. *Am J Clin Nutr.* 1989;49 5 Suppl:1115–23.
21. Church T, Earnest C, Blair S. Dietary overcompensation across different doses of exercise. *Obesity.* 2007;15 Suppl:A17.
22. Shai I, Schwarzfuchs D, Henkin Y, Shahar DR, Witkow S, Greenberg I, et al. Weight loss with a low-carbohydrate, Mediterranean, or low-fat diet. *N Engl J Med.* 2008;359(3):229–41.
23. Sacks FM, Bray GA, Carey VJ, Smith SR, Ryan DH, Anton SD, et al. Comparison of weight loss diets with different compositions of fat, protein, and carbohydrates. *N Engl J Med.* 2009;360(9):859–73.
24. Cornier MA, Donahoo WT, Pereira R, Gurevich I, Westergren R, Enerback S, et al. Insulin sensitivity determines the effectiveness of dietary macronutrient composition on weight loss in obese women. *Obes Res.* 2005;13(4):703–9.
25. Foster GD, Wyatt HR, Hill JO, Mcguckin BG, Brill C, Mohammed BS, et al. A randomized trial of a low-carbohydrate diet for obesity. *N Engl J Med.* 2003;348(21):2082–90.
26. Ebbeling CB, Leidig MM, Feldman HA, Lovesky MM, Ludwig DS. Effects of a low-glycemic load vs low-fat diet in obese young adults: A randomized trial. *JAMA.* 2007;297(19):2092–102.
27. Orentreich N, Matias JR, Defelice A, Zimmerman JA. Low methionine ingestion by rats extends life span. *J Nutr.* 1993;123(2):269–74.
28. Hasek BE, Stewart LK, Henagan TM, Boudreau A, Lenard NR, Black C, et al. Dietary methionine restriction enhances metabolic flexibility and increases uncoupled respiration in both fed and fasted states. *Am J Physiol Regul Integr Comp Physiol* 2010;299(3):R728–39.
29. Epner DE, Morrow S, Wilcox M, Houghton JL. Nutrient intake and nutritional indexes in adults with metastatic cancer on a phase 1 clinical trial of dietary methionine restriction. *Nutr Cancer.* 2002;42(2):158–66.
30. Plaisance EP, Greenway FL, Boudreau A, Hill KL, Johnson WD, Krajcik RA, et al. Dietary methionine restriction increases fat oxidation in obese adults with metabolic syndrome. *J Clin Endocrinol Metab.* 2011;96(5):E836–40.
31. Perrone CE, Mattocks DA, Plummer JD, Chittur SV, Mohney R, Vignola K, et al. Genomic and metabolic responses to methionine-restricted and methionine-restricted, cysteine-supplemented diets in Fischer 344 rat inguinal adipose tissue, liver and quadriceps muscle. *J Nutrigenet Nutrigenomics.* 2012;5(3):132–57.
32. Wadden TA, Berkowitz RI, Womble LG, Sarwer DB, Phelan S, Cato RK, et al. Randomized trial of lifestyle modification and pharmacotherapy for obesity. *N Engl J Med.* 2005;353(20):2111–20.
33. Lichtman SW, Pisarska K, Berman ER, Pestone M, Dowling H, Offenbacher E, et al. Discrepancy between self-reported and actual caloric intake and exercise in obese subjects. *N Engl J Med.* 1992;327(27):1893–8.
34. Martin CK, Nicklas T, Gunturk B, Correa JB, Allen HR, Champagne C. Measuring food intake with digital photography. *J Hum Nutr Diet.* 2014;27 Suppl 1:72–81.
35. Martin CK, Correa JB, Han H, Allen HR, Rood JC, Champagne CM, et al. Validity of the remote food photography method (RFPM) for estimating energy and nutrient intake in near real-time. *Obesity (Silver Spring).* 2012;20(4):891–9.

36. Thomas DM, Martin CK, Heymsfield S, Redman LM, Schoeller DA, Levine JA. A Simple model predicting individual weight change in humans. *J Biol Dyn.* 2011;5(6):579–99.

37. Thomas DM, Martin CK, Lettieri S, Bredlau C, Kaiser K, Church T, et al. Can a weight loss of one pound a week be achieved with a 3500-kcal deficit? Commentary on a commonly accepted rule. *Int J Obes (Lond).* 2013;37(12):1611–13.

38. Hall KD, Sacks G, Chandramohan D, Chow CC, Wang YC, Gortmaker SL, et al. Quantification of the effect of energy imbalance on bodyweight. *Lancet.* 2011;378(9793):826–37.

39. Zhang K, Pi-Sunyer FX, Boozer CN. Improving energy expenditure estimation for physical activity. *Med Sci Sports Exerc.* 2004;36(5):883–9.

40. Ryan J, Gormley J. An evaluation of energy expenditure estimation by three activity monitors. *Eur J Sport Sci.* 2013;13(6):681–8.

41. Johannsen DL, Calabro MA, Stewart J, Franke W, Rood JC, Welk GJ. Accuracy of armband monitors for measuring daily energy expenditure in healthy adults. *Med Sci Sports Exerc.* 2010;42(11):2134–40.

42. US FDA. Dietary Supplement Health And Education Act of 1994. http://wwwfdagov/regulatoryinformation/legislation/federalfooddrugandcosmeticactfdcact/significantamendmentstothefdcact/ucm148003htm

43. Congressional hearing investigates Dr. Oz 'miracle' weight loss claims. 2014. http://wwwcnncom/2014/06/17/health/senate-grills-dr-oz/, accessed December 8, 2014.

44. Authors retract green coffee bean diet paper touted by Dr. Oz. 2014. http://retractionwatchcom/2014/10/20/authors-retract-green-coffee-bean-diet-paper-touted-by-dr-oz/, accessed December 8, 2014.

45. Greenway FL. The safety and efficacy of pharmaceutical and herbal caffeine and ephedrine use as a weight loss agent. *Obes Rev.* 2001;2(3):199–211.

46. Cockey CD. Ephedra banned. *Awhonn Lifelines.* 2004;8(1):19–25.

47. Shekelle PG, Hardy ML, Morton SC, Maglione M, Mojica WA, Suttorp MJ, et al. Efficacy and safety of ephedra and ephedrine for weight loss and athletic performance: A meta-analysis. *JAMA.* 2003;289(12):1537–45.

48. United States Drug Enforcement Administration. 2014. http://www.justice.gov/dea/druginfo/concern_thebaine.shtml

49. Maeda H, Tsukui T, Sashima T, Hosokawa M, Miyashita K. Seaweed carotenoid, fucoxanthin, as a multi-functional nutrient. *Asia Pac J Clin Nutr.* 2008;17 Suppl 1:196–9.

50. Abidov M, Ramazanov Z, Seifulla R, Grachev S. The effects of Xanthigen in the weight management of obese premenopausal women with non-alcoholic fatty liver disease and normal liver fat. *Diabetes Obes Metab* 2010;12(1):72–81.

51. Maeda H, Hosokawa M, Sashima T, Funayama K, Miyashita K. Effect of medium-chain triacylglycerols on anti-obesity effect of fucoxanthin. *J Oleo Sci.* 2007;56(12):615–21.

52. Maeda H, Hosokawa M, Sashima T, Miyashita K. Dietary combination of fucoxanthin and fish oil attenuates the weight gain of white adipose tissue and decreases blood glucose in obese/diabetic kk-ay mice. *J Agric Food Chem.* 2007;55(19):7701–6.

53. Maclean DB, Luo LG. Increased ATP content/production in the hypothalamus may be a signal for energy-sensing of satiety: Studies of the anorectic mechanism of a plant steroidal glycoside. *Brain Res.* 2004;1020(1–2):1–11.

54. Blom WA, Abrahamse SL, Bradford R, Duchateau GS, Theis W, Orsi A, et al. Effects of 15-d repeated consumption of *Hoodia gordonii* purified extract on safety, ad libitum energy intake, and body weight in healthy, overweight women: A randomized controlled trial. *Am J Clin Nutr.* 2011;94(5):1171–81.

55. Oben J, Kuate D, Agbor G, Momo C, Talla X. The use of a *Cissus quadrangularis* formulation in the management of weight loss and metabolic syndrome. *Lipids Health Dis.* 2006;5:24.

56. Oben JE, Enyegue DM, Fomekong GI, Soukontoua YB, Agbor GA. The effect of *Cissus quadrangularis* (CQR-300) and a Cissus formulation (CORE) on obesity and obesity-induced oxidative stress. *Lipids Health Dis.* 2007;6:4.

57. Oben JE, Ngondi JL, Momo CN, Agbor GA, Sobgui CS. The use of a *Cissus quadrangularis/Irvingia gabonensis* combination in the management of weight loss: A double-blind placebo-controlled study. *Lipids Health Dis.* 2008;7:12.

58. Sullivan AC, et al. Factors Influencing the *in vivo* Rates of Lipogenesis in Rat Liver. *J Nutr.* 1971;101:265–272.

59. Sullivan AC. Inhibition of lipogenesus in rat liver by (–)hydroxycitrate. *Arch Biochem. Biophys.* 1972;150 (1):183–190.

60. Sullivan AC, et al. Effect of (–) hydroxycitrate upon the accumulation of lipik in the rat: I. Lipogenesis. *Lipids.* 1974;9(2):121–128.

61. Sullivan AC, et al. Effect of (–) hydroxycitrate upon the accumulation of lipik in the rat: II. Appetite. *Lipids.* 1974;9(2):129–134.

62. Heymsfield SB, Allison DB, Vasselli JR, Pietrobelli A, Greenfield D, Nunez C. *Garcinia cambogia* (hydroxycitric acid) as a potential antiobesity agent: A randomized controlled trial. *JAMA.* 1998;280(18):1596–600.

63. Preuss HG, Garis RI, Bramble JD, Bagchi D, Bagchi M, Rao CV, et al. Efficacy of a novel calcium/potassium salt of (-)-hydroxycitric acid in weight control. *Int J Clin Pharmacol Res.* 2005;25(3):133–44.

64. Stern JS, Peerson J, Mishra AT, Sadasiva Rao MV, Rajeswari KP. Efficacy and tolerability of a novel herbal formulation for weight management. *Obesity (Silver Spring).* 2013;21(5):921–7.

65. Keenan MJ, Zhou J, Mccutcheon KL, Raggio AM, Bateman HG, Todd E, et al. Effects of resistant starch, a non-digestible fermentable fiber, on reducing body fat. *Obesity (Silver Spring).* 2006;14(9):1523–34.

66. Zhou J, Hegsted M, Mccutcheon KL, Keenan MJ, Xi X, Raggio AM, et al. Peptide Yy and proglucagon mRNA expression patterns and regulation in the gut. *Obesity (Silver Spring).* 2006;14(4):683–9.

67. Greenway F, O'Neil CE, Stewart L, Rood J, Keenan M, Martin R. Fourteen weeks of treatment with viscofiber increased fasting levels of glucagon-like peptide-1 and peptide-yy. *J Med Food.* 2007;10(4):720–4.

68. Rudkowska I, Roynette CE, Demonty I, Vanstone CA, Jew S, Jones PJ. Diacylglycerol: Efficacy and mechanism of action of an anti-obesity agent. *Obes Res.* 2005;13(11):1864–76.

69. Taguchi H, Nagao T, Watanabe H, Onizawa K, Matsuo N, Tokimitsu I, et al. Energy value and digestibility of dietary oil containing mainly 1,3-diacylglycerol are similar to those of triacylglycerol. *Lipids.* 2001;36(4):379–82.

70. Kamphuis MM, Mela DJ, Westerterp-Plantenga MS. Diacylglycerols affect substrate oxidation and appetite in humans. *Am J Clin Nutr.* 2003;77(5):1133–9.

71. Matsuyama T, Shoji K, Watanabe H, Shimizu M, Saotome Y, Nagao T, et al. Effects of diacylglycerol oil on adiposity in obese children: Initial communication. *J Pediatr Endocrinol Metab*. 2006;19(6):795–804.

72. Chorvat RJ, Berbaum J, Seriacki K, Mcelroy JF. Jd-5006 and Jd-5037: Peripherally restricted (pr) cannabinoid-1 receptor blockers related to slv-319 (ibipinabant) as metabolic disorder therapeutics devoid of CNS liabilities. *Bioorg Med Chem Lett*. 2012;22(19):6173–80.

73. Chorvat RJ. Peripherally restricted cb1 receptor blockers. *Bioorg Med Chem Lett*. 2013;23(17):4751–60.

74. Fitzgerald LW, Burn TC, Brown BS, Patterson JP, Corjay MH, Valentine PA, et al. Possible role of valvular serotonin 5-ht(2b) receptors in the cardiopathy associated with fenfluramine. *Mol Pharmacol*. 2000;57(1):75–81.

75. Smith SR, Weissman NJ, Anderson CM, Sanchez M, Chuang E, Stubbe S, et al. Multicenter, placebo-controlled trial of lorcaserin for weight management. *N Engl J Med*. 2010;363(3):245–56.

76. Clinicaltrials.Gov. A multicenter pilot study of 12-week duration to assess the short-term safety and tolerability of lorcaserin plus two doses of immediate-release phentermine-HCL compared with lorcaserin alone in overweight and obese adults. 2013. https://clinicaltrials.gov/ct2/results?term=lorcaserin+and+phentermine&search=search

77. Kopelman P, Bryson A, Hickling R, Rissanen A, Rossner S, Toubro S, et al. Cetilistat (ATL-962), a novel lipase inhibitor: A 12-week randomized, placebo-controlled study of weight reduction in obese patients. *Int J Obes (Lond)*. 2007;31(3):494–9.

78. Astrup A, Meier DH, Mikkelsen BO, Villumsen JS, Larsen TM. Weight loss produced by tesofensine in patients with Parkinson's or Alzheimer's disease. *Obesity (Silver Spring)*. 2008;16(6):1363–9.

79. Sjodin A, Gasteyger C, Nielsen A-LH, Madsbad S, Breum L, Kroustrup JP, et al. The effects of tesofensine on body composition in obese subjects. *Int J Obes*. 2008;32 Suppl 1:S83.

80. Astrup A, Madsbad S, Breum L, Jensen TJ, Kroustrup JP, Larsen TM. Effect of tesofensine on bodyweight loss, body composition, and quality of life in obese patients: A randomised, double-blind, placebo-controlled trial. *Lancet*. 2008;372(9653):1906–13.

81. Greenway FL, Fujioka K, Plodkowski RA, Mudaliar S, Guttadauria M, Erickson J, et al. Effect of naltrexone plus bupropion on weight loss in overweight and obese adults (COR-I): A multicentre, randomised, double-blind, placebo-controlled, phase 3 trial. *Lancet*. 2010;376(9741):595–605.

82. Greenway FL, Anderson JW, Atkinson RL, Fujioka K, Gadde KM, Gupta AK, et al. Bupropion and zonisamide for the treatment of obesity. *Obes Res*. 2006;14 Suppl:A17.

83. Gadde KM, Allison DB, Ryan DH, Peterson CA, Troupin B, Schwiers ML, et al. Effects of low-dose, controlled-release, phentermine plus topiramate combination on weight and associated comorbidities in overweight and obese adults (conquer): A randomised, placebo-controlled, phase 3 trial. *Lancet*. 2011;377(9774):1341–52.

84. Astrup A, Rossner S, Van Gaal L, Rissanen A, Niskanen L, Al Hakim M, et al. Effects of liraglutide in the treatment of obesity: A randomised, double-blind, placebo-controlled study. *Lancet*. 2009;374(9701):1606–16.

85. FDA Committee Recommends Approval For Liraglutide As Anti-Obesity Drug. http://formularyjournalmodernmedicinecom/formulary-journal/content/tags/liraglutide/FDA-Committee-Recommends-Approval-Liraglutide-Anti-Obesit?Page=Full, accessed December 8, 2014.

86. Fiercebiotech. *Zafgen Announces Initial Results from Phase 2a Study of Beloranib in Patients with Prader-Willi Syndrome.* 2014. http://www.Fiercebiotech.Com/Press-Releases/Zafgen-Announces-Initial-Results-Phase-2a-Study-Beloranib-Patients-Prader-W

87. Businesswire. Research And Markets: Obesity Velneperit (S-2367)—Forecast and Market Analysis To 2022. 2014. http://www.Businesswire.Com/News/Home/20140403005650/En/Research-Markets-Obesity-Velneperit-S-2367---Forecast

88. Sjostrom L, Narbro K, Sjostrom CD, Karason K, Larsson B, Wedel H, et al. Effects of bariatric surgery on mortality in Swedish obese subjects. *N Engl J Med.* 2007;357(8):741–52.

89. Chang SH, Stoll CR, Song J, Varela JE, Eagon CJ, Colditz GA. The effectiveness and risks of bariatric surgery: An updated systematic review and meta-analysis, 2003–2012. *JAMA Surg.* 2014;149(3):275–87.

90. Stimac D, Majanovic SK. The position of endoscopic procedures in the treatment of obesity. *Curr Clin Pharmacol.* 2013;8(3):238–46.

91. WebMD. *FDA Panel Backs Appetite-Curbing Implant For Severely Obese.* 2014. http://www.Webmd.Com/Diet/News/20140617/Fda-Considers-Appetite-Curbing-Implant-For-Severely-Obese?Page=2

92. Obalon.Com. *The Obalon Balloon. The Power of Innovation Applied to Weight Loss.* 2014. http://www.Obalon.Com/Hcp/En/

93. Society of American Gastrointestinal & Endoscopic Surgeons. 2014. http://www.Sages.Org/Meetings/Annual-Meeting/Abstracts-Archive/First-Clinical-Experience-With-The-Transpyloric-Shuttle-Tpsr-Device-A-Non-Surgical-Endoscopic-Treatment-For-Obesity-Results-From-A-3-Month-And-6-Month-Study/

94. Patel SR, Mason J, Hakim N. The duodenal-jejunal bypass sleeve (endobarrier gastrointestinal liner) for weight loss and treatment of type II diabetes. *Indian J Surg.* 2012;74(4):275–7.

95. Golden RL. William Osler at 150: An overview of a life. *JAMA.* 1999;282(23):2252–8.

96. Health implications of obesity. National Institutes of Health Consensus Development Conference Statement. *Ann Intern Med.* 1985;103(1):147–51.

97. The New York Times. A.M.A. Recognizes Obesity As A Disease. 2013. http://www.Nytimes.Com/2013/06/19/Business/Ama-Recognizes-Obesity-As-A-Disease.Html?_R=0

98. Banting FG. Pancreatic extracts in the treatment of diabetes mellitus: Preliminary report. *Can Med Assoc J.* 1922;12(3):141–6.

99. Kempner W. Treatment of hypertensive disease with rice diet. *Am J Med.* 1948;3:545.

100. Platt R, Gilchrist R, Wilson C, Cooke W. Discussion on sympathectomy in hypertension. *Br Heart J.* 1948;10(4):293–7.

101. Gliedman ML, Tellis VA, Soberman R, Rifkin H, Veith FJ. Long-term effects of pancreatic transplant function in patients with advanced juvenile-onset diabetes. *Diabetes Care.* 1978;1(1):1–9.

102. Song YB, On YK, Kim JH, Shin DH, Kim JS, Sung J, et al. The effects of atorvastatin on the occurrence of postoperative atrial fibrillation after off-pump coronary artery bypass grafting surgery. *Am Heart J.* 2008;156(2):373. E9–16.

103. Karamanakos SN, Vagenas K, Kalfarentzos F, Alexandrides TK. Weight loss, appetite suppression, and changes in fasting and postprandial ghrelin and peptide-yy levels after Roux-en-Y gastric bypass and sleeve gastrectomy: A prospective, double blind study. *Ann Surg*. 2008;247(3):401–7.

104. Dequattro V, Li D. Sympatholytic therapy in primary hypertension: A user friendly role for the future. *J Hum Hypertens*. 2002;16 Suppl 1:S118–23.

105. Rapoport A, Evans BM, Wong H. Some short-term metabolic effects of chlorothiazide in hypertensives on a rice diet. *Can Med Assoc J*. 1959;81:984–90.

106. McMahon FG. Efficacy of an antihypertensive agent. comparison of methyldopa and hydrochlorothiazide in combination and singly. *JAMA*. 1975;231(2):155–8.

107. Putnam J. Cases of myxoedema and acromegalia treated with benefit by sheep's thyroids. *Am J Med Sci*. 1893;106(2):125–48.

108. Gardner DF, Kaplan MM, Stanley CA, Utiger RD. Effect of tri-iodothyronine replacement on the metabolic and pituitary responses to starvation. *N Engl J Med*. 1979;300(11):579–84.

109. Masserman J. Dinotrophenol. Its therapeutic and toxic actions in certain types of psychobiologic underactivity. *JAMA*. 1934;102:523.

110. Colman E. Dinitrophenol and obesity: An early twentieth-century regulatory dilemma. *Regul Toxicol Pharmacol*. 2007;48(2):115–17.

111. Bartholomew AA. Amphetamine addiction. *Med J Aust*. 1970;1(24):1209–14.

112. Kramer MS, Lane DA. Aminorex, dexfenfluramine, and primary pulmonary hypertension. *J Clin Epidemiol*. 1998;51(4):361–4.

113. Connolly HM, Crary JL, McGoon MD, Hensrud DD, Edwards BS, Edwards WD, et al. Valvular heart disease associated with fenfluramine-phentermine. *N Engl J Med*. 1997;337(9):581–8.

114. Kernan WN, Viscoli CM, Brass LM, Broderick JP, Brott T, Feldmann E, et al. Phenylpropanolamine and the risk of hemorrhagic stroke. *N Engl J Med*. 2000;343(25):1826–32.

115. James WP, Caterson ID, Coutinho W, Finer N, Van Gaal LF, Maggioni AP, et al. Effect of sibutramine on cardiovascular outcomes in overweight and obese subjects. *N Engl J Med*. 2010;363(10):905–17.

116. Sharma AM, Kushner RF. A proposed clinical staging system for obesity. *Int J Obes (Lond)*. 2009;33(3):289–95.

117. Padwal RS, Pajewski NM, Allison DB, Sharma AM. Using the Edmonton Obesity Staging System to predict mortality in a population-representative cohort of people with overweight and obesity. *CMAJ*. 2011;183(14):E1059–66.

118. Stafford RS, Radley DC. National trends in antiobesity medication use. *Arch Intern Med*. 2003;163(9):1046–50.

119. Andres R, Muller DC, Sorkin JD. Long-term effects of change in body weight on all-cause mortality. A review. *Ann Intern Med*. 1993;119(7 Pt 2):737–43.

120. Pi-Sunyer FX. A review of long-term studies evaluating the efficacy of weight loss in ameliorating disorders associated with obesity. *Clin Ther*. 1996;18(6):1006–35; Discussion 5.

121. Allison DB, Zannolli R, Faith MS, Heo M, Pietrobelli A, Vanitallie TB, et al. Weight loss increases and fat loss decreases all-cause mortality rate: Results from two independent cohort studies. *Int J Obes Relat Metab Disord*. 1999;23(6):603–11.

122. Troiano RP, Frongillo EA, Jr., Sobal J, Levitsky DA. The relationship between body weight and mortality: A quantitative analysis of combined information from existing studies. *Int J Obes Relat Metab Disord*. 1996;20(1):63–75.

123. Kissebah AH, Krakower GR. Regional adiposity and morbidity. *Physiol Rev.* 1994;74(4):761–811.

124. Coleman DL, Hummel KP. Effects of parabiosis of normal with genetically diabetic mice. *Am J Physiol.* 1969;217(5):1298–304.

125. Halaas JL, Gajiwala KS, Maffei M, Cohen SL, Chait BT, Rabinowitz D, et al. Weight-reducing effects of the plasma protein encoded by the obese gene. *Science.* 1995;269(5223):543–6.

126. Cone RD, Cowley MA, Butler AA, Fan W, Marks DL, Low MJ. The Arcuate nucleus as a conduit for diverse signals relevant to energy homeostasis. *Int J Obes Relat Metab Disord.* 2001;25 Suppl 5:S63–7.

127. Greenway FL, Whitehouse MJ, Guttadauria M, Anderson JW, Atkinson RL, Fujioka K, et al. Rational design of a combination medication for the treatment of obesity. *Obesity (Silver Spring).* 2009;17(1):30–9.

128. Manolio TA, Brooks LD, Collins FS. A HapMap harvest of insights into the genetics of common disease. *J Clin Invest.* 2008;118(5):1590–605.

129. Wang S, Sparks LM, Xie H, Greenway FL, De Jonge L, Smith SR. Subtyping obesity with microarrays: Implications for the diagnosis and treatment of obesity. *Int J Obes (Lond).* 2009;33(4):481–9.

130. Novik KL, Nimmrich I, Genc B, Maier S, Piepenbrock C, Olek A, et al. Epigenomics: Genome-wide study of methylation phenomena. *Curr Issues Mol Biol.* 2002;4(4):111–28.

131. Weaver IC, Cervoni N, Champagne FA, D'alessio AC, Sharma S, Seckl JR, et al. Epigenetic programming by maternal behavior. *Nat Neurosci.* 2004;7(8):847–54.

132. Griffin JL, Vidal-Puig A. Current challenges in metabolomics for diabetes research: A vital functional genomic tool or just a ploy for gaining funding? *Physiol Genomics.* 2008;34(1):1–5.

133. Lawton KA, Berger A, Mitchell M, Milgram KE, Evans AM, Guo L, et al. Analysis of the adult human plasma metabolome. *Pharmacogenomics.* 2008;9(4):383–97.

134. Psychogios N, Hau DD, Peng J, Guo AC, Mandal R, Bouatra S, et al. The human serum metabolome. *PLoS One.* 2011;6(2):E16957.

135. Gross RW, Han X. Lipidomics in diabetes and the metabolic syndrome. *Methods Enzymol.* 2007;433:73–90.

136. Ptitsyn A, Hulver M, Cefalu W, York D, Smith SR. Unsupervised clustering of gene expression data points at hypoxia as possible trigger for metabolic syndrome. *BMC Genomics.* 2006;7:318.

137. Segal E, Friedman N, Kaminski N, Regev A, Koller D. From signatures to models: Understanding cancer using microarrays. *Nat Genet.* 2005;37 Suppl:S38–45.

138. Raetz EA, Moos PJ. Impact of microarray technology in clinical oncology. *Cancer Invest.* 2004;22(2):312–20.

139. Ginsburg GS, McCarthy JJ. Personalized medicine: Revolutionizing drug discovery and patient care. *Trends Biotechnol.* 2001;19(12):491–6.

140. Redman LM, De Jonge L, Fang X, Gamlin B, Recker D, Greenway FL, et al. Lack of an effect of a novel beta3-adrenoceptor agonist, TAK-677, on energy metabolism in obese individuals: A double-blind, placebo-controlled randomized study. *J Clin Endocrinol Metab.* 2007;92(2):527–31.

141. Martin CK, Redman LM, Zhang J, Sanchez M, Anderson CM, Smith SR, et al. Lorcaserin, a 5-HT(2C) receptor agonist, reduces body weight by decreasing energy intake without influencing energy expenditure. *J Clin Endocrinol Metab.* 2011;96(3):837–45.

142. Fountaine RJ, Taylor AE, Mancuso JP, Greenway FL, Byerley LO, Smith SR, et al. Increased food intake and energy expenditure following administration of olanzapine to healthy men. *Obesity (Silver Spring)*. 2010;18(8):1646–51.

143. Smith SR, Blundell JE, Burns C, Ellero C, Schroeder BE, Kesty NC, et al. Pramlintide treatment reduces 24-h caloric intake and meal sizes and improves control of eating in obese subjects: A 6-wk translational research study. *Am J Physiol Endocrinol Metab*. 2007;293(2):E620–7.

144. Napolitano A, Miller SR, Murgatroyd PR, Coward WA, Wright A, Finer N, et al. Validation of a quantitative magnetic resonance method for measuring human body composition. *Obesity (Silver Spring)*. 2008;16(1):191–8.

145. Zhou L, Sutton GM, Rochford JJ, Semple RK, Lam DD, Oksanen LJ, et al. Serotonin 2c Receptor agonists improve type 2 diabetes via melanocortin-4 receptor signaling pathways. *Cell Metab*. 2007;6(5):398–405.

Appendix A: Notes on nutrition for obesity medicine

JEFFREY D. LAWRENCE

A full discussion of human nutrition is beyond the scope of this book. However, it is important to emphasize that obesity medicine specialists must have a good understanding of basic nutritional science. It does not make any sense to just reduce caloric intake without any regard to maintaining adequate levels of the various essential nutrients. Although obesity has been shown to be an important factor for many medical conditions, nutritional deficiencies alone can cause many medical problems. Many of these conditions are life-altering or -threatening. The following outline covers some basic nutritional information. I suggest checking one of the many nutrition textbooks for a more complete discussion.

The information below is basic normal nutrition. When we manipulate the macronutrients to achieve weight loss, we must adjust all of the micronutrients. With very-low calorie, protein-sparing diets, for example, micronutrient supplementation is required. With low-fat diets, there must be adequate amounts of essential fatty acids (FAs) and fat-soluble vitamins. Low-carbohydrate diets must have adequate water-soluble vitamins, minerals, and fiber.

ENERGY REQUIREMENTS

Recommended dietary allowance (RDA) for men is 2300 to 2900 kcal/day and for women is 1900 to 2200 kcal/day.

Basal

Resting metabolic rate (RMR)—Energy expended resting in bed, in the morning, fasting, ambient conditions. Correlates with sex (women lower), lean body mass (more muscle = higher RMR), slight decline with age, correlates with body temperature. Largest component of energy needs (60%–70%).

Resting energy expenditure (REE)—Energy expended at rest, ambient conditions (not necessarily fasting, in a.m.). Used by World Health Organization, differs less than 10% from RMR, used interchangeably.

Physical activity

Energy expenditure due to occupation has declined; recreational activity is now an important determinant. Energy requirement is proportional to body weight; however, obesity is associated with lower activity level. Second largest component of energy requirements (20%–40%).

Thermic effect of food

Metabolic rate increases after eating, maximum at 1 hour. Energy expenditure small (10%–15% of total).

Other determinants of energy needs

Age—Lean body mass declines beyond early adulthood at 2% to 3% per decade, one factor in calculating REE.

Sex—Ten percent difference of REE per unit weight between men (higher) and women due to increased muscle mass of men.

Growth—Except for first year of life, small component.

Body size—Large bodies require more energy per unit of time for activities that involve moving mass over distance (e.g., walking).

Climate—Requirements increase when physically active in extreme heat. Exposure to cold conditions may also increase needs due to increased muscle activity or shivering.

Special requirements

Pregnancy—Increased need of 300 kcal/day

Lactation—Increased need of 500 kcal/day

Disease states—Malabsorption, infection, trauma, surgery will increase needs variably

Calorie

Kilocalorie—The amount of heat necessary to raise 1 kg of water from 15°C to 16°C. Note: We do not eat calories, we eat food. All food is not burned for energy.

DIETARY STANDARDS

Recommended daily allowances

The levels of intake of essential nutrients that, on the basis of scientific knowledge, are judged by the Food and Nutrition Board of the National Research Council to be adequate to meet the known nutrient needs of 97% to 98% of healthy persons. They are amounts intended to be consumed as part of a normal diet. If they are met through diets with a variety of foods from diverse food groups rather than by supplementation, such diets are likely to be adequate in other nutrients for which RDAs cannot currently be established. RDAs are neither minimal requirements nor necessarily optimal levels of intake. Rather, RDAs are safe and adequate levels of intake (with built in margins of safety to account for the variability in requirements among people) with regard to the knowledge about a nutrient. RDAs generally allow substantial storage to cover periods of reduced intake or increased needs. The RDAs are set to meet the needs of 97% to 98% of individuals in that group. The RDA values for nutrients were, in the past, revised on a regular basis by the Food and Nutrition Board of the National Research Council and published in book form. It was last done in 1989.

US recommended dietary allowances

Started in 1974 by the Food and Drug Administration to be used for labeling only. Unlike the RDA, it used a single standard for everyone over the age of 4 years old. There were separate values for infants, toddlers, and pregnant and lactating women. They are dated and no longer used.

Daily values and percent daily values

The daily value (DV) was introduced for labeling purposes only. The purpose was to allow people to compare processed foods. Data for the macronutrients, fat, carbohydrates, and protein that are the sources of energy and for cholesterol, sodium, potassium, and vitamins A and C, which do not contribute calories. In 2006, the amount of trans-FAs was added. The DV is based on a 2000 calorie daily intake.

Dietary reference intake

The dietary reference intake (DRI) is a system of nutrition recommendations. This standard is an ongoing effort by the National Research Council to create a set of reference values that can be used for planning and assessing diets for healthy populations and for many other purposes. They will replace the periodic revisions of the RDAs. Their first report, "Dietary Reference Intakes for Calcium, Phosphorus, Magnesium, Vitamin D, and Fluoride," was published by the National Academies Press in March 1998. The dietary reference intakes refer to daily intakes averaged over time and are classified as follows:

Estimated average requirement (EAR)—Intake that meets the nutrient need of 50% of individuals in that group.

Adequate intake (AI)—Average observed or experimentally derived intake by a defined population or subgroup that appears to sustain a defined nutritional state, such as normal circulating nutrient values, growth, or other functional indicators of health. AI is expected to exceed the EAR and possibly the RDA.

RDA—See definition above; this is the value to be used in guiding individuals to achieve adequate nutrient intake. It is a "target" intake. Remember that nutrient intake less than the RDA does not necessarily mean that the criterion for adequacy has not been met. RDA is generally defined as EAR + 2 standard deviations.

Tolerable upper intake level—The maximum intake by an individual that is unlikely to pose risks of adverse health effects in almost all (97%–98%) individuals.

Acceptable macronutrient distribution ranges—Healthy range of intake for carbohydrates, fat, and protein (expressed as percentage of total daily calories) that are sufficient to provide adequate nutrients while reducing the risk of chronic disease.
45% to 65% of daily calories from carbohydrate
10% to 35% of daily calories from protein
20% to 35% of daily calories from fat
5% to 10% of daily calories from linoleic acid (omega-6)
0.6% to 1.2% of daily calories from α-linolenic acid (omega-3)

There are DRIs for water, all vitamins, minerals, electrolytes, antioxidants, protein, fats, and carbohydrates. The DRI can be seen at https://fnic.nal.usda.gov/dietary-guidance/dietary-reference-intakes/dri-tables-and-application-reports

NUTRIENTS

Macronutrients

Defined as the principal dietary sources of energy.

PROTEINS

1. RDA—Men, 63 g/day and women, 50 g/day. Furnish amino acids required to build and maintain body tissues. Several times more protein is turned over daily within the body than is ordinarily consumed, indicating reuse of amino acids is a major feature of protein metabolism. As an energy source, they are equivalent to carbohydrates, providing 4 kcal/g.
2. Dietary sources—Meat, poultry, fish, milk, legumes (soybeans, peanuts, peas, beans, lentils), and cereals (lesser amount, but important because of quantity consumed)
3. Digestion
   a. Stomach: (Pepsin) proteins → polypeptides
   b. Small intestine:
      i. (Carboxypeptidase) polypeptides, dipeptides → amino acids
      ii. (Trypsin, chymotrypsin) proteins, polypeptides → amino acids
      iii. (Enterokinase) activates trypsinogen
      iv. (Aminopeptidase) polypeptides, dipeptides → amino acids
      v. (Dipeptidase) dipeptides → amino acids
4. Requirements—based on nitrogen balance. The difference between measured nitrogen intake and the amount excreted in urine, feces, sweat, and other minor losses is measured and data are extrapolated to zero balance point for adults or to defined positive balance for children to allow for growth.
5. Essential amino acids
   a. Leucine
   b. Isoleucine
   c. Valine
   d. Tryptophan
   e. Phenylalanine
   f. Methionine
   g. Threonine
   h. Lysine
   i. Histidine (in infants only, adults can synthesis it)
6. Deficiency—Rarely occurs as an isolated condition. It usually accompanies energy and other nutrient deficiencies from insufficient food intake.
   a. Primary
      i. Protein/calorie malnutrition (marasmus)
      ii. Protein malnutrition with adequate calories (kwashiorkor)
   b. Secondary—Illness
      i. Inflammatory bowel disease
      ii. Chronic renal failure
      iii. Intestinal malabsorption
      iv. Malignancy
7. Excess—No current firm evidence that increased levels are harmful, other than obesity.

8. High-protein diets can be an important part of weight management programs. Current literature suggests increased satiety, increased thermogenesis, and protection of lean body mass with 30% protein diets.

CARBOHYDRATES

1. RDA—≥50% of daily calories, 250 g in a 2000-calorie diet. As a macronutrient, it is an important source of energy. Provides 4 kcal/g, as does protein.
2. Sugar
   a. Monosaccharides—Glucose, fructose
   b. Disaccharides—Sucrose = glucose + fructose (table sugar)
   c. Maltose = glucose + glucose
   d. Lactose = glucose + galactose (milk sugar)
3. Complex carbohydrates
   a. Starches—Polymers of glucose
   b. Dietary fiber
      i. Soluble—Pectins, gums, mucilages; found primarily in fruits and vegetables; can hold water and form gels; can act as substrate for fermentation by colonic bacteria (apples, oranges, carrots, oats)
      ii. Insoluble—Cellulose and some hemicellulose (bran layer of cereal)
      iii. Lignin—A noncarbohydrate that is often included in fiber determinations; provides structure to the woody parts of plants
4. Dietary sources—Most originate in foods of plant origin, lactose is an exception (milk); plants such as cereal grains are major source
5. Digestion
   a. Mouth: (Salivary amylase) starch → disaccharides
   b. Small intestine: (Pancreatic amylase) starch → maltose
      i. (Sucrase) sucrose → glucose + fructose
      ii. (Maltase) maltose → glucose
      iii. (Lactase) lactose → glucose + galactose
6. Deficiency in dietary fiber—Constipation, possible increase in incidence of colon cancer
7. The fructose problem
   a. There has been a large increase in the amount of dietary fructose consumption, coming largely from added sucrose (glucose + fructose) and HFCS to foods and drinks.
   b. This increase of fructose load to the liver disturbs glucose metabolism and the glucose uptake pathways and leads to an enhanced rate of de novo lipogenesis and triglyceride synthesis. These changes may underlie the induction of insulin resistance and metabolic syndrome.

FATS

1. RDA—Five percent to 30% of daily calories, <67 g in a 2000-calorie diet. Aid in transport and absorption of the fat-soluble vitamins, depress gastric secretion, slow gastric emptying, add palatability to the diet, and reduce feeling of satiety. Energy-dense source of fuel, with 9 kcal/g.
2. Dietary sources—More than one-third of the calories consumed by most people in the United States is provided by fat. Animal products, in particular, contribute more than

half of the fat, three-fourths of the saturated fat, and all of the cholesterol. Ground beef has been found to be the single largest contributor to fat in the US diet. Eggs supply the most cholesterol. Grains, nuts, and animal and vegetable oils are some of the good sources of fats.

3. Nonpolar sources—Mainly esters of FAs, insoluble in water, enter metabolic pathways only after hydrolysis
   a. *Triglycerides*: Three FAs + glycerol
4. Polar sources
   a. FAs—Polar component is a negatively charged carboxyl ion; more than 90% have even number of carbons. Classification:
      i. Short-chain FAs: <6 carbons
      ii. Medium-chain FAs: 6 to 10 carbons
      iii. Long-chain FAs: ≥12 carbons
      iv. Saturated: No double bonds
         A. RDA ≤10% of daily calories
         B. Palmitic acid and stearic acid are major FAs
      v. Monounsaturated: Single double bond
      vi. Polyunsaturated: More than one double bond
      vii. Essential FAs: Prevent deficiency symptoms and cannot be synthesized by humans; they carry fat-soluble vitamins
         A. Linoleic acid: The primary omega-6 FA; does not have the properties of the omega-3 FAs. Deficiency causes dermatitis and poor growth.
         B. α-Linolenic acid: The primary omega-3 FA; converted to a hormone-like substances that reduce inflammation. Deficiency causes neurologic changes (numbness, paresthesia, weakness, inability to walk, blurring of vision)
         (both are 18-carbon unsaturated FAs)
   b. Cholesterol—Polar component is an alcohol; RDA <300 mg/day. With phospholipids, it is a major component of all cell membranes; a precursor to steroid hormones of adrenal and gonadal origin, and of the bile acids. Amount of fat ingested, especially saturated FAs, affects serum levels. Cholesterol intake in the diet has a lesser, if any effect.
   c. Phospholipids—See above.
   d. Olestra—This is not a fat. It is a sucrose polyester that has the taste and properties of fat and is not absorbed in the gastrointestinal (GI) tract.
5. Digestion
   a. Stomach: (Gastric lipase) emulsified fats → glycerol + FAs
   b. Small intestine: (Pancreatic lipase) fats → glycerol + mono- and diglycerides + FAs
   c. (Intestinal lipase) fats → glycerol + glycerides + FAs
   d. (Bile) accelerates action of pancreatic lipase, emulsifies fat, neutralizes chyme, and stabilizes emulsions
6. Deficiencies (essential FAs)—Dermatitis, alopecia, fat-soluble vitamin deficiencies
7. Trans-FAs—Hydrated polyunsaturated fats. Created by food chemists to solidify liquid fats, increase shelf life of fat-containing processed food (e.g., cookies, 90%; fatty snacks, 50%). Have been related to cardiovascular disease. Should be eliminated or at least markedly reduced in the diet.

Micronutrients

VITAMINS

Thirteen organic molecules needed in the diet in tiny amounts. They can serve two functions in the body. In small amounts, they serve as catalysts, increasing the speed of a chemical reaction without being used up by that reaction. In large doses (above a body's demand), they can act like drugs or chemicals, causing other, sometimes significant, effects. Original theory as "vital amines" has been discredited.

1. Fat soluble—Absorbed with other lipids; need bile and pancreatic juice for efficient absorption; are stored in various body tissues, notably fat
   a. Vitamin A (retinol, β-carotene) (retinoids)
      i. *RDA*—Men, 1000 retinol equivalents (RE)/day and women, 800 RE/day; 1/2 cup cooked spinach, 1/2 carrot; carotenoids are provitamins, converted by the body to vitamin A
      ii. *Dietary sources*: Preformed vitamin A from foods of animal origin (liver, fat from milk and eggs). Carotenoids from carrots. Dark green leafy vegetables. Fortified foods. Cooking increases bioavailability, but overcooking decreases bioavailability.
      iii. *Digestion*:
         A. Absorption: small intestine
         B. Storage: 90% in liver
      iv. *Deficiency*:
         A. Ocular—Night blindness, corneal lesions (xerophthalmia).
         B. Cutaneous—follicular hyperkeratosis "goose flesh" (keratin plugs), dry, scaly, rough skin
      v. *Excess*: Nausea, vomiting, fatigue, diplopia, alopecia, dryness of mucous membranes, desquamation, and death; carotenoids, even in large amounts, are safe because of limited conversion to vitamin A; skin may turn yellow, however
   b. Vitamin D (calciferol)
      i. *RDA*—400 IU. There is a strong suggestion that the RDA for vitamin D in the far northern and southern hemispheres should be 50 µg = 2000 IU due to the lack of exposure to ultraviolet (UV) light.
      ii. Calcitriol (most active form of vitamin D) stimulates synthesis of calcium binding protein in the intestines, promoting calcium absorption.
      iii. *Dietary sources*: Vitamin D (cholecalciferol) is a provitamin formed in the skin by the action of UV rays from sunlight. It is also found in fish liver oils. Milk and many dairy products are fortified with vitamin D2 (ergosterol). It is remarkably stable and does not deteriorate with heating.
      iv. *Absorption*: Small intestine
      v. *Storage*: Liver, skin, brain, bones
      vi. *Deficiency*: Children—rickets; adults—osteomalacia
      vii. *Excess*: Calcification of soft tissues like kidney (including stones), lungs, tympanic membrane (deafness), also headache, nausea
   c. Vitamin E (tocopherols, tocotretinols)
      i. *RDA*—Men, 10 IU and women, 8 IU; 1 tbsp corn oil, 1.5 cups milk, two avocados
      ii. An antioxidant, vitamin E protects cellular and subcellular membranes from deterioration by scavenging free radicals that contain oxygen. Is currently under study

in preventing aging effects of environmental toxins and the triggering of some forms of carcinogenesis.

   iii. *Dietary sources*: Seed oils, especially wheat germ oil; stable with cooking (in water), except deep fat frying; freezing also destroys
   iv. *Absorption*: Small intestine (inefficiently)
   v. *Storage*: Liver and fat
   vi. *Deficiency*: Uncommon; peripheral neuropathy
   vii. *Excess*: Low toxicity, possibly bleeding associated with warfarin use

d. Vitamin K (phyloquinone, methaquinone)

   i. *RDA*—Men, 80 µg/day and women, 65 µg/day; 50 g broccoli, 66 g cabbage, 200 g green beans. Antihemorrhagic factor: acts as a cofactor for carboxylase in the liver in the formation of prothrombin, among other proteins. Warfarin drugs antagonize the action of vitamin K.
   ii. *Dietary sources*: Green leafy vegetables, especially broccoli, cabbage, turnip greens, lettuce. A significant amount is formed by the intestinal flora of the lower intestinal tract. Fairly resistant to heat, not destroyed by ordinary cooking methods.
   iii. *Absorption*: Small intestine, requires bile and pancreatic juice
   iv. *Storage*: Liver
   v. *Deficiency*: Associated with lipid malabsorption or destruction of intestinal flora by antibiotics. Liver disease that prevents use produces deficiency. Newborns susceptible because of poor placental transfer and failure to establish intestinal bacteria that produce vitamin K.
   vi. *Excess*: Excessive doses of synthetic vitamin K have produced kernicterus in infants.

2. Water soluble—Most are components of essential enzyme systems, are not normally stored in the body in appreciable amounts, and are excreted in the urine.

a. Thiamin (B_1)

   i. *RDA*—Men, 1.5 mg/day and women, 1.1 mg/day; 3 oz lean pork, 1.5 cups roasted peanuts
   ii. Coenzyme in phosphate forms vital to tissue respiration. Strongly linked to carbohydrate metabolism.
   iii. *Dietary sources*: Lean pork, wheat germ, organ meats. Cooking losses highly variable, depending on cooking time, temperature, and quantity of water.
   iv. *Absorption*: Actively transported in the acid medium of the proximal duodenum. Can be inhibited by alcohol.
   v. *Storage*: Liver
   vi. *Deficiency*: Seen most frequently in alcoholics, clinical signs most often involve nervous (dementia) and cardiovascular systems. Beriberi includes mental confusion, muscle wasting (dry beriberi), edema (wet beriberi), peripheral paralysis, tachycardia, and enlarged heart.
   vii. *Excess*: No known toxic effects.

b. Riboflavin (B_2)

   i. *RDA*—Men, 1.7 mg/day and women, 1.3 mg/day; 1.5 oz beef liver, 3 cups fruit-flavored low-fat yogurt
   ii. Discovered as a yellow-green fluorescent pigment in milk, is a component of the coenzyme (FAD) important in energy production.

      iii. *Dietary sources*: Milk, cheddar cheese, cottage cheese, organ meats, eggs. Heat, oxidation, and acid stable, but disintegrates in alkali or UV light. Little lost in the cooking and processing of food.

      iv. *Absorption*: Actively absorbed in the proximal small intestine.

      v. *Storage*: Not stored in any great amount, must be supplied in the diet regularly.

      vi. *Deficiency*: Usually associated with deficiencies of other water-soluble vitamins. Photophobia, lacrimation, burning-itching eyes, soreness and burning of the lips and tongue. Cheilosis (fissuring of lips), angular stomatitis (cracks in the skin at the corners of the mouth).

      vii. *Excess*: No known toxicity.

c. Niacin (nicotinic acid and nicotinamide) (B_3)

      i. *RDA*—Men, 19 mg NE/day and women, 15 mg NE/day; average daily intake, 41 mg NE (men), 27 mg NE (women); acts as a coenzyme in oxidation–reduction.

      ii. *Dietary sources*: Lean meats, poultry, fish, and peanuts. Resistant to heat, light, air, acids, and alkalis—small amount may be lost in cooking water.

      iii. Niacin can be synthesized from tryptophan with vitamin B_6 as a cofactor.

      iv. *Absorption*: Small intestine

      v. *Storage*: Very little storage

      vi. *Deficiency*: Pellagra—(4 D's = dermatitis, dementia, diarrhea, and death), tremors, and sore tongue. Seen on highly inadequate diets with little niacin and inadequate protein.

      vii. *Excess*: Large doses of niacin (1–2 g three times a day) can cause histamine release with flushing, also liver toxicity.

d. Vitamin B_6 (pyridoxine, pyridoxal, pyridoxamine)

      i. *RDA*—Men, 2.0 mg/day and women, 1.6 mg/day; 5 oz liver, 12 oz chicken

      ii. Coenzyme in transamination and other reactions related to protein metabolism

      iii. *Dietary sources*: Yeast, wheat germ, pork, glandular meats, whole-grain cereals, oatmeal. Unstable in light; losses in freezing, 36% to 55%.

      iv. *Absorption*: Upper small intestine

      v. *Storage*: Muscle (up to 50% of stores)

      vi. *Deficiency*: Rare, medications (isoniazid, oral contraceptive pills) can interfere with metabolism. Malaise, depression, glucose intolerance. With severe deficiency, convulsions.

      vii. *Excess*: Seen in premenstrual syndrome treatment studies; ataxia and severe sensory neuropathy.

e. Folic acid

      i. *RDA*—Men, 200 µg/day and women, 180 µg per day; 3 oz fried beef liver, 3/4 cup white baked beans; women of reproductive age planning to conceive, 400 µg/day to prevent neural tube defects.

      ii. Important role in RNA and DNA synthesis.

      iii. *Dietary sources*: Liver, kidney beans, lima beans, fresh dark green leafy vegetables (spinach, asparagus, broccoli). Losses occur with storage of vegetables at room temperature, and during processing at high temperatures.

      iv. *Absorption*: Folate broken down and then actively absorbed in the small intestine.

      v. *Storage*: In the form of methyltetrahydrofolic acid.

      vi. *Deficiency*: Alteration of DNA metabolism, therefore affects rapidly dividing cells—red blood cells, leukocytes; epithelium of stomach, intestine, vagina, cervix. See poor growth, megaloblastic anemia, glossitis, GI tract disturbances.

      vii. *Excess*: No toxicity reported in adults.

   f. Vitamin B_{12} (cobalamin)

      i. *RDA*—2.0 pg/day; 2 oz canned tuna, 4 oz beef hamburger

      ii. Essential for the normal function of all cells, DNA synthesis, affects myelin formation.

      iii. *Dietary sources*: Animal protein foods, liver, kidney, milk, eggs, cheese, fish, and muscle meats.

      iv. *Absorption*: Hydrochloric acid in the stomach releases cobalamin from its peptide bonds, binds with the intrinsic factor, and then is absorbed in the ileum. There is a problem of poor absorption in patients after certain bariatric surgeries because of reduced gastric HCl.

      v. *Storage*: Liver and kidney before release to bone marrow and other tissues.

      vi. *Deficiency*: Megaloblastic anemia, glossitis, hypospermia, degeneration of central and peripheral nerves (seen as numbness, tingling, burning of the feet with stiffness and weakness of the legs)

      vii. *Excess*: No known toxic effects.

   g. Pantothenic acid

      i. *RDA*—Level not determined, but 4 to 7 mg estimated; 3 oz beef liver, 6 cups low-fat yogurt with fruit

      ii. Constituent of coenzyme A essential to many areas of cellular metabolism.

      iii. *Dietary sources*: Present in all plant and animal tissues, egg yolk, kidney, liver, and yeast; 33% lost in cooking; 50% lost in milling of flour

      iv. *Absorption*: Small intestine

      v. *Storage*: Little known

      vi. *Deficiency*: No deficiency disease observed in humans

      vii. *Excess*: No serious toxic effects known

   h. Biotin

      i. *RDA*—Not known, but 30 to 100 µg/day estimated

      ii. Coenzyme for reactions involving gluconeogenesis, synthesis and oxidation of fatty acids, and purine synthesis

      iii. *Dietary sources*: Protein bound in most natural foods; significant amount synthesized by intestinal bacteria. Kidney, liver, egg yolk, soybeans, and yeast. Stable to heat, soluble in water and alcohol.

      iv. *Absorption*: Readily absorbed; taken up by liver, muscle, and kidney

      v. *Storage*: Little is known.

      vi. *Deficiency*: Dry scaly dermatitis, pallor, alopecia, nausea; long-term anticonvulsant drugs interfere with biotin transport.

      vii. *Excess*: No known toxic effects.

   i. Vitamin C (ascorbic acid)

      i. *RDA*—75 mg (female); 90 mg (male)

      ii. Antiscorbutic vitamin that has multiple functions as either a coenzyme or cofactor can lose and take on hydrogen, helps iron absorption, involved in collagen formation; promotes resistance to infection via immunological function of leukocytes, interferon production, or integrity of the mucous membrane. Findings related to prevention and cure of the common cold are controversial. Is an important antioxidant.

      iii. *Dietary sources*: Fresh acidic fruits and vegetables (citrus fruits, fresh leafy vegetables, tomatoes). It is easily destroyed by oxidation particularly with heat and alkali. Cooking should be rapid, in little water, and food served immediately. Refrigeration and quick freezing help retain vitamin.

     iv. *Absorption*: Small intestine; between 20 and 120 mg of absorption 90%; at high intakes (12 g) only 16%.

     v. *Storage*: Adrenals, kidney, liver, spleen, in equilibrium with serum.

     vi. *Deficiency*: Scurvy, swollen and inflamed gums, loosening teeth, dryness of the mouth and eyes, loss of hair, dry itchy skin, failure of wound healing, possible gallstone formation.

     vii. *Excess*: Diarrhea from osmotic effect of unabsorbed vitamin; excreted in the urine, can give a false-positive test for sugar. In amount greater than 10 times the normal amount, may inhibit absorption of vitamin B_{12}.

j. Vitamin-like factors

     i. Other food factors that have some but not all of the characteristic of vitamins. Their role is unclear. Requirements are unclear.

     ii. Choline: As phophatidylcholine is a structural element of membranes, a precursor of sphingolipids, and a promoter of lipid transport. As acetylcholine, it functions as a neurotransmitter and as a component of platelet-activating factor. DRI varies with age. Has been used in very high doses to alleviate symptoms of tardive dyskinesia and Huntington's disease. Has been used with some success to diminish short-term memory loss in Alzheimer's disease.

     iii. Others: Carnitine, *myo*-inositol, pyrroloquinoline, quinone, ubiquinones, and the bioflavonoids.

MINERALS

Constitute 4% to 5% of body weight (40% calcium)

1. Calcium
   a. *RDA*—1200 mg/day through age 24; 800 to 1200 mg thereafter; 4 cups milk, 3 cups yogurt with fruit.
   b. Functions in building and maintaining bone and teeth, roles in cell membrane stabilization and membrane transport, important in nerve transmission and blood clotting.
   c. *Dietary sources*: Dairy products, dark green leafy vegetables, sardines, canned salmon.
   d. *Absorption*: Duodenum and proximal jejunum in acidic medium; vitamin D stimulates absorption.
   e. *Storage*: Nonexchangable skeletal pool, exchangeable pool in trabeculae of bone; stored in the form of hydroxyapatite crystals.
   f. *Deficiency*: Bone deformities (osteoporosis, osteomalacia), tetany, hypertension.
   g. *Excess*: With high levels of vitamin D, may lead to excessive calcification of bone and soft tissues; can interfere with iron absorption if taken at same time.
2. Magnesium
   a. *RDA*—Men, 350 mg/day and women, 280 mg/day; 3 cups chili with beans, 1 cup roasted cashews; intracellular cation.
   b. *Dietary sources*: Seeds, nuts, legumes, unmilled cereal grains; lost during refining and processing.
   c. *Absorption*: Most in jejunum, but all along small intestine.
   d. *Storage*: Sixty percent in bone, 26% in muscle.
   e. *Deficiency*: Tremor, muscle spasms, personality changes, anorexia, possible cardiac arrhythmias.

f. *Excess*: With normal renal function, is excreted; with compromised renal function, can see nausea, vomiting, hypotension, and hypotonia; may progress to respiratory depression and asystolic arrest.

3. Phosphorus
   a. *RDA*—Same as calcium, 800 to 1200 mg/day; 4 cups milk, two grilled cheese sandwiches.
   b. One of the most essential elements; 80% bound as calcium phosphate crystals in bone and teeth; many functions—DNA, RNA, ATP, cAMP.
   c. *Dietary sources*: Meat, poultry, fish, eggs, and dairy.
   d. *Absorption*: Mostly as inorganic phosphate; organic phosphate hydrolyzed in the acid environment of the proximal jejunum for absorption; vegetarian diets contain mainly phytate, which is poorly digested in humans.
   e. *Storage*: Bone, every cell in body.
   f. *Deficiency*: From decreased production of ATP; see neuromuscular, skeletal, hematological, and renal abnormalities.
   g. *Excess*: Can lower blood calcium level.

4. Iron
   a. *RDA*—Men, 10 mg/day and women, 15 mg/day; 6 oz beef liver, 1/4 cup clams.
   b. Constituent of hemoglobin, myoglobin.
   c. *Dietary sources*: Liver, oysters, shellfish, kidney, heart, lean meat.
   d. *Absorption*: Small intestine; heme iron highly absorbed, nonheme iron absorption can be influenced by the presence of vitamin C.
   e. *Storage*: Ferritin and hemosiderin (spleen, liver, bone marrow).
   f. *Deficiency*: Most common nutritional deficiency; most common cause of anemia among children and women of child-bearing age; manifested by a hypochromic, microcytic anemia, corrected by iron supplementation.
   g. *Excess*: Seen with hereditary hemochromatosis; recent studies do not support relationship between high serum ferritin and risk of heart disease.

5. Zinc
   a. *RDA*—Men, 15 mg/day and women, 12 mg/day; 1/4 cup Pacific oysters, 9 oz ground beef.
   b. Known to participate in reactions involving synthesis or degradation of major metabolites.
   c. *Dietary sources*: Meat, fish, poultry, milk.
   d. *Absorption*: Small intestine; not well understood.
   e. *Storage*: All tissues.
   f. *Deficiency*: Short stature, hypogonadism, mild anemia; delayed wound healing, alopecia, skin lesions; zinc-responsive night blindness.

6. Iodine
   a. *RDA*—150 µg/day; 1/2 tsp iodized salt, four slices bread.
   b. Integral part of thyroid hormone.
   c. *Dietary sources*: Seafood, iodized salt.
   d. *Absorption*: Easily in small intestine.
   e. *Storage*: Primarily in the thyroid gland; also in mammary tissue.
   f. *Deficiency*: Cretinism (severe deficiency during gestation and early postnatal growth), goiter.
   g. *Excess*: Goiter can be seen in long-term excesses.

7. Selenium
   a. An antioxidant; no comprehensive table for content in food; present in Brazil nuts, seafood, kidney.

8. Copper
   a. Normal constituent of blood; component of many enzymes.
   b. *Deficiency*: Causes microcytic, hemochromic anemia followed by neutropenia, leukopenia, and bone demineralization; Wilson's disease is characterized by the accumulation of excess copper in body tissues from genetic defect in liver synthesis of ceruloplasmin.

9. Manganese
   a. Found in tissues rich in mitochondria; a component of many enzymes.
   b. *Dietary sources*: Whole grains, legumes, nuts, tea.
   c. *Deficiency*: Causes weight loss, transient dermatitis, slow growth of hair.

10. Fluoride
    a. Essential because of its beneficial effect on tooth enamel; resisting dental caries.
    b. Major source is fluoridated drinking water, and tea leaves.

11. Chromium
    a. *RDA*—50 to 200 µg/day; in self-selected diet of 2300 kcal, average intake is 33 µg/day.
    b. Chromium potentates insulin action and therefore influences carbohydrate, lipid, and protein metabolism; in 1977, patients receiving total parenteral nutrition exhibited abnormalities of glucose metabolism reversed by chromium supplementation; proposed role as "glucose tolerance factor" is controversial.
    c. *Dietary sources*: Difficult to assess because biologically available and inorganic chromium cannot be distinguished from each other; Brewer's yeast, oysters, liver, and potatoes have high concentrations.
    d. *Absorption*: Organic and inorganic forms are absorbed differently. Organic is easily absorbed, but quickly passes out of the body; less than 2% of trivalent chromium consumed is absorbed; appears to be a commonality with iron absorption pathways; is carried by transferrin.
    e. Strenuous exercise increases excretion of chromium.
    f. *Deficiency*: Mertz (1)
       i. Chromium deficiency results in insulin resistance.
       ii. Insulin resistance caused by chromium deficiency can be ameliorated by chromium supplementation.
       iii. Chromium deficiency does occur in populations in the United States and may be an important cause of insulin resistance.
       iv. In animals, deficiency signs include impaired growth, elevated serum cholesterol and triglyceride concentrations, increased aortic plaques, corneal lesions, and decreased fertility and sperm count.
       v. Chromium for weight loss: In a study by Grant et al. (2) using 43 obese women, the women on 400 µg of chromium picolinate gained weight, whereas those on chromium nicotinate lost weight if they were engaged in exercise as well. Recent meta-analyses of studies of chromium suggest only minimal effects on weight loss. It has been shown to be toxic in bacterial cultures.

12. Molybdenum
    a. Required in enzymes that catalyze oxidation–reduction reactions.
    b. Distributed widely in commonly used foods, such as legumes, whole-grain cereals, milk, and milk products.

Vegetarianism

Lacto-ovo-vegetarian—Eats no meat, fish, or poultry; does include milk, cheese, dairy products, and eggs

Lacto-vegetarian—Eats no meat, fish, poultry, or eggs; does include milk, cheese, and other dairy products

Vegan—Eats no food of animal origin

The only variety of vegetarianism that incorporates any real risk of inadequate nutrition. This can be avoided with careful planning.

1. Iron—Assimilation of nonheme iron in fruits, vegetables, and unrefined cereals aided with ascorbic acid
2. Calcium—Without dairy products, calcium and vitamin D intake may be low
3. Vitamin B_{12}—Megaloblastic anemia may develop in long standing vegans. Vitamin B_{12} occurs only in foods of animal origin. High levels of folate may mask the neurologic damage of this deficiency. Vegans need a reliable source, such as fortified cereals, soy beverages, or supplements.
4. Protein—Lower content than most omnivores. Usually results in lower intake of dietary fat. Sources should be varied (cereals plus legumes) to ensure complimentary proteins.

BARIATRIC SURGERY–RELATED NUTRITIONAL PROBLEMS

Bariatric surgery–related nutritional problems are highly dependent on the type of surgery done. In the Roux-en-Y procedure, the duodenum and part of the jejunum are eliminated. The absorption of calcium, iron, and vitamin B_{12} is depressed. This can result in anemia from lack of iron and vitamin B_{12} and osteoporosis from lack of calcium.

Dumping syndrome results from rapid passage of food into the small intestine, shifting fluid too quickly into the intestine. The result is often diarrhea and dehydration. Cramping, sweating, flushed appearance, dizziness, weakness, and headaches characterize dumping syndrome. This results in electrolyte imbalance and reduced fat-soluble vitamin absorption.

REFERENCES

1. Mertz W. Essential trace metals: new definitions based on new paradigms. *Nutr Rev.* 1993;51:287–95.
2. Grant KE, Chandler RM, Castle AL, Ivy JL. Chromium and exercise training: Effect on obese women. *Med Sci Sports Exerc.* 1997;29(8):992–8.

ADDITIONAL RESOURCES

1. Mahan L, Escott-Stump S. *Krause's Food, Nutrition, & Diet Therapy*, 12th ed. Philadelphia, PA: Saunders; 2005. An up-to-date comprehensive text for nutrition professionals. An in depth look at nutrition in health and disease. Despite its size, very readable.

2. Food and Nutrition Board—National Research Council. *Recommended Dietary Allowances*, 10th ed. Washington, DC: National Academy Press; 1989. Published by the National Research Council, the basics on RDAs. Now out of print, will be replaced by the various reports of DRIs released in a serial fashion.
3. Food and Nutrition Board—National Research Council. *Dietary Reference Intakes*. Washington, DC: National Academy Press. www.nin.ca/Comsumer/dri_p.html. A series of reports on Dietary Reference Intakes the last published in 2002.
4. Rinzler CA. *Nutrition for Dummies*, 2nd ed. New York: Hungry Minds; 1999. Fun, easy book on basic nutrition.
5. Barrett S, Herbert V. *The Vitamin Pushers*. Amherst, NY: Prometheus; 1994. Written by two physicians respected for their work in exposing quackery in medicine. Reviews many of the common myths regarding vitamins and supplementation. Old but still of interest.
6. Mahan LK, Escott-Stump S. *Nutritional Concepts and Controversies*, 11th ed. Saunders; 2008.
7. Van Way CW III, Ireton-Jones C. *Nutrition Secrets*. Hanley and Belfus; 2003.

Appendix B: Behavioral modification attachments

Form 1   Medical history form
Form 2   Weight loss questionnaire
Form 3   Assessment of patient readiness form
Form 4   Food and activity diary
Form 5   Keeping a food diary
Form 6   Food/Activity and Behavior diary
Form 7   AIM to Change journal
Form 8   Quality of Life Self-Assessment
Form 9   Diet readiness test questionnaire
Form 10 Diet readiness test scoring
Form 11 Food addiction questionnaire

Medical History Form

Name: _____ Age: _____ Sex: M   F

Family Physician: _____ Phone: _____

<u>Present Status:</u>

1. Are you in good health at the present time to the best of your knowledge?   Yes   No

2. Are you under a doctor's care at the present time?   Yes   No
    If yes, for what? _____

3. Are you taking any medications at the present time?   Yes   No
    What: _____ Dosages: _____
    What:_____ Dosages: _____

4. Any allergies to any medications?   Yes   No
    _____

5. History of high blood pressure?   Yes   No

6. History of diabetes?   Yes   No
    At what age: _____

7. History of heart attack or chest pain?   Yes   No

8. History of swelling feet   Yes   No

9. History of frequent headaches?   Yes   No
    Migraines?   Yes   No   Medications for headaches: _____

10. History of constipation (difficulty in bowel movements)?   Yes   No

11. History of glaucoma?   Yes   No

12. Gynecologic History:
    Pregnancies: Number: _____ Dates: _____
    Natural Delivery or C-Section (specify): _____
    Menstrual: Onset: _____
                     Duration: _____
                     Are they regular: Yes   No
                     Pain associated: Yes   No
                     Last menstrual period: _____
    Hormone Replacement Therapy: Yes   No
                     What: _____
    Birth Control Pills: Yes   No
                     Type: _____
    Last Checkup: _____

13. Serious Injuries: Yes   No
    Specify: _____ Date: _____

Form 1 Medical history form.   *(Continued)*

14. Any Surgery: Yes   No

    Specify: _____ Date: _____

    Specify: _____ Date: _____

15. Family History:

	Age	Health	Disease	Cause of Death	Overweight?
Father:					
Mother:					
Brothers:					
Sisters:					

    Has any blood relative ever had any of the following:

Glaucoma:	Yes	No	Who:	_____
Asthma:	Yes	No	Who:	_____
Epilepsy:	Yes	No	Who:	_____
High Blood Pressure	Yes	No	Who:	_____
Kidney Disease:	Yes	No	Who:	_____
Diabetes:	Yes	No	Who:	_____
Tuberculosis:	Yes	No	Who:	_____
Psychiatric Disorder	Yes	No	Who:	_____
Heart Disease/Stroke	Yes	No	Who:	_____

Past Medical History: (check all that apply)

_____ Polio	_____ Measles	_____ Tonsillitis
_____ Jaundice	_____ Mumps	_____ Pleurisy
_____ Kidneys	_____ Scarlet Fever	_____ Liver Disease
_____ Lung Disease	_____ Whooping Cough	_____ Chicken Pox
_____ Rheumatic Fever	_____ Bleeding Disorder	_____ Nervous Breakdown
_____ Ulcers	_____ Gout	_____ Thyroid Disease
_____ Anemia	_____ Heart Valve Disorder	_____ Heart Disease
_____ Tuberculosis	_____ Gallbladder Disorder	_____ Psychiatric Illness
_____ Drug Abuse	_____ Eating Disorder	_____ Alcohol Abuse
_____ Pneumonia	_____ Malaria	_____ Typhoid Fever
_____ Cholera	_____ Cancer	_____ Blood Transfusion
_____ Arthritis	_____ Osteoporosis	_____ Other: _____

Nutrition Evaluation:

1. Present weight: _____ Height (no shoes): _____ Desired weight: _____

2. In what time frame would you like to be at your desired weight? _____

3. Birth weight: _____ Weight at 20 years of age: _____ Weight one year ago: _____

4. What is the main reason for your decision to lose weight? _____

5. When did you begin gaining excess weight? (Give reasons, if known): _____

    _____

Form 1 (Continued) Medical history form.   *(Continued)*

6. What has been your maximum lifetime weight (non-pregnant) and when?_____

7. Previous diets you have followed: Give dates and results of your weight loss:

   _____   _____

   _____   _____

8. Is your spouse, fiancee or partner overweight?   Yes   No

9. By how much is he or she overweight? _____

10. How often do you eat out? _____

11. What restaurants do you frequent? _____

12. How often do you eat "fast foods?" _____

13. Who plans meals? _____ Cooks? _____ Shops? _____

14. Do you use a shopping list?   Yes   No

15. What time of day and on what day do you shop for groceries? _____

16. Food allergies: _____

17. Food dislikes: _____

18. Food you crave: _____

19. Any specific time of the day or month do you crave food? _____

20. Do you drink coffee or tea?   Yes   No   How much daily? _____

21. Do you drink cola drinks?   Yes   No   How much daily? _____

22. Do you drink alcohol?   Yes   No
    What? _____ How much? _____ Weekly? _____

23. Do you use a sugar substitute? _____ Butter? _____ Margarine? _____

24. Do you awaken hungry during the night?   Yes   No
    What do you do? _____

25. What are your worst food habits? _____

26. Snack Habits:
    What? _____ How much? _____ When? _____

    _____   _____   _____

27. When you are under a stressful situation at work or family related, do you tend to eat more? Explain:

    _____

    _____

28. Do you thing you are currently undergoing a stressful situation or an emotional upset? Explain:

    _____

    _____

Form 1 (Continued) Medical history form.   (Continued)

29. Smoking Habits: **(answer only one)**

   _____ You have never smoked cigarettes, cigars or a pipe.

   _____ You quit smoking _____ years ago and have not smoked since.

   _____ You have quit smoking cigarettes at least one year ago and now smoke cigars or a pipe without inhaling smoke.

   _____ You smoke 20 cigarettes per day (1 pack).

   _____ You smoke 30 cigarettes per day (1-1/2 packs).

   _____ You smoke 40 cigarettes per day (2 packs).

30.

Typical Breakfast	Typical Lunch	Typical Dinner
_____	_____	_____
_____	_____	_____
_____	_____	_____
_____	_____	_____
Time eaten: _____	Time eaten: _____	Time eaten: _____
Where: _____	Where: _____	Where: _____
With whom: _____	With whom: _____	With whom: _____

31. Describe your usual energy level: _____

32. Activity Level: **(answer only one)**

   _____ Inactive—no regular physical activity with a sit-down job.

   _____ Light activity—no organized physical activity during leisure time.

   _____ Moderate activity—occasionally involved in activities such as weekend golf, tennis, jogging, swimming, or cycling.

   _____ Heavy activity—consistent lifting, stair climbing, heavy construction, etc., or regular participation in jogging, swimming, cycling or active sports at least three times per week.

   _____ Vigorous activity—participation in extensive physical exercise for at least 60 minutes per session 4 times per week.

33. Behavior style: **(answer only one)**

   _____ You are always calm and easygoing.

   _____ You are usually calm and easygoing.

   _____ You are sometimes calm with frequent impatience.

   _____ You are seldom calm and persistently driving for advancement.

   _____ You are never calm and have overwhelming ambition.

   _____ You are hard-driving and can never relax.

34. Please describe your general health goals and improvements you wish to make: _____
_____
_____
_____

This information will assist us in assessing your particular problem areas and establishing your medical management. Thank you for your time and patience in completing this form.

Form 1 (Continued) Medical history form. (Reprinted from Obesity Medicine Association [formerly American Society of Bariatric Physicians]. With permission.)

Weight Loss Questionnaire

Name_____Date_____

Please complete this questionnaire, which will help you and your physician develop the best management plan for you.

1. Is there a reason you are seeking treatment at this time? _____

2. What are your goals about weight control and management? _____

3. Your level of interest in losing weight is:

| Not interested | 1 | 2 | 3 | 4 | 5 | Very interested |

4. Are you ready for lifestyle changes to be a part of your weight control program?

| Not ready | 1 | 2 | 3 | 4 | 5 | Very ready |

5. How much support can your family provide?

| Not support | 1 | 2 | 3 | 4 | 5 | Much support |

6. How much support can your friends provide?

| Not support | 1 | 2 | 3 | 4 | 5 | Much support |

7. What is the hardest part about managing your weight? _____

8. What do you believe will be of most help to assist you in losing weight? _____

9. How confident are you that you can lose weight at this time?

| Not interested | 1 | 2 | 3 | 4 | 5 | Very interested |

Weight history

10. As best as you can recall, what was your body weight at each of the following time points (if they apply)?
    Grade school _____ High school _____ College _____ Ages 20–29 _____ 30–39 _____ 40–49 _____ 50–59 _____

11. What has been your lowest body weight as an adult?_____ What has been your heaviest body weight as an adult? _____

12. At what age did you start trying to lose weight? _____

13. Please check all previous programs you have tried in order to lose weight. Include dates and your length of participation.

Program	Date	Weight (lost or gained)	Length of participation
• TOPS	_____	_____	_____
• Weight Watchers	_____	_____	_____
• Overeaters Anonymous	_____	_____	_____
• Liquid diets (eg, Optifast)	_____	_____	_____
• Diet pills: Meridia, Xenical	_____	_____	_____
• Diet pills: phen-fen, Redux	_____	_____	_____
• NutriSystem / Jenny Craig	_____	_____	_____
• OTC diet pills	_____	_____	_____
• Obesity Surgery	_____	_____	_____
• Registered Dietitian	_____	_____	_____
• Other	_____	_____	_____

14. Have you maintained any weight loss for up to 1 year on any of these programs?   Yes ☐   No ☐

15. What did you learn from these programs regarding your weight? _____

16. What did not work about these programs? _____

17. Have you been involved in physical activity programs to help with weight loss?   Yes ☐   No ☐
    Which ones or in what way? _____

Adapted with permission from the Wellness Institute, Northwestern Memorial Hospital.

This project was funded by the American Medical Association and The Robert Wood Johnson Foundation. • November 2003   SEE:03-0107:4M:11/03

Form 2 Weight loss questionnaire. (Reprinted from Roadmaps for Clinical Practice: Case Studies in Disease Prevention and Health Promotion, *Assessment and Management of Adult Obesity: A Primer for Physicians*. With permission from American Medical Association.)

Assessment of Patient Readiness

Patient Readiness Checklist

Motivation/support
- ☐ How important is it that you lose weight at this time?
- ☐ Have you tried to lose weight before? What factors have led to your success and what has made weight loss difficult? (For example, cost, peer pressure, family, etc.)
- ☐ Is your decision to lose weight your own, or for someone else?
- ☐ Is your family supportive?
- ☐ Who, if anyone, is supportive of your decision to begin a weight loss program?
- ☐ What do you consider the benefits of weight loss?
- ☐ What would you have to sacrifice? What are the down sides?

Stressful life events
- ☐ Are there events in your life right now that might make losing weight especially difficult? (For example, work responsibilities, family commitments)
- ☐ If now is not a convenient time for weight loss, what would it take for you to be ready to lose weight? When do you think you might be ready to begin losing weight?

Psychiatric issues
- ☐ What is your mood like most of the time? Do you feel you have the needed energy to lose weight? (may need to assess for depression)
- ☐ Do you feel that you eat what most people would consider a large amount of food in a short period of time? Do you feel out of control during this time? (may need to assess for binge eating disorders)
- ☐ Do you ever forcibly vomit, use laxatives, or engage in excessive physical activity as a means of controlling weight? (may need to assess for bulimia nervosa)

Time availability/constraints
- ☐ How much time are you able to devote to physical activity on a weekly basis?
- ☐ Do you believe that you can make time to record your caloric intake?
- ☐ Can you take time out of your schedule to relax and engage in personal activities?

Weight-loss goals/expectations
- ☐ How much weight do you expect to lose?
- ☐ How fast do you expect to lose weight?
- ☐ What other benefits do you expect to experience as a result of weight loss?

Adapted with permission from the Wellness Institute, Northwestern Memorial Hospital.

This project was funded by the American Medical Association and The Robert Wood Johnson Foundation. • November 2003   SEE:03-0107:2M:11/03

Form 3 Assessment of patient readiness form. (Reprinted from Roadmaps for Clinical Practice: Case Studies in Disease Prevention and Health Promotion, *Assessment and Management of Adult Obesity: A Primer for Physicians*. With permission from American Medical Association.)

Food and Activity Diary

As part of your dietary management plan, you may want to utilize a Food and Activity Diary. This sample log is a good tool to help you keep track of what you are eating and doing and when. Be sure to record the following information each day and review it with your health care provider at your next visit.

1. Date, time, and place of your meals, snacks, or nibbles.
2. Describe the foods eaten and estimate the portion size.
   - Meat, poultry, fish, and cheese are best described in ounces (3 oz. is approximately equal to the size of a deck of cards)
   - Vegetables and cut fruit are best described in relation to cups (1 cup is approximately the size of a woman's fist)
   - Beverages are best described in terms of fluid ounces (1 cup = 8 fluid ounces)
3. Rate your hunger before eating:
   0 = Not hungry and uninterested in eating
   1 = Not hungry but could still be interested
   2 = Neutral
   3 = Mild to moderately hungry
   4 = Moderately to extremely hungry
4. List, describe, and estimate the time spent on any physical activity performed throughout the day. Be specific.
5. Remember to also record the following:
   - All condiments (1 t. butter, 1 T. mayonnaise, 3 T. sour cream, etc.)
   - Combination foods by breaking them down (eg. 2 c. noodles, 1/2 c. marinara sauce)
   - How food is prepared (home, restaurant, fast food — baked, broiled, fried, etc.)

Time	Amount	Food selection	Hunger rating
12:30	1 large	onion pita	3
ite	3 oz.	turkey, white	ite
	2 oz.	American cheese	
	1 c.	lettuce	
	1 slice	tomato	
	8 oz.	yogurt, custard style	
	1 large	banana	
	16 oz.	root beer	

Type of activity (10 minutes per circle)

Laundry, cleaning house ● ● ○

Adapted with permission from the Wellness Institute, Northwestern Memorial Hospital

Food and Activity Log (front)

Enlarge the activity log 127% from letter (8 1/2" × 11") to legal size (8 1/2" × 14") on a copy machine. You may make copies of this sheet to record information weekly.

__/__/__ Sunday

Time	Amount	Food selection	Hunger rating

Type of activity (10 minutes per circle)
○○○ ○○○
○○○ ○○○
○○○ ○○○
○○○ ○○○
○○○ ○○○

Water (8 fluid oz per circle)
○○○○○○○○○○

__/__/__ Monday

Time	Amount	Food selection	Hunger rating

Type of activity (10 minutes per circle)
○○○
○○○
○○○
○○○
○○○

Water (8 fluid oz per circle)
○○○○○○○○○○

__/__/__ Tuesday

Time	Amount	Food selection	Hunger rating

Type of activity (10 minutes per circle)
○○○
○○○
○○○
○○○
○○○

Water (8 fluid oz per circle)
○○○○○○○○○○

This project was funded by the American Medical Association and The Robert Wood Johnson Foundation. · November 2003   SEE03-0107:4M:11/03

(Continued)

Form 4 Food and activity diary.

Wednesday _/_ _/_

Time	Amount	Food selection	Hunger rating

Type of activity (10 minutes per circle)

Water (8 fluid oz per circle)
○ ○ ○ ○ ○ ○ ○ ○ ○ ○

Food and Activity Log (back)

Enlarge the activity log 127% from letter (8 1/2" × 11") to legal size (8 1/2" × 14") on a copy machine. You may make copies of this sheet to record information weekly.

Thursday _/_ _/_

Time	Amount	Food selection	Hunger rating

Type of activity (10 minutes per circle)

Water (8 fluid oz per circle)
○ ○ ○ ○ ○ ○ ○ ○ ○ ○

Friday _/_ _/_

Time	Amount	Food selection	Hunger rating

Type of activity (10 minutes per circle)

Water (8 fluid oz per circle)
○ ○ ○ ○ ○ ○ ○ ○ ○ ○

Saturday _/_ _/_

Time	Amount	Food selection	Hunger rating

Type of activity (10 minutes per circle)

Water (8 fluid oz per circle)
○ ○ ○ ○ ○ ○ ○ ○ ○ ○

Record your weight

Form 4 (Continued) Food and activity diary. (Reprinted from Roadmaps for Clinical Practice: Case Studies in Disease Prevention and Health Promotion, Assessment and Management of Adult Obesity: A Primer for Physicians. With permission from American Medical Association.)

READ THIS FIRST

Keeping a Food Diary

Keeping a food diary will help your doctor individualize your food for maximum success. Tell the truth. There's nothing to be gained by trying to look good on your diary. Your doctor can only help you if you record what you typically eat. Be sure to bring your completed food diary to your next appointment.

The "How-Much" Column:

Write down the amount of the food item you ate, such as, the size (in inches or deck of cards), volume (1/2 cup), weight (1 ounce=1 finger), and/or number of items of that food. If the item is packaged write down the amount that is a serving.

What Kind:

Write down the specific type of food you ate. Don't forget to write down "extras" like salad dressings, mayonnaise, butter, sour cream, sugar, ketchup, and gravies.

Time:

Write down the time you wake, exercise (what kind and how much), when you eat, and when you go to sleep.

Where:

Write down what part of the house, what restaurant, in the car, etc.

Along or With Someone:

If you ate alone, write "alone." If you ate with other people write who.

Paired With:

List any activity that you were doing while you were eating (e.g. watching TV, working, ironing).

Mood:

How were you feeling when you were eating? (happy, sad, etc.)

Symptoms:

Write down if you have any symptoms such as headaches, tired, light headed, hungry, craving sweets, etc.

BASIC RULES TO REMEMBER

Write everything down that you put in your mouth including liquids and medications.

Do it now. Your weight loss results will be better. If you forget to write everything down during the day, don't go to sleep before you write down as much as possible.

Form 5 Keeping a food diary. (Reprinted with permission from *Nutrition: Keeping a Food Diary 2009*. Available at: http://familydoctor/org/online/famdocen/home/general-nutrition/299.html. Copyright 2009 American Acadamy of Family Physicians. All rights reserved.)

American Weight Loss Center Food/Activity and Behavior Diary

TIME														
	Wake-Up	Amounts	Carbs	Protein	Fat	Calorie	Location	Why Trigged	Mood	W/Whom	How Long	Meds	Symptoms BP/BS, etc.	Solution
	Breakfast													
	Liquid													
	Snack													
	Exercise													
	Liquid													
	Lunch													
	Liquid													
	Snack													
	Exercise													
	Liquid													
	Dinner													
	Exercise													
	TV, other													
	Bed													

Record all items placed in mouth, including fluids, condiments, vitamins/meds. Type and how many minutes spent on physical activity

Record why you ate; i.e., hunger, tired, bored, anxious, persuasion, someone told you to eat, the item was around trigger, item was present, sugar or comfort craving, planned for it

Record any physical symptoms and the time; i.e., lightheaded, nausea, tired, headache, depressed, and blood pressure/sugars

Record possible solutions; ways to avoid the trigger event that led to a less healthy food choice or avoid getting too hungry, tired, bored, etc.

Form 6 Food/Activity and Behavior diary. (Courtesy of Erin Chamberlin, MD, FAAFP.)

AIM to CHANGE

DAY ONE

Date:_____

TIME	Food and Drink (type and amount)	Physical Symptoms, Thoughts, Feelings	Am I hungry?

WHAT DID I DO TO BE ACTIVE TODAY?   (Include time)

WHAT DID I DO FOR MYSELF TODAY?   ("Me time")

FOOD FOR THOUGHT   (Notes, goals, insights, challenges, reminders, questions)

Form 7 AIM to Change journal.

(Continued)

AIM to CHANGE

DAY TWO

Date:_____

TIME	Food and Drink (type and amount)	Physical Symptoms, Thoughts, Feelings	Am I hungry?

WHAT DID I DO TO BE ACTIVE TODAY?   (Include time)

WHAT DID I DO FOR MYSELF TODAY?   ("Me time")

FOOD FOR THOUGHT   (Notes, goals, insights, challenges, reminders, questions)

Form 7 (Continued) AIM to Change journal.   *(Continued)*

AIM to CHANGE

DAY THREE

Date:_____

TIME	Food and Drink (type and amount)	Physical Symptoms, Thoughts, Feelings	Am I hungry?

WHAT DID I DO TO BE ACTIVE TODAY? (Include time)

WHAT DID I DO FOR MYSELF TODAY? ("Me time")

FOOD FOR THOUGHT (Notes, goals, insights, challenges, reminders, questions)

Form 7 (Continued) AIM to Change journal.

(Continued)

AIM to CHANGE

DAY FOUR

Date:_____

TIME	Food and Drink (type and amount)	Physical Symptoms, Thoughts, Feelings	Am I hungry?

WHAT DID I DO TO BE ACTIVE TODAY?   (Include time)

WHAT DID I DO FOR MYSELF TODAY?   ("Me time")

FOOD FOR THOUGHT   (Notes, goals, insights, challenges, reminders, questions)

Form 7 (Continued) AIM to Change journal.   *(Continued)*

AIM to CHANGE

DAY FIVE

Date:_____

TIME	Food and Drink (type and amount)	Physical Symptoms, Thoughts, Feelings	Am I hungry?

WHAT DID I DO TO BE ACTIVE TODAY?   (Include time)

WHAT DID I DO FOR MYSELF TODAY?   ("Me time")

FOOD FOR THOUGHT   (Notes, goals, insights, challenges, reminders, questions)

Form 7 (Continued) AIM to Change journal. (Available at: http://familydoctor.org/dam/familydoctor/documents/aim_blank_journal.pdf)

Quality of Life Self-Assessment

Please use the following scale to rate how satisfied you feel now about different aspects of your daily life. Choose any number from this list (1 to 9) and indicate your choice on the questions below.

1 = Extremely Dissatisfied	6 = Somewhat Satisfied
2 = Very Dissatisfied	7 = Moderately Satisfied
3 = Moderately Dissatisfied	8 = Very Satisfied
4 = Somewhat Dissatisfied	9 = Extremely Satisfied
5 = Neutral	

1. _____ Mood (feelings of sadness, worry, happiness, etc.)

2. _____ Self-esteem

3. _____ Confidence, self-assurance, and comfort in social situations

4. _____ Energy and feeling healthy

5. _____ Health problems (diabetes, high blood pressure, etc.)

6. _____ General appearance

7. _____ Social life

8. _____ Leisure and recreational activities

9. _____ Physical mobility and physical activity

10. _____ Eating habits

11. _____ Body image

12. _____ Overall quality of life

Form 8 Quality of Life Self-Assessment. (Reprinted with permission from the LEARN [Lifestyle, Exercise, Attitudes, Relationships and Nutrition] Program director, Kelly Brownell, PhD. Yale University.)

DIET READINESS TEST QUESTIONNAIRE

For each question, circle the answer that best describes how you feel.

Section 1: Goals and Attitudes

1. Compared to previous attempts, how motivated to lose weight are you this time?

1	2	3	4	5
Not At All Motivated	Slightly Motivated	Somewhat Motivated	Quite Motivated	Extremely Motivated

2. How certain are you that you will stay committed to a weight loss program for the time it will take to reach your goal?

1	2	3	4	5
Not At All Certain	Slightly Certain	Somewhat Certain	Quite Certain	Extremely Certain

3. Consider all outside factors at this time in your life (the stress you're feeling at work, your family obligations, etc.). To what extent can you tolerate the effort required to stick to a diet?

1	2	3	4	5
Cannot Tolerate	Can Tolerate Somewhat	Uncertain	Can Tolerate Well	Can Tolerate Easily

4. Think honestly about how much weight you hope to lose and how quickly you hope to lose it. Figuring a weight loss of 1 to 2 pounds per week, how realistic is your expectation?

1	2	3	4	5
Very Unrealistic	Somewhat Unrealistic	Moderately Unrealistic	Somewhat Realistic	Very Realistic

5. While dieting, do you fantasize about eating a lot of your favorite foods?

1	2	3	4	5
Always	Frequently	Occasionally	Rarely	Never

6. While dieting, do you feel deprived, angry and/or upset?

1	2	3	4	5
Always	Frequently	Occasionally	Rarely	Never

Section 1 — TOTAL Score _____

> 6–16
> 17–23
> 24–30

Section 2: Hunger and Eating Cues

7. When food comes up in conversation or in something you read, do you want to eat even if you are not hungry?

1	2	3	4	5
Never	Rarely	Occasionally	Frequently	Always

8. How often do you eat because of **physical hunger**?

1	2	3	4	5
Always	Frequently	Occasionally	Rarely	Never

9. Do you have trouble controlling your eating when your favorite foods are around the house?

1	2	3	4	5
Never	Rarely	Occasionally	Frequently	Always

Section 2 — TOTAL Score _____

> 3–6
> 7–9
> 10–15

Form 9 Diet readiness test questionnaire.   (Continued)

Section 3: Control Over Eating

If the following situations occurred while you were on a diet, would you be likely to eat more or less immediately afterward and for the rest of the day?

10. Although you planned on skipping lunch, a friend talks you into going out for a midday meal.

1	2	3	4	5
Would Eat Much Less	Would Eat Somewhat Less	Would Make No Difference	Would Eat Somewhat More	Would Eat Much More

11. You "break" your diet by eating a fattening, "forbidden" food.

1	2	3	4	5
Would Eat Much Less	Would Eat Somewhat Less	Would Make No Difference	Would Eat Somewhat More	Would Eat Much More

12. You have been following your diet faithfully and decide to test yourself by eating something you consider a treat.

1	2	3	4	5
Would Eat Much Less	Would Eat Somewhat Less	Would Make No Difference	Would Eat Somewhat More	Would Eat Much More

Section 3 — TOTAL Score _____

3–7

8–11

12–15

Section 4: Binge Eating and Purging

13. Aside from holiday feasts, have you ever eaten a large amount of food rapidly and felt afterward that this eating incident was excessive and out of control?

2	0
Yes	No

14. If you answered yes to #13 above, how often have you engaged in this behavior during the last year?

1	2	3	4	5	6
Less Than Once A Month	About Once A Month	A Few Times A Month	About Once A Week	About Three Times A Week	Daily

15. Have you ever purged (used laxatives, diuretics or induced vomiting) to control your weight?

5	0
Yes	No

16. If you answered yes to #15 above, how often have you engaged in this behavior during the last year?

1	2	3	4	5	6
Less Than Once A Month	About Once A Month	A Few Times A Month	About Once A Week	About Three Times A Week	Daily

Section 4 — TOTAL Score _____

0–1

2–11

12–19

Section 5: Emotional Eating

17. Do you eat more than you would like to when you have negative feelings such as anxiety, depression, anger, or loneliness?

1	2	3	4	5
Never	Rarely	Occasionally	Frequently	Always

Form 9 (Continued) Diet readiness test questionnaire.   (Continued)

18. Do you have trouble controlling your eating when you have positive feelings—do you celebrate feeling good by eating?

1	2	3	4	5
Never	Rarely	Occasionally	Frequently	Always

19. When you have unpleasant interactions with others in your life, or after a difficult day at work, do you eat more than you'd like?

1	2	3	4	5
Never	Rarely	Occasionally	Frequently	Always

Section 5 — TOTAL Score _____

3–8
9–11
12–15

Section 6: Exercise Patterns and Attitudes

20. How often do you exercise?

1	2	3	4	5
Never	Rarely	Occasionally	Somewhat	Frequently

21. How confident are you that you can exercise regularly?

1	2	3	4	5
Not At All Confident	Slightly Confident	Somewhat Confident	Highly Confident	Completely Confident

22. When you think about exercise, do you develop a positive or negative picture in your mind?

1	2	3	4	5
Completely Negative	Somewhat Negative	Neutral	Somewhat Positive	Completely Positive

23. How certain are you that you can work regular exercise into your daily schedule?

1	2	3	4	5
Not At All Certain	Slightly Certain	Somewhat Certain	Quite Certain	Extremely Certain

Section 6 — TOTAL Score _____

4–10
11–16
17–20

Form 9 (Continued) Diet readiness test questionnaire. (Reprinted with permission from the LEARN [Lifestyle, Exercise, Attitudes, Relationships and Nutrition] Program director, Kelly Brownell, PhD. Yale University.)

THE DIET READINESS TEST SCORING GUIDE
(For use with the Diet Readiness Test)

After the patient completes each of the six sections, add the numbers of answers and compare them with the scoring guide below:

Section 1: Goals and Attitudes

TOTAL Score _____

If you scored:

6 to 16: This may not be a good time for you to start a weight loss program. Inadequate motivation and commitment together with unrealistic goals could block your progress. Think about those things that contribute to this, and consider changing them before undertaking a diet program.

17 to 23: You may be close to being ready to begin a program but should think about ways to boost your preparedness before you begin.

24 to 30: The path is clear with respect to goals and attitudes.

Section 2: Hunger and Eating Cues

TOTAL Score _____

If you scored:

3 to 6: You might occasionally eat more than you would like, but it does not appear to be a result of high responsiveness to environmental cues. Controlling the attitudes that make you eat may be especially helpful.

7 to 9: You may have a moderate tendency to eat just because food is available. Dieting may be easier for you if you try to resist external cues and eat only when you are physically hungry.

10 to 15: Some or most of your eating may be in response to thinking about food or exposing yourself to temptations to eat. Think of ways to minimize your exposure to temptations, so that you eat only in response to physical hunger.

Section 3: Control Over Eating

TOTAL Score _____

If you scored:

3 to 7: You recover rapidly from mistakes. However, if you frequently alternate between eating out of control and dieting strictly, you may have a serious eating problem and should get professional help.

8 to 11: You do not seem to let unplanned eating disrupt your program. This is a flexible, balanced approach.

12 to 15: You may be prone to overeat after an event breaks your control or throws you off track. Your reaction to these problem-causing eating events can be improved.

Form 10 Diet readiness test scoring.   *(Continued)*

Section 4: Binge Eating and Purging

TOTAL Score _____

If you scored:

0 to 1:   It appears that binge eating and purging is not a problem for you.

2 to 11:   Pay attention to these eating patterns. Should they arise more frequently, get professional help.

12 to 19:   You show signs of having a potentially serious eating problem. See a counselor experienced in evaluating eating disorders right away.

Section 5: Emotional Eating

TOTAL Score _____

If you scored:

3 to 8:   You do not appear to let your emotions affect your eating.

9 to 11:   You sometimes eat in response to emotional highs and lows. Monitor this behavior to learn when and why it occurs and be prepared to find alternative activities.

12 to 15:   Emotional ups and downs can stimulate your eating. Try to deal with feelings that trigger the eating and find other ways to express them.

Section 6: Exercise Patterns and Attitudes

TOTAL Score _____

If you scored:

4 to 10:   You're probably not exercising as regularly as you should. Determine whether your attitudes about exercise are blocking your way, then change what you must and put on those walking shoes.

11 to 16:   You need to feel more positive about exercise so you can do it more often. Think of ways to be more active that are fun and fit your lifestyle.

17 to 20:   It looks like the path is clear for you to be active. Now think of ways to get motivated.

Form 10 (Continued) Diet readiness test scoring. (Reprinted with permission from the LEARN [Lifestyle, Exercise, Attitudes, Relationships and Nutrition] Program director, Kelly Brownell, PhD. Yale University.)

Food Addiction Questionnaire
Do you see yourself in some of these questions?

1. Has anyone expressed concern about your thoughts and/or behavior around your eating, body, or weight?

2. Do you think or obsess about food, your eating, your body, and/or your weight much of the time?

3. Do you binge on a regular basis, eating a relatively large quantity of food at one sitting?

4. Do you eat to relieve unpleasant emotions?

5. Do you eat when you are not hungry?

6. Do you hide food for yourself or eat in secret?

7. Can you stop eating without difficulty after one or two bites of a snack food or sweets?

8. Do you often eat more than you originally planned to eat?

9. Do you have feelings of guilt, shame, or embarrassment when you eat—or afterwards?

10. Do you spend a lot of time calculating the calories you ate and the calories you burned?

11. Do you feel anxious about your weight, body, or eating?

12. Are you fearful of gaining weight?

13. Do you tell yourself you'll be happy when you achieve a certain weight?

14. Do you feel like your whole life is a struggle with food and your weight?

15. Do you feel hopeless about your behavior with food, and/or your obsession with your body and weight?

16. Do you entertain yourself with thoughts of food and what you are going to eat next?

17. Do you weigh yourself once, twice, or more daily?

18. Do you exercise excessively to control your weight?

19. Do you avoid eating or severely limit the amount of food you will eat?

20. Being totally honest with yourself, do you think you have a problem with food?

Form 11 Food addiction questionnaire. (Reprinted with permission from Obesity Action Coalition. Available at: http://www.obesityaction.org/educational-resources/resource-articles-2/weight-loss-surgery/food-addiction-and-the-weight-loss-surgery-patient)

Appendix C: ASBP algorithm

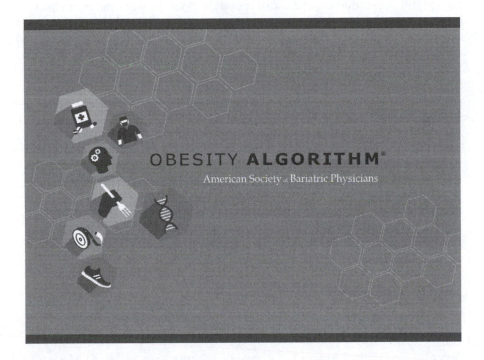

OBESITY ALGORITHM

Disclaimer

The Obesity Algorithm, originally presented by the American Society of Bariatric Physicians (ASBP) in 2013, was developed to assist health care professionals in medical decision making in the management and care of patients with overweight and obesity. However, the Obesity Algorithm is not intended to be a substitute for a medical professional's independent judgment and should not be considered medical advice. Most of the content herein is based on the medical literature and the clinical experience of obesity medicine specialists. In areas regarding inconclusive or insufficient scientific evidence, the authors used their professional judgment.

The Obesity Algorithm is a working document that represents the state of obesity medicine at the time of publication. The ASBP encourages medical professionals to use this information in conjunction with, and not as a replacement for, their best clinical judgment. The presented recommendations may not be appropriate in all situations. Any decision by practitioners to apply these guidelines must be made in light of local resources and individual patient circumstances.

Permissions

The ASBP owns the copyright to the Obesity Algorithm but invites you to use the slide set. Access to the Obesity Algorithm content and permission for extensive quoting or reproducing excerpts and for the reproduction and use of copyrighted text, images, or entire slides will not be granted until the requestor has signed the copyright consent and permission agreement available at www.ObesityAlgorithm.org. The ASBP reserves the right to deny a request for permission to use the Obesity Algorithm.

AUTHORS AND CITATION

- Cochair persons of the Obesity Algorithm Committee
  - Jennifer Seger, MD and Deborah Bade Horn, DO, MPH, FASBP
- Coauthors
  - Eric C. Westman, MD, MHS
  - Craig Primack, MD, FACP, FAAP
  - Stacy L. Schmidt, PhD
  - Debra Ravasia, MD, FACOG, FPMRS
  - William McCarthy, MD
  - Ursula Ferguson, DO, FACOI
  - Brian Sabowitz, MD, MS, FACP
  - Wendy Scinta, MD, MS
  - Harold E. Bays, MD, FTOS, FACC, FACE, FNLA
- Administrative assistance
  - Laurie Traetow, CAE, CPA
- Citation
  - Seger JC, Horn DB, Westman EC, Primack C, Schmidt SL, Ravasia D, McCarthy W, Ferguson U, Sabowitz BN, Scinta W, Bays HE. Obesity Algorithm, presented by the American Society of Bariatric Physicians. 2014–2015 www.obesityalgorithm.org (accessed January 01, 2016)

PURPOSE

To provide clinicians an overview of principles important to the care of patients with increased and/or dysfunctional body fat, based upon scientific evidence, supported by the medical literature, and derived from the clinical experiences of members of the ASBP.

ASBP DEFINITION OF OBESITY

"Obesity is defined as a chronic, relapsing, multi-factorial, neurobehavioral disease, wherein an increase in body fat promotes adipose tissue dysfunction and abnormal fat mass physical forces, resulting in adverse metabolic, biomechanical, and psychosocial health consequences."

Obesity as a Multifactorial Disease

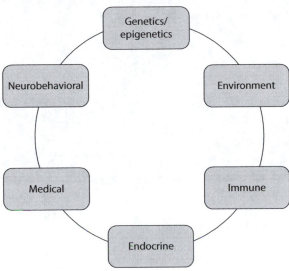

Two Subsets of Morbidity in Patients with Overweight and/or Obesity

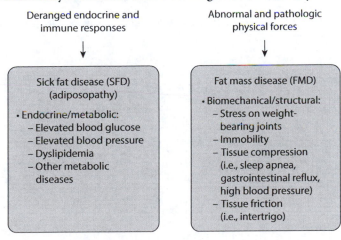

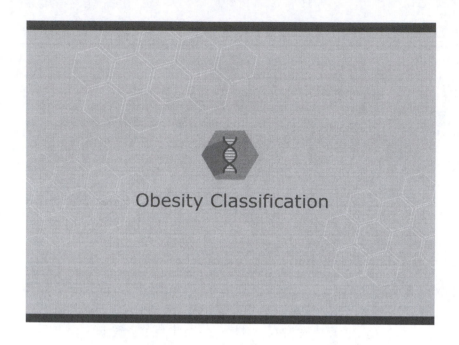

Body Mass Index: Increased Body Fat (Adiposity)

Overweight and Obesity Classification:
Body mass index (BMI) in kg/m²*

Normal weight 18.5–24.9	Overweight 25.0–29.9	Class I obesity 30.0–34.9	Class II obesity 35.0–39.9	Class III obesity ≥40

* Different BMI cutoff points may be more appropriate for women versus men, those of different races, and individuals.

Percent Body Fat: Increased Body Fat (Adiposity)

American Council on Exercise Classification:
Percent body fat*

Essential fat Women: 10–13% Men: 2–5%	Athletes Women: 14–20% Men: 6–13%	Fitness Women: 21–24% Men: 14–17%	Acceptable Women: 25–31% Men: 18–24%	Obesity Women: ≥ 32% Men: ≥ 25%

* Based on "expert opinion"; cutoff points not scientifically validated.

Percent Body Fat: Increased Body Fat (Adiposity)

US Army Regulations:
Percent body fat (%BF)

Men %BF calculator (height, neck, and waist)	Women %BF calculator (height, neck, waist, and hip)
Maximum allowable %BF to join Army	**Maximum allowable %BF to join Army**
• Age 17–20 24%	• Age 17–20 30%
• Age 21–27 26%	• Age 21–27 32%
• Age 28–39 28%	• Age 28–39 34%
• Age 40+ 30%	• Age 40+ 36%
Maximum allowable %BF after entry	**Maximum allowable %BF after entry**
• Age 17–20 20%	• Age 17–20 30%
• Age 21–27 22%	• Age 21–27 32%
• Age 28–39 24%	• Age 28–39 34%
• Age 40+ 26%	• Age 40+ 36%

Waist Circumference: Increased Body Fat (Adiposity)

Overweight and Obesity Classification:
Waist circumference (WC)*

Men abdominal obesity	Women abdominal obesity
≥ 40 in.	≥ 35 in.
≥ 102 cm	≥ 88 cm

* Different WC abdominal obesity cut-off points are appropriate for different races (i.e., ≥ 90 cm for Asian men and ≥ 80 cm for Asian women).

Which is the "Best" Measure of Obesity?

- Population assessment
  - BMI, waist circumference (WC), and percent body fat (%BF) similarly correlate with prevalence of metabolic syndrome.
- Individual assessment
  - BMI is a reasonable initial screening measurement for most patients.
  - WC provides additional information regarding adipose tissue function/dysfunction and predisposition to metabolic disease among individuals with BMI <35 kg/m^2.
  - %BF may be useful in patients with extremes in muscle mass (i.e., individuals with sarcopenia or substantial increases in muscle mass) and thus may be a more accurate measure of body composition when assessing the efficacy of interventions directed toward change in muscle mass.

Index